Antibiotic Residues, Antimicrobial Resistance and Intervention Strategies of Foodborne Pathogens

Antibiotic Residues, Antimicrobial Resistance and Intervention Strategies of Foodborne Pathogens

Editors

Yongning Wu
Zhenling Zeng

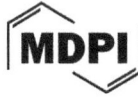

Basel • Beijing • Wuhan • Barcelona • Belgrade • Novi Sad • Cluj • Manchester

Editors

Yongning Wu
NHC Key Laboratory of Food
Safety Risk Assessment
China National Center for
Food Safety Risk Assessment
Beijing
China

Zhenling Zeng
College of Veterinary
Medicine
South China Agricultural
University
Guangzhou
China

Editorial Office
MDPI
St. Alban-Anlage 66
4052 Basel, Switzerland

This is a reprint of articles from the Special Issue published online in the open access journal *Antibiotics* (ISSN 2079-6382) (available at: www.mdpi.com/journal/antibiotics/special_issues/foodborne_antimicrobial).

For citation purposes, cite each article independently as indicated on the article page online and as indicated below:

Lastname, A.A.; Lastname, B.B. Article Title. *Journal Name* **Year**, *Volume Number*, Page Range.

ISBN 978-3-7258-0924-0 (Hbk)
ISBN 978-3-7258-0923-3 (PDF)
doi.org/10.3390/books978-3-7258-0923-3

© 2024 by the authors. Articles in this book are Open Access and distributed under the Creative Commons Attribution (CC BY) license. The book as a whole is distributed by MDPI under the terms and conditions of the Creative Commons Attribution-NonCommercial-NoDerivs (CC BY-NC-ND) license.

Contents

About the Editors vii

Yongning Wu and Zhenling Zeng
Antibiotic Residues, Antimicrobial Resistance and Intervention Strategies of Foodborne Pathogens
Reprinted from: *Antibiotics* 2024, 13, 321, doi:10.3390/antibiotics13040321 1

Ning Han, Jie Li, Peng Wan, Yu Pan, Tiantian Xu and Wenguang Xiong et al.
Co-Existence of Oxazolidinone Resistance Genes *cfr*(D) and *optrA* on Two *Streptococcus parasuis* Isolates from Swine
Reprinted from: *Antibiotics* 2023, 12, 825, doi:10.3390/antibiotics12050825 8

Patrick Muinde, John Maina, Kelvin Momanyi, Victor Yamo, John Mwaniki and John Kiiru
Antimicrobial Resistant Pathogens Detected in Raw Pork and Poultry Meat in Retailing Outlets in Kenya
Reprinted from: *Antibiotics* 2023, 12, 613, doi:10.3390/antibiotics12030613 18

Nicholas Bor, Alessandro Seguino, Derrick Noah Sentamu, Dorcas Chepyatich, James M. Akoko and Patrick Muinde et al.
Prevalence of Antibiotic Residues in Pork in Kenya and the Potential of Using Gross Pathological Lesions as a Risk-Based Approach to Predict Residues in Meat
Reprinted from: *Antibiotics* 2023, 12, 492, doi:10.3390/antibiotics12030492 29

Yi-Yun Liu, Zong-Hua Qin, Hui-Ying Yue, Phillip J. Bergen, Li-Min Deng and Wan-Yun He et al.
Synergistic Effects of Capric Acid and Colistin against Colistin-Susceptible and Colistin-Resistant *Enterobacterales*
Reprinted from: *Antibiotics* 2022, 12, 36, doi:10.3390/antibiotics12010036 40

Shaofei Yan, Xiaofan Zhang, Xiaofang Jia, Jiguo Zhang, Xiaomin Han and Chang Su et al.
Characterization of the Composition Variation of Healthy Human Gut Microbiome in Correlation with Antibiotic Usage and Yogurt Consumption
Reprinted from: *Antibiotics* 2022, 11, 1827, doi:10.3390/antibiotics11121827 46

Dennis Carhuaricra, Carla G. Duran Gonzales, Carmen L. Rodríguez Cueva, Yennifer Ignacion León, Thalia Silvestre Espejo and Geraldine Marcelo Monge et al.
Occurrence and Genomic Characterization of *mcr-1*-Harboring *Escherichia coli* Isolates from Chicken and Pig Farms in Lima, Peru
Reprinted from: *Antibiotics* 2022, 11, 1781, doi:10.3390/antibiotics11121781 55

Xin Mao, Xiaozhen Zhou, Jun He, Gongzhen Liu, Huihui Liu and Han Zhao et al.
Metabolism Profile of Mequindox in Sea Cucumbers In Vivo Using LC-HRMS
Reprinted from: *Antibiotics* 2022, 11, 1599, doi:10.3390/antibiotics11111599 65

Tingting Cao, Yajie Guo, Dan Wang, Zhiyang Liu, Suli Huang and Changfeng Peng et al.
Effect of Phorate on the Development of Hyperglycaemia in Mouse and Resistance Genes in Intestinal Microbiota
Reprinted from: *Antibiotics* 2022, 11, 1584, doi:10.3390/antibiotics11111584 75

Zhixin Fei, Shufeng Song, Xin Yang, Dingguo Jiang, Jie Gao and Dajin Yang
Occurrence and Risk Assessment of Fluoroquinolone Residues in Chicken and Pork in China
Reprinted from: *Antibiotics* 2022, 11, 1292, doi:10.3390/antibiotics11101292 85

Huixian Liang, Xinhui Li and He Yan
Identification of a Novel IncHI1B Plasmid in MDR *Klebsiella pneumoniae* 200 from Swine in China
Reprinted from: *Antibiotics* **2022**, *11*, 1225, doi:10.3390/antibiotics11091225 . . . . **96**

Alvin C. Alvarado, Samuel M. Chekabab, Bernardo Z. Predicala and Darren R. Korber
Impact of Raised without Antibiotics Measures on Antimicrobial Resistance and Prevalence of Pathogens in Sow Barns
Reprinted from: *Antibiotics* **2022**, *11*, 1221, doi:10.3390/antibiotics11091221 . . . . **107**

Weishuai Zhai, Yingxin Tian, Dongyan Shao, Muchen Zhang, Jiyun Li and Huangwei Song et al.
Fecal Carriage of *Escherichia coli* Harboring the *tet*(X4)-IncX1 Plasmid from a Tertiary Class-A Hospital in Beijing, China
Reprinted from: *Antibiotics* **2022**, *11*, 1068, doi:10.3390/antibiotics11081068 . . . . **120**

Qiyan Chen, Zhiyu Zou, Chang Cai, Hui Li, Yang Wang and Lei Lei et al.
Characterization of bla_{NDM-5}-and $bla_{CTX-M-199}$-Producing ST167 *Escherichia coli* Isolated from Shared Bikes
Reprinted from: *Antibiotics* **2022**, *11*, 1030, doi:10.3390/antibiotics11081030 . . . . **132**

Zengfeng Zhang, Xiaorong Tian and Chunlei Shi
Global Spread of MCR-Producing *Salmonella enterica* Isolates
Reprinted from: *Antibiotics* **2022**, *11*, 998, doi:10.3390/antibiotics11080998 . . . . **142**

Senlin Zhang, Honghu Sun, Guangjie Lao, Zhiwei Zhou, Zhuochong Liu and Jiong Cai et al.
Identification of Mobile Colistin Resistance Gene *mcr-10* in Disinfectant and Antibiotic Resistant *Escherichia coli* from Disinfected Tableware
Reprinted from: *Antibiotics* **2022**, *11*, 883, doi:10.3390/antibiotics11070883 . . . . **153**

Jing Cao, Yajie Wang, Guanzhao Wang, Pingping Ren, Yongning Wu and Qinghua He
Effects of Typical Antimicrobials on Growth Performance, Morphology and Antimicrobial Residues of Mung Bean Sprouts
Reprinted from: *Antibiotics* **2022**, *11*, 807, doi:10.3390/antibiotics11060807 . . . . **168**

About the Editors

Yongning Wu

Prof Dr Wu is the Chief Technical Officer of the China National Center for Food Safety Risk Assessment (CFSA), a Professor and Director of the Research Unit on Food Safety in the Chinese Academy of Medical Science (2019RU014) and the Department of Nutrition and Food Safety at Peking Union Medical College, the Director of the Key Lab for Food Safety Risk Assessment, and the head of the WHO Collaborating Center of Food Contamination Monitoring (China). He graduated from Nanjing Medical College in 1983, then from Chinese Academy of Preventive Medicine for MPH, and earned a Ph D degree in Nutrition and Food Hygiene in 1997. Prof Dr. WU has held several positions on the Food Safety Committee, including: 1. a member of the WHO Technical Advisory Group on Food Safety (TAG – Food Safety, 2021–24); 2. a member of the WHO Strategic and Technical Advisory Group on Antimicrobial Resistance (STAG – AMR 2018–2020); 3. the FAO/WHO Joint Expert Committee on Food Additives (JECFA), roster list of FAO/WHO Dietary Exposure in Chemical (2012–) and roster list of FAO roster list (2007–); 4. the Food Safety Commission and the State Council in China; a member of the Scientific Committee; 5. the Chief Technology Advisor of The National Expert Committee of Food Safety Risk Assessment, National Health Commission, China; 6. a member (2015–2020) and Advisor (2021–2025) of the USP Food Ingredient Expert Committee (FIEP); and finally, a member of the Food Ingredient Intentional Adulteration Expert Panel (2011-2015; 2016-2020). He is member of several journals' Editorial Advisory Boards for food and environment science, as well as preventive medicine, and he has published more than 500 papers, with an H index of 70.

Zhenling Zeng

Prof. Zeng is the Director of the National Veterinary Drug Residue Baseline Laboratory (SCAU), head of the National Veterinary Drug Safety Assessment Laboratory (SCAU), and Director of the Veterinary Drug Innovation Engineering Technology Research Center in Guangdong Province. He is also the Honorary Chairman of the Veterinary Pharmacology and Toxicology Branch of the China Association of Animal Husbandry and Veterinary Medicine, the Vice Chairman of the Animal Toxicology Branch of the China Association of Animal Husbandry and Veterinary Medicine, and a member of the Second and Third Veterinary Drug Residue Expert Committee of the Ministry of Agriculture. Prof. Zeng has been awarded the National Science and Technology Progress Second Prize and Guangdong Province Ministerial Science and Technology Progress First Prize. He presided over the 14th Five-Year National Key R & D Program Key Special Project (Chief Scientist), the 13th Five-Year National Key R & D Program Project, and 973 Projects. Prof. Zeng graduated from South China Agricultural University in 1984 with a bachelor's degree in agronomy. In 1987 and 1996, he graduated from the School of Veterinary Medicine of South China Agricultural University with a master's degree in agronomy and a doctorate in pharmacology and toxicology, respectively. From 2002 to 2003, he travelled to the United States as a Senior Visiting Scholar at UIUC. Prof. Zeng is a renowned teacher at South China Agricultural University, and has been awarded the honorary titles of National Candidate of the Thousand Hundred and Ten Project of Guangdong Provincial Colleges and Universities, Outstanding Teacher of Southern Guangdong, and Outstanding Doctoral Dissertation Supervisor of Guangdong Province. He has published more than 150 SCI papers, and 10 monographs, textbooks and popular science books. He has had more than 20 invention patents authorized and 3 certificates of a new national veterinary drug.

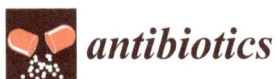

Editorial

Antibiotic Residues, Antimicrobial Resistance and Intervention Strategies of Foodborne Pathogens

Yongning Wu [1,2,*] and Zhenling Zeng [3,4,*]

1. NHC Key Laboratory of Food Safety Risk Assessment, China National Center for Food Safety Risk Assessment, Beijing 100021, China
2. Research Unit of Food Safety (2019RU014), Chinese Academy of Medical Sciences and Peking Union Medical College, Beijing 100021, China
3. Guangdong Provincial Key Laboratory of Veterinary Pharmaceutics Development and Safety Evaluation, College of Veterinary Medicine, South China Agricultural University, Guangzhou 510642, China
4. National Risk Assessment Laboratory for Antimicrobial Resistance of Animal Original Bacteria, South China Agricultural University, Guangzhou 510642, China
* Correspondence: wuyongning@cfsa.net.cn (Y.W.); zlzeng@scau.edu.cn (Z.Z.)

1. Introduction

The primary determinant of human health is undoubtedly safe food. Nevertheless, unsafe foodstuffs, containing hazardous substances, such as bacteria, chemical, and physical contaminants, at harmful levels can lead to various acute and chronic illnesses, including over 200 diseases ranging from diarrhea to cancers, and even permanent disabilities or death. Alarmingly, an estimated 600 million individuals worldwide—almost one in ten people—suffer from illnesses caused by contaminated food, resulting in a global annual burden of 33 million disability-adjusted life years (DALYS) and 420,000 premature deaths [1].

Given the significance of this issue, it is imperative to monitor potential food safety concerns associated with global changes in food systems, as appropriate, to determine exposure to both new and existing hazards. Food safety science and risk assessment should be used to determine the likelihood of foodborne illnesses. In recognition of this, the World Health Organization (WHO) has updated the Global Strategy for Food Safety, while China has also issued the national roadmap with the One Health Approach [2,3].

The high volume of antibiotics in food-producing animals significantly contributes to the emergence of antibiotic-resistant bacteria (ARB), particularly in scenarios of intense animal husbandry. Notably, in some countries, the total quantity of antibiotics administered to animals surpasses that used in humans by four times. A significant portion of antibiotic use in animals in many countries is aimed at promoting growth and preventing disease, rather than treating sick animals. Resilient bacteria can be transferred from animals to humans through direct contact or via the food chain and the environment. Antimicrobial resistance (AMR) infections in humans can result in prolonged illnesses, increased frequency of hospitalization, and treatment failures that can even lead to death. Tragically, some types of bacteria that cause severe infections in humans have already developed resistance to most or all available therapeutics, leaving us with dwindling treatment options for certain types of infections [4].

Food products are increasingly being recognized as important contributors to antibiotic usage, leading to the presence of veterinary drug residues and the transmission of ARB, AMR and their associated ARGs. These unexplained transmission mechanisms pose a significant public health threat to the general population, highlighting the urgent need for effective measures to address this issue.

Increasing cross-sector connectivity has fueled the global dissemination of ARGs. The concept of 'One Health' represents an integrated, unifying framework aimed at harmonizing and optimizing the health of humans, animals and the environment. This approach necessitates collaboration among the public health, veterinary, and public health and environmental sectors. It holds particular significance in ensuring food and water safety, controlling zoonotic diseases, managing pollution from veterinary drug residues, and combating AMR. In recognition of this urgent need, the WHO initiated a Global Action Plan in 2015 [4], urging for AMR surveillance across these three sectors as well as integrating data to gain insights into the transmission and cross-sectoral connectivity of AMR. Against this global background, China submitted the National Action Plan in 2016–2020 and updated it for 2022–2025, embracing the One Health Approach to tackle AMR surveillance effectively [5] The National Nature Science Foundation of China has kicked off several Major Programs (No 22193060, 32141000, 42021000, 81991535) with the One Health Approach. These efforts are crucial in the global fight against AMR, safeguarding the health and well-being of all. This Special Issue devotes particular attention to the interfaces among humans, animals, plants, food, and the environment, seeking to delve into the intervention strategies used to combat foodborne pathogens. Furthermore, it aims to characterize the composition variations within the healthy human gut microbiome, particularly in relation to antibiotic usage and food consumption. The focus of this Special Issue is to explore food safety intervention strategies involving antibiotics used in animals and plants, while also identifying ARB and ARGs. Through this comprehensive approach, we strive to gain a deeper understanding of these complex interactions and their potential implications for food safety and public health.

2. An Overview of Published Articles

Conventional single-level and single-perspective approaches have proven inadequate for the effective prevention and control of AMR and antimicrobial-resistant pathogens. To effectively address this problem, it is necessary to use multidisciplinary and multisectoral cooperation approaches that encompass human, animal, and environmental dimensions. The "One Health" approach offers a comprehensive and systematic framework for tackling AMR and foodborne pathogens from a multidimensional and multifaceted perspective. In this Special Issue of *Antibiotics (Basel)*, a total of 16 papers were published based on the concept and method of "One Health" to control antibiotic residues, AMR and foodborne pathogens. The research fields of these papers cover antibiotic residue detection, AMR generation and spreading, antibiotic pharmacodynamic evaluation and metabolism, discussing various facets of the prevention and control of threats posed by antibiotics and AMR to food safety.

The investigation of antibiotic residue detection includes chloramphenicol, nitrofuran and fluoroquinolone residue on plants and animals. Cao et al. reported that antimicrobials not only affect the production and morphology of mung bean sprouts, but also produce an antimicrobial residue. Additionally, chloramphenicol, enrofloxacin, and furazolidone residue was also found in commercial mung bean sprouts. In a Chinese nation-wide survey, Fei et al. found that the levels of fluoroquinolone residues in chicken were higher than those in pork, with detection frequencies of 3.99% and 1.69%, respectively. Enrofloxacin and its metabolite ciprofloxacin were found to be the most predominant fluoroquinolones. Bor et al. examined pig carcasses for gross pathological lesions and collected pork samples for antibiotic residue testing. Their result showed that the prevalence of antibiotic residues was 41.26% (95% CI, 34.53–48.45%) in Kenya, posing potential public health risks to pork consumers.

The large-scale use of antimicrobials in farms not only increases the potential presence of their residues in food and the environment, but also leads to a greater probability of AMR generation and spread. A major factor in the prevalence of ARGs in the food chain is the presence of ARB in food animals, which poses a potential risk to public health and safety. Han et al. reported the co-occurrence of *optrA* and *cfr*(D) operons in *Streptococcus parasuis* collected from pig farms. The presence of Tn554–*optrA* in *Enterococcus* spp., *Staphylococcus* spp., and *Streptococcus* spp. with various genetic and source backgrounds demonstrated that the Tn554 element plays an important role in the dissemination of *optrA*.

This study extended the current knowledge of the genetic background of *optrA* and *cfr*(D) and indicated that Tn*554* and IS*1202* may play an important role in the transmission of *optrA* and *cfr*(D) originating from pig farms. Based on whole-genome sequencing (WGS), a novel plasmid pYhe2001 from swine-origin *Klebsiella pneumoniae* 200 is reported for the first time, suggesting that the plasmids may act as reservoirs for various ARGs and transport multiple resistance genes in *K. pneumoniae* of both animal and human origin.

Colistin is a last-line antibiotic against Gram-negative pathogens. However, the emergence of colistin resistance has substantially reduced the clinical effectiveness of this antimicrobial. In the study of Carhuaricra et al., the occurrence of *mcr-1*-harboring *Escherichia coli* was determined for the first time in chicken farms and pig farms in Lima, Peru. The genomic analysis showed diverse lineages of *E. coli* carrying the *mcr-1* gene mobilized by the IncI2 and IncHI1A:IncHI1B plasmids, including the presence of ISApl1 copies enhancing the dissemination of *mcr-1*. The elevated prevalence of multidrug-resistant (MDR) strains in farms in Lima could serve as a reservoir of ARGs that can be disseminated by farmers or food, impacting public health. A study in Kenya found that poultry meat and pork were contaminated with high levels of bacteria with MDR, potentially spreading foodborne illnesses. This resistance was noted for critically essential antimicrobials (according to the WHO) such as rifampicin (96%), ampicillin (35%), cefotaxime (9%), cefepime (6%), and ciprofloxacin (6%).

The global epidemiological investigation of the AMR of pathogenic bacteria is crucial for clinical therapy and the mitigation of this threat. Colistin resistance in bacteria has become a significant threat to food safety and public health, and its development was mainly attributed to the plasmid-mediated *mcr* genes. Twenty *mcr* variants were identified from 2279 *mcr*-producing *Salmonella* genomes, and the most common ones were *mcr-9.1* (65.2%) and *mcr-1.1* (24.4%). Phylogenetic results indicated that *mcr*-producing *Salmonella* fell into nine lineages (Lineages I–IX), and *Salmonella* Typhimurium, 1,4,[5],12:i:- and 4,[5],12:i:- isolates from different countries were mixed into Lineages I, II and III, suggesting that international spread occurred in *Salmonella*-bearing *mcr* genes. Liu et al. examined the synergy between colistin and capric acid against twenty-one Gram-negative bacterial isolates. Checkerboard and time–kill assays showed that capric acid can enhance the bacterial killing of colistin-resistant Gram-negative bacteria when combined with colistin.

The widespread escalation of bacterial resistance threatens the safety of the food chain. While investigating the resistance characteristics of *E. coli* strains isolated from disinfected tableware against both disinfectants and antibiotics, a recently described mobile colistin resistance gene *mcr-10* present on the novel IncFIB-type plasmid was found to be able to successfully transform the resistance. This work warned that continuous monitoring of ARGs in the catering industry is essential to understand and respond to the transmission of ARGs from the environment and food to humans and clinics. Shared bikes act as a potential vector for ARB and ARGs. Two ST167 *E. coli* isolated from shared bikes show high similarities in their core genomes and plasmid profiles with strains from hospital inpatients and farm animals. This study indicated that vectors such as shared bikes may contribute to the dissemination of these ARB in the environment. There is a need to take measures to assess the risk of ARB in the environment and cut off transmission.

The emergence of the mobile tigecycline-resistance gene, *tet*(X4), poses a significant threat to public health. The study of Zhai investigates the prevalence and genetic characteristics of the *tet*(X4)-positive *E. coli* in clinical human stool samples. The clonal spread of *tet*(X4)-positive isolates indicated the risk of intra-hospital transmission of the *tet*(X4) gene. Furthermore, these strains and plasmids of clinical patient origin showed a strong genetic resemblance to some animal-origin strains, implying a potential risk of transmission between animals and humans.

The growing concern over the emergence of AMR in animal production as a result of extensive and inappropriate antibiotic use has prompted many swine farmers in Canada to raise their animals without antibiotics (RWA). Alvarado et al. investigates the impact of implementing an RWA approach in sow barns on actual on-farm antibiotic use, the emergence of AMR, and the abundance of pathogens. Metagenomic analyses demonstrated an increased abundance of pathogenic *Actinobacteria*, *Firmicutes*, and *Proteobacteria* in the nasopharynx microbiome of RWA sows relative to non-RWA sows. WGS analyses revealed that the nasal microbiome of sows raised under RWA production exhibited a significant increase in the frequency of resistance genes coding for β-lactams, MDR, and tetracycline.

Antibiotic usage and yogurt consumption are the major interventions for gut microbiota. Yan et al. found that antibiotic usage and yogurt consumption demonstrated significant changes in specific bacterial groups (*Streptococcaceae*, *Enterococcaceae* and so on) in healthy human gut microbiomes, sharing more identical changes in the healthy human gut microbiome than disparities, especially ARG-related bacteria groups that could induce an intensification of ARG transfer processes from commensal bacteria to pathogens in the human gut.

Phorate is a systemic, broad-spectrum organophosphorus insecticide. Cao et al. assessed the blood glucose concentrations of high-fat-diet-fed mice exposed to phorate and the distribution characteristics of the resistance genes in the intestinal microbiota of these mice. The result revealed that phorate can affect the abundance of the intestinal microbiota and therefore alter the expression of drug-resistance genes. This study indicates that changes in the abundance of the intestinal microbiota are closely related to the presence of ARB in the intestinal tract and the metabolic health of the host.

In the study of Mao et al., the metabolism behavior of mequindox (MEQ) in sea cucumber in vivo was investigated using LC-HRMS. This work first reported 3-methyl-2-quinoxalinecarboxylic acid (MQCA) as a metabolite of MEQ, and carboxylation is a major metabolic pathway of MEQ in sea cucumber. This work revealed that the metabolism of MEQ in marine animals is different from that in land animals. The metabolism results in this work could facilitate the accurate risk assessment of MEQ in sea cucumber and related marine foods.

3. Conclusions

AMR poses a significant threat to human health. This compilation of articles dedicated to the field of retailing encompasses a comprehensive overview of a diverse range of research, elucidative of the richness of the research field. The articles showcase a range of methodologies that were adopted for the studies of occurrence and genomic characterization of AMR, ranging from qualitative approaches based on in situ observations and interviews to quantitative studies using omics and artificial intelligence (AI) tools to trace the evolution of bacteria harboring certain emerging ARGs or/and mobile genes. Case studies focus on specific ARGs and plasmids, such as the colistin resistance gene *mcr-X*, *bla*$_{NDM-5}$ and *bla*$_{CTX-M-199}$, *tet(X4)-IncX1*, *cfr*(D) and *optrA*, providing insights into their dissemination and health impact. Notably, many bacteria carried by animals (such as *Salmonella*, *Campylobacter* and *E. coli*, and *K. pneumoniae*) can also cause diseases in humans. These bacteria, often harboring ARGs, can contaminate our food supply throughout the entire production chain, from farm to fork, during slaughtering and processing. Vegetables, including mung bean sprouts, as described in this Special Issue, are susceptible to contamination by harmful bacteria, either at the farm or subsequently through cross-contamination. This knowledge is derived from our ability to trace the origin of ARB isolated from ill individuals back to agricultural sources using DNA fingerprinting techniques. This underscores the importance of vigilant monitoring and sanitary practices throughout the entire food production chain to ensure food safety and protect public health.

Annually, over 400,000 people die from foodborne diseases, with children under five years old accounting for over a third of these tragic deaths. According to estimates by the WHO, microbes, including bacteria, cause the vast majority of foodborne illnesses [1]. Alarmingly, if these bacteria develop resistance to antibiotics, effective treatments will become limited, leading to an increase in deaths from foodborne diseases. Therefore, optimizing the use of antibiotics in both human medicine and animal husbandry is crucial to mitigate the emergence and spread of ARB and ARGs, thereby safeguarding public health. To address the critical public health threat, the WHO has developed several guidelines aimed at preserving the effectiveness of antibiotics vital for human health. Our recommendations align with the WHO's list of critically important antimicrobials for humans, especially critically important antibiotics, to treat multidrug-resistant infections in humans. When considering antibiotics used in food-producing animals, it is essential to prioritize those with the least significance for human health. This means starting with antimicrobial classes that are not used in humans, and then proceeding with those listed on the WHO's list of critically important antimicrobials for human medicine, followed by those classified as highly important. Antibiotics categorized by the WHO as critically important for human medicine should be used in animals only when the most recent culture and sensitivity results of bacteria known to have caused the disease indicate that this critically important antimicrobial is the sole viable option. Competent authorities may require a cross-disciplinary "One Health" approach when evaluating new hazards emerging at the human–animal–environmental interface [6]. This approach can be instrumental in minimizing the use of antibiotics in food animal production by enhancing husbandry and management practices for disease prevention and control, as well as strengthening AMR surveillance within the food chain. By adopting these strategies, we can work towards mitigating the threat of AMR and safeguarding public health.

The WHO has established a "One Health Initiative" to integrate efforts in humans, animals, and environmental health across its organization. Given the interconnectedness of human and animal health, it is crucial to incorporate information gathered from pathogens in animals and the food chain into AMR surveillance programs, which falls under the umbrella of the One Health framework. The WHO is collaborating with the Food and Agriculture Organization of the United Nations (FAO), the United Nations Environment Program (UNEP), and the World Organization for Animal Health (WOAH) as part of a One Health quadripartite [7]. This quadripartite promotes multi-sectoral approaches aimed at reducing health threats at the intersection of humans, animals, and the ecosystem. The quadripartite One Health Joint Plan of Action (OH-JPA) outlines the necessary transformations to prevent and mitigate the impact of current and future health challenges at the global, regional, and country levels. Notably, AMR and food safety are included in this plan. However, according to the latest global database from the Tracking AMR Country Self-Assessment Survey (TrACSS, 2023) [8], which has been executed in 177 countries, only 16 countries have formalized multi-sectoral coordination mechanisms with functional working groups, and only 25 countries possess adequate technical capacity, resources, and established systems to gather data across the "One Health" sectors. This highlights the urgent need for further development and coordination to fully realize the potential of the "One Health" approach in addressing AMR and other critical health challenges.

In high-income countries, trends in AMR in animals and food are monitored via systematic surveillance by organizations such as the European Food Safety Authority (EFSA) in Europe [9], the National Antimicrobial Resistance Monitoring System for Enteric Bacteria (NARMS) in the United States [10], or the Canadian Integrated Program for Antimicrobial Resistance Surveillance (CIPARS) in Canada [11]. The One Health approach can also be found in a UK report [12]. However, in low- and middle-income countries (LMICs), where demand for meat (and antimicrobials) is rising, rapid systematic surveillance systems remain largely absent. This Special Issue seeks to promote this approach further.

Conflicts of Interest: The author declares no conflicts of interest.

List of Contributions:

1. Cao, J.; Wang, Y.; Wang, G.; Ren, P.; Wu, Y.; He, Q. Effects of Typical Antimicrobials on Growth Performance, Morphology and Antimicrobial Residues of Mung Bean Sprouts. *Antibiotics* **2022**, *11*, 807. https://doi.org/10.3390/antibiotics11060807.
2. Zhang, S.; Sun, H.; Lao, G.; Zhou, Z.; Liu, Z.; Cai, J.; Sun, Q. Identification of Mobile Colistin Resistance Gene mcr-10 in Disinfectant and Antibiotic Resistant Escherichia coli from Disinfected Tableware. *Antibiotics* **2022**, *11*, 883. https://doi.org/10.3390/antibiotics11070883.

3. Zhang, Z.; Tian, X.; Shi, C. Global Spread of MCR-Producing Salmonella enterica Isolates. *Antibiotics* **2022**, *11*, 998. https://doi.org/10.3390/antibiotics11080998.
4. Chen, Q.; Zou, Z.; Cai, C.; Li, H.; Wang, Y.; Lei, L.; Shao, B. Characterization of blaNDM-5-and blaCTX-M-199-Producing ST167 Escherichia coli Isolated from Shared Bikes. *Antibiotics* **2022**, *11*, 1030. https://doi.org/10.3390/antibiotics11081030.
5. Zhai, W.; Tian, Y.; Shao, D.; Zhang, M.; Li, J.; Song, H.; Sun, C.; Wang, Y.; Liu, D.; Zhang, Y. Fecal Carriage of Escherichia coli Harboring the tet(X4)-IncX1 Plasmid from a Tertiary Class-A Hospital in Beijing, China. *Antibiotics* **2022**, *11*, 1068. https://doi.org/10.3390/antibiotics11081068.
6. Alvarado, A.; Chekabab, S.; Predicala, B.; Korber, D. Impact of Raised without Antibiotics Measures on Antimicrobial Resistance and Prevalence of Pathogens in Sow Barns. *Antibiotics* **2022**, *11*, 1221. https://doi.org/10.3390/antibiotics11091221.
7. Liang, H.; Li, X.; Yan, H. Identification of a Novel IncHI1B Plasmid in MDR Klebsiella pneumoniae 200 from Swine in China. *Antibiotics* **2022**, *11*, 1225. https://doi.org/10.3390/antibiotics11091225.
8. Fei, Z.; Song, S.; Yang, X.; Jiang, D.; Gao, J.; Yang, D. Occurrence and Risk Assessment of Fluoroquinolone Residues in Chicken and Pork in China. *Antibiotics* **2022**, *11*, 1292. https://doi.org/10.3390/antibiotics11101292.
9. Cao, T.; Guo, Y.; Wang, D.; Liu, Z.; Huang, S.; Peng, C.; Wang, S.; Wang, Y.; Lu, Q.; Xiao, F.; et al. Effect of Phorate on the Development of Hyperglycaemia in Mouse and Resistance Genes in Intestinal Microbiota. *Antibiotics* **2022**, *11*, 1584. https://doi.org/10.3390/antibiotics11111584.
10. Mao, X.; Zhou, X.; He, J.; Liu, G.; Liu, H.; Zhao, H.; Luo, P.; Wu, Y.; Li, Y. Metabolism Profile of Mequindox in Sea Cucumbers In Vivo Using LC-HRMS. *Antibiotics* **2022**, *11*, 1599. https://doi.org/10.3390/antibiotics11111599.
11. Carhuaricra, D.; Duran Gonzales, C.; Rodríguez Cueva, C.; Ignacion León, Y.; Silvestre Espejo, T.; Marcelo Monge, G.; Rosadio Alcántara, R.; Lincopan, N.; Espinoza, L.; Maturrano Hernández, L. Occurrence and Genomic Characterization of mcr-1-Harboring Escherichia coli Isolates from Chicken and Pig Farms in Lima, Peru. *Antibiotics* **2022**, *11*, 1781. https://doi.org/10.3390/antibiotics11121781.
12. Yan, S.; Zhang, X.; Jia, X.; Zhang, J.; Han, X.; Su, C.; Zhao, J.; Gou, W.; Xu, J.; Zhang, B. Characterization of the Composition Variation of Healthy Human Gut Microbiome in Correlation with Antibiotic Usage and Yogurt Consumption. *Antibiotics* **2022**, *11*, 1827. https://doi.org/10.3390/antibiotics11121827.
13. Liu, Y.; Qin, Z.; Yue, H.; Bergen, P.; Deng, L.; He, W.; Zeng, Z.; Peng, X.; Liu, J. Synergistic Effects of Capric Acid and Colistin against Colistin-Susceptible and Colistin-Resistant Enterobacterales. *Antibiotics* **2023**, *12*, 36. https://doi.org/10.3390/antibiotics12010036.
14. Bor, N.; Seguino, A.; Sentamu, D.; Chepyatich, D.; Akoko, J.; Muinde, P.; Thomas, L. Prevalence of Antibiotic Residues in Pork in Kenya and the Potential of Using Gross Pathological Lesions as a Risk-Based Approach to Predict Residues in Meat. *Antibiotics* **2023**, *12*, 492. https://doi.org/10.3390/antibiotics12030492.
15. Muinde, P.; Maina, J.; Momanyi, K.; Yamo, V.; Mwaniki, J.; Kiiru, J. Antimicrobial Resistant Pathogens Detected in Raw Pork and Poultry Meat in Retailing Outlets in Kenya. *Antibiotics* **2023**, *12*, 613. https://doi.org/10.3390/antibiotics12030613.
16. Han, N.; Li, J.; Wan, P.; Pan, Y.; Xu, T.; Xiong, W.; Zeng, Z. Co-Existence of Oxazolidinone Resistance Genes cfr(D) and optrA on Two Streptococcus parasuis Isolates from Swine. *Antibiotics* **2023**, *12*, 825. https://doi.org/10.3390/antibiotics12050825.

References

1. World Health Organization. Food Safety. 2022. Available online: https://www.who.int/news-room/fact-sheets/detail/food-safety (accessed on 19 May 2022).
2. World Health Organization. WHO Global Strategy for Food Safety 2022–2030: Towards Stronger Food Safety Systems and Global Cooperation. 2022. Available online: https://www.who.int/publications/i/item/9789240057685 (accessed on 12 October 2022).
3. Wu, Y. Global Food Safety Strategies: Need to Develop Roadmap of Implementation in China. *China CDC Wkly.* **2022**, *4*, 478–482. [PubMed]
4. World Health Organization. Antimicrobial Resistance: The Food Chain. 2017. Available online: https://www.who.int/news-room/questions-and-answers/item/antimicrobial-resistance-in-the-food-chain (accessed on 1 November 2017).
5. World Health Organization. Global Action Plan on Antimicrobial Resistance. 2015. Available online: https://www.who.int/publications/i/item/9789241509763 (accessed on 1 January 2016).

6. Chen, S.; Zhang, J.; Wu, Y. National Action Plan in Antimicrobial Resistance Using Framework Analysis for China. *China CDC Wkly.* **2023**, *5*, 492–498. [CrossRef]
7. World Health Organization. One Health Joint Plan of Action (2022–2026): Working Together for the Health of Humans, Animals, Plants and the Environment. 2022. Available online: https://www.who.int/publications/i/item/9789240059139 (accessed on 14 October 2022).
8. World Health Organization. Global Antimicrobial Resistance and Use Surveillance System (GLASS) Report: 2022. 2022. Available online: https://www.who.int/publications/i/item/9789240062702 (accessed on 9 December 2022).
9. European Centre for Disease Prevention and Control (ECDC) ; European Food Safety Authority (EFSA); European Medicines Agency (EMA). *Fourth Joint Inter-Agency Report on Integrated Analysis of Consumption of Antimicrobial Agents and Occurrence of Antimicrobial Resistance in Bacteria from Humans and Food-Producing Animals in the EU/EEA*; ECDC: Stockholm, Sweden; EFSA: Parma, Italy; EMA: Amsterdam, The Netherlands, 2024. [CrossRef]
10. Centers for Disease Control and Prevention. National Antimicrobial Resistance Monitoring System for Enteric Bacteria (NARMS). Available online: https://www.cdc.gov/narms/index.html (accessed on 18 March 2024).
11. Karp, B.E.; Tate, H.; Plumblee, J.R.; Dessai, U.; Whichard, J.M.; Thacker, E.L.; Hale, K.R.; Wilson, W.; Friedman, C.R.; Griffin, P.M.; et al. National antimicrobial resistance monitoring system: Two decades of advancing public health through integrated surveillance of antimicrobial resistance. *Foodborne Pathog. Dis.* **2017**, *14*, 545–557. [CrossRef]
12. Veterinary Medicines Directorate. *Third UK One Health Report—Joint Report on Antibiotic Use, Antibiotic Sales and Antibiotic Resistance*; Veterinary Medicines Directorate: Addlestone, UK, 2023.

Disclaimer/Publisher's Note: The statements, opinions and data contained in all publications are solely those of the individual author(s) and contributor(s) and not of MDPI and/or the editor(s). MDPI and/or the editor(s) disclaim responsibility for any injury to people or property resulting from any ideas, methods, instructions or products referred to in the content.

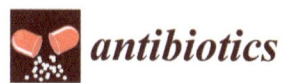

Article

Co-Existence of Oxazolidinone Resistance Genes *cfr*(D) and *optrA* on Two *Streptococcus parasuis* Isolates from Swine

Ning Han [1,2,3], Jie Li [1,2,3], Peng Wan [1,2,3], Yu Pan [1,2,3], Tiantian Xu [1,2,3], Wenguang Xiong [1,2,3,*] and Zhenling Zeng [1,2,3,*]

1. Guangdong Provincial Key Laboratory of Veterinary Pharmaceutics Development and Safety Evaluation, College of Veterinary Medicine, South China Agricultural University, Guangzhou 510642, China
2. National Laboratory of Safety Evaluation (Environmental Assessment) of Veterinary Drugs, College of Veterinary Medicine, South China Agricultural University, Guangzhou 510642, China
3. National Risk Assessment Laboratory for Antimicrobial Resistance of Animal Original Bacteria, College of Veterinary Medicine, South China Agricultural University, Guangzhou 510642, China
* Correspondence: xiongwg@scau.edu.cn (W.X.); zlzeng@scau.edu.cn (Z.Z.)

Abstract: This study was performed to investigate the presence and characteristics of the oxazolidinone resistance genes *optrA* and *cfr*(D) in *Streptococcus parasuis*. In total, 36 *Streptococcus* isolates (30 *Streptococcus suis* isolates, 6 *Streptococcus parasuis* isolates) were collected from pig farms in China in 2020–2021, using PCR to determine the presence of *optrA* and *cfr*. Then, 2 of the 36 *Streptococcus* isolates were further processed as follows. Whole-genome sequencing and de novo assembly were employed to analyze the genetic environment of the *optrA* and *cfr*(D) genes. Conjugation and inverse PCR were employed to verify the transferability of *optrA* and *cfr*(D). The *optrA* and *cfr*(D) genes were identified in two *S. parasuis* strains named SS17 and SS20, respectively. The *optrA* of the two isolates was located on chromosomes invariably associated with the *araC* gene and Tn554, which carry the resistance genes *erm*(A) and *ant*(9). The two plasmids that carry *cfr*(D), pSS17 (7550 bp) and pSS20-1 (7550 bp) have 100% nucleotide sequence identity. The *cfr*(D) was flanked by GMP synthase and IS1202. The findings of this study extend the current knowledge of the genetic background of *optrA* and *cfr*(D) and indicate that Tn554 and IS1202 may play an important role in the transmission of *optrA* and *cfr*(D), respectively.

Keywords: *cfr*(D); *optrA*; oxazolidinones; resistance; *Streptococcus parasuis*

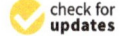

Citation: Han, N.; Li, J.; Wan, P.; Pan, Y.; Xu, T.; Xiong, W.; Zeng, Z. Co-Existence of Oxazolidinone Resistance Genes *cfr*(D) and *optrA* on Two *Streptococcus parasuis* Isolates from Swine. *Antibiotics* 2023, 12, 825. https://doi.org/10.3390/antibiotics12050825

Academic Editor: Thierry Vernet

Received: 20 March 2023
Revised: 13 April 2023
Accepted: 19 April 2023
Published: 28 April 2023

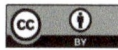

Copyright: © 2023 by the authors. Licensee MDPI, Basel, Switzerland. This article is an open access article distributed under the terms and conditions of the Creative Commons Attribution (CC BY) license (https://creativecommons.org/licenses/by/4.0/).

1. Introduction

Oxazolidinones, such as linezolid and tedizolid, are regarded as the last-resort antibacterial compounds used to treat serious clinical infections caused by multidrug-resistant (MDR) Gram-positive bacteria, specifically methicillin-resistant strains of *Staphylococcus aureus* (MRSA) and vancomycin-resistant *Enterococci* (VRE) infections [1,2]. Statistics show that MRSA causes approximately 95,000 invasive infections and 19,000 deaths each year in the United States, which is a higher mortality rate than human immunodeficiency virus, viral hepatitis, tuberculosis and influenza combined [3,4]. Enterococci are of major importance in central line-associated bloodstream infections, catheter-associated urinary tract infections, ventilator-associated pneumonia and surgical site infections [5]. The target site of linezolid is the 50S large subunit of ribosomal proteins, especially the ribosomal proteins L3 and L4 that are encoded by the *rplC* and *rplD* genes, respectively [6]. However, with the widespread use of oxazolidinone antibiotics in livestock and poultry, many oxazolidinone-resistant bacteria have recently been reported [7–10]. The existence of transferable resistance genes, such as *optrA*, *poxtA*, *cfr*, and *cfr*-like genes, is considered to be one of the causes of oxazolidinone resistance [11,12].

The transferable oxazolidinone resistance genes, *optrA* and *cfr*, have been identified in considerable bacterial species worldwide. Since the *optrA* gene was first discovered in the *Enterococcus* spp. of human and animal origin in 2015 in China, numerous reports have indicated that the *optrA* genes exist in Gram-positive bacteria, such as *Enterococcus faecalis* and *Staphylococcus sciuri* [13]. The *optrA* gene confers transferable resistance to oxazolidinones and phenols by encoding an ATP-binging cassette (ABC-F) protein [14]. The *cfr* gene, initially isolated from *S. sciuri*, mainly confers multidrug resistance to lincosamides, oxazolidinones, phenols, and pleuromutilins by mediating methylation at position 2503 of the 23S rRNA gene [15]. The *cfr* and *cfr*-like genes (e.g., *cfr*(B), *cfr*(C) and *cfr*(D)) have been discovered in various Gram-positive and Gram-negative pathogens, such as *Staphylococcus*, *Enterococcus*, *Streptococcus suis*, *Escherichia coli*, and *Micrococcus caseolyticus* [16,17].

Streptococcus parasuis, once taxonomically classified as serotypes 20, 22, and 26 of *S. suis*, is rarely reported in clinics compared with *S. suis* because of the lack of appropriate detection methods that can be used to distinguish it from *S. suis* [18]. Given the lack of clinical isolates, the significance of *S. parasuis* for public health is underestimated [19]. The presence of *S. parasuis* has recently been reported in a few countries, such as China, Japan, Canada, and Switzerland [20–23]. The *S. parasuis* strain that harbors *optrA* and *cfr*(D) genes was first discovered in Qinghai Province, China, in 2018 [21]. Then, we accidentally isolated two *S. parasuis* strains that carry a chromosomal *optrA* gene and a plasmid-borne *cfr*(D) gene during drug-resistance monitoring on a pig farm in Guangdong Province, China, in 2021. Furthermore, the two *S. parasuis* isolates showed different sequence types. The strain has spread across a large geographic area among livestock and poultry. Here, we report two *S. parasuis* strains with *cfr*(D) and *optrA* from a Chinese pig farm.

2. Materials and Methods

2.1. Sample Collection and Bacterial Strains

A total of 912 samples (762 pig lung samples and 150 pig nasal swab samples) were collected from abattoir and pig farms in three provinces of China (i.e., Guangdong, Jiangxi, and Hunan) during 2020–2021. All samples were incubated in tryptic soy broth (TSB, 5% fetal bovine serum) and then streaked onto tryptic soy agar (TSA) with 5% defibrinated sheep blood. The rifampicin-resistant *E. faecalis* JH2-2 served as the recipient strain in the transfer experiments.

2.2. Antimicrobial Susceptibility Testing

Antimicrobial susceptibility testing for meropenem, rifampicin, linezolid, florfenicol, tetracycline, erythromycin, clindamycin, penicillin, ceftiofur, ampicillin, amoxicillin, enrofloxacin, cotrimoxazole, and vancomycin was performed using the broth microdilution method according to the guidelines of the Clinical and Laboratory Standards Institute (VET01-S2 and M100-S26) [24,25]. *Streptococcus pneumoniae* ATCC 49,619 was used as a quality control strain to determine the minimum inhibitory concentration.

2.3. PCR Analysis

The *optrA* and *cfr* genes were detected in all strains by using polymerase chain reaction (PCR), as described previously [26,27]. The presence of circular intermediates was detected by inverse PCR using the primers in-*optrA*-F, GGGAACAGTTGATGAGAGAA, and in-*optrA*-R, CCAACACCATATTACCATCAT (annealing temperature of 51 °C). Sanger sequencing was used for all PCR products.

2.4. Whole-Genome Sequencing (WGS) and Analysis

The genomic DNA of the *S. parasuis* strains SS17 and SS20 that carry both *optrA* and *cfr* genes was extracted using a HiPure Bacterial DNA Kit (Magen, Shanghai, China). The WGS was performed on an Illumina HiSeq TM2000 sequence platform (Novogene, Beijing, China) and PacBio RS III sequencing platform (Tianjin Biochip Company, Tianjin, China). Draft genomes of Illumina HiSeq sequences were assembled using the CLC Genomics Workbench 10.0.1 (CLC Bio, Aarhus, Denmark) [28]. HGAP4 analysis was used to generate assemblies de novo and data statistics for the original genome data that was measured using Pacbio sequel technology [29]. The Rapid Annotation using the Subsystem Technology (RAST) (https://rast.nmpdr.org/, accessed on 7 August 2021) server was accessed for genome annotation. Antimicrobial resistance genes, virulence genes, and mobile genetic elements were identified using CGE ResFinder 3.2 (https://cge.cbs.dtu.dk/services/ResFinder/, accessed on 7 August 2021), Virulence Finder 2.0 (https://cge.cbs.dtu.dk/services/VirulenceFinder/accessed on 7 August 2021), and MGE (https://cge.cbs.dtu.dk/services/MobileElementFinder/, accessed on 7 August 2021), respectively. The genetic environments of *optrA* and *cfr* were analyzed using the BLAST program (http://blast.ncbi.nlm.nih.gov/Blast.cgi, accessed on 7 August 2021) and Easyfig 2.2.5 (developed by the Beatson Microbial Genomics Lab, Brisbane, Australia) [30].

2.5. Phylogenetic Analyses of S. parasuis Isolates

To construct the phylogeny of *S. parasuis*, all of the genomes of *S. parasuis* ($n = 9$, collected from NCBI) were extracted compared with the genomes of the *S. parasuis* isolates in this study. The phylogenic tree was constructed by RAxML, with the genome of SS20 used as a reference [31]. Snippy was employed to calculate the single nucleotide polymorphism (SNP) among the various genomes. The phylogenic tree was illustrated using iTOL [32].

2.6. Transfer Experiments

Conjugation experiments were performed by filter mating using rifampicin-resistant *E. faecalis* JH2-2 as the recipient strain and the two isolates, which carried the *cfr* gene on the plasmids and *optrA* in the chromosome, as donors [33]. Transconjugants were selected on brain–heart infusion agar plates containing 100 mg/L rifampicin and 32 mg/L florfenicol or 10 mg/L chloramphenicol, 20 mg/L chloramphenicol, and 30 mg/L chloramphenicol [1].

2.7. Nucleotide Sequence Accession Numbers

The complete genomes of *S. parasuis* SS17 and SS20 have been deposited in GenBank and assigned the nucleotide sequence accession numbers CP090522 and CP086728.

3. Results

3.1. Identification of cfr(D) and optrA in the Streptococcus Isolates

A total of 30 strains of *S. suis* (3.29%, 30/912) and 6 strains of *S. parasuis* (0.66%, 6/912) were isolated and identified from 912 samples. Among the pig lung samples, 26 *S. suis* isolates (3.41%, 26/762) and 4 *S. parasuis* isolates (0.52%, 4/762) were isolated from 762 samples, but none of these were positive for *optrA* or *cfr*(D). From the 150 pig nasal swab samples, 4 *S. suis* and 2 *S. parasuis* strains were isolated. The coexistence of *optrA* and *cfr*(D) in the two *S. parasuis* isolates, SS17 and SS20, was detected.

3.2. Antibiotic Resistance and Resistance Determinants

The resistance rate to erythromycin and clindamycin was over 90% among 36 Streptococcus strains, followed by tetracycline. Most strains remain susceptible to florfenicol, meropenem, and enrofloxacin. Antibiotic susceptibility tests showed that *S. parasuis* SS17 and SS20 demonstrated a multidrug resistance profile. They were resistant to florfenicol, erythromycin, clindamycin, tetracycline, penicillin, ampicillin, and enrofloxacin, but remained susceptible to meropenem, vancomycin, linezolid, amoxicillin, and ceftiofur. Acquired drug resistance gene test results showed that *S. parasuis* SS17 contained *ant*(6)-*la*, *optrA*, *aac*(6')-*aph*(2''), *erm*(B), *tet*(M), and *cfr*(D), while *S. parasuis* SS20 contained *ant*(6)-*la*, *optrA*, *erm*(B), *tet*(M), *msr*(D), *mef*(A), and *cfr*(D) (Table 1).

Table 1. Minimum inhibitory concentrations of 13 antimicrobial agents and ARGs among 2 *Streptococcus parasuis* isolates carrying both *optrA* and a *cfr*(D).

Isolate	Species	Source	MLST	MIC (mg/L)													Resistance Genes
				ERY	CLI	MEM	CEF	LZD	VAN	TET	PEN	AMP	ENR	SXT	FFC	AMO	
SS17	S. parasuis	nasal swab	NA	32	>32	≤0.03	0.5	1	0.12	64	2	1	4	32	64	0.5	ant(6)-Ia, aac(6′)-aph(2″), optrA, erm(B), tet(M), cfr(D)
SS20	S. parasuis	nasal swab	NA	32	>32	≤0.03	0.5	1	0.12	64	2	1	4	64	>64	1	erm(B), ant(6)-Ia, optrA, mef(A), tet(M), cfr(D)

MLST, multi-locus sequence type; MIC, minimum inhibitory concentration; ERY, erythromycin; CLI, clindamycin; MEM, meropenem; CEF, ceftiofur; LZD, linezolid; VAN, vancomycin; TET, tetracycline; PEN, penicillin; AMP, ampicillin; ENR, enrofloxacin; SXT, cotrimoxazole; FFC, florfenicol; AMO, amoxicillin; NA, not available.

3.3. WGS Analyses

The whole-genome sequence analysis showed that the chromosomes of SS17 and SS20 were 1,959,737 bp and 2,083,983 bp in size with GC contents of 39.6% and 39.5%, respectively. The genome of SS17 contained 2066 coding sequences and 46 RNA genes shown by RAST, while the SS20 contained 2275 coding sequences and 46 RNA genes. *S. parasuis* SS17 harbored a chromosomal *optrA* and a *cfr*(D)-carrying plasmid named pSS17. *S. parasuis* SS20 contained a chromosomal *optrA* and two plasmids named pSS20-1 and pSS20-2. The plasmid pSS20-1 carried a *cfr*(D) gene, while another plasmid, pSS20-1, was associated with no antimicrobial resistance gene.

3.4. Characterization of Plasmids Carrying cfr(D)

The plasmids pSS17 and pSS20-1, which carry *cfr*(D), had a 100% nucleotide sequence identity. They were 7550 bp in length with 37.8% GC content and have nine coding sequences and no RNAs. Except for the four open reading frames (ORFs) that encode hypothetical proteins, the remaining five ORF coding proteins were identified as *cfr*(D), GMP synthase, replication protein, IS1202, and IS431mec (Figure 1a,b). The nucleotide sequences of *cfr*(D) in pSS17 and pSS20-1 showed 100% (1074 of 1074) identity with the corresponding *cfr*(D) sequence from plasmid pH35-cfrD, which was from the *S. parasuis* strain H35 (GenBank accession no.CP076722.1) of porcine origin. The *cfr*(D) genes of pSS17 and pSS20-1 were flanked by GMP synthase, IS1202, and IS431mec. BLASTn analysis showed that pSS17 and pSS20-1 shared 99% (5334 of 5335) nucleotide sequence identity with the pH35-cfrD plasmid of the *S. parasuis* strain H35 isolated from a lung sample of a pig in Qinghai province, China, in 2018. In addition, SS17, SS20 and H35 had 100% identity in the *cfr*(D) gene sequences. This result indicated the possibility of a similar origin for pSS17, pSS20-1, and pH35-cfrD [21]. To identify the ability of the *cfr*(D) plasmid to conjugate, filter matings were performed using graded levels of chloramphenicol (10, 20, and 30 mg/L) or 32 mg/L florfenicol with the *E. faecalis* JH2-2 as the recipient strain. Nevertheless, no transconjugant was obtained in the triplicate assays.

3.5. Genetic Environment of optrA in the Chromosomal DNA

The *optrA* genes from SS17 and SS20 had 100% nucleotide sequence identity. Genetic environment analysis indicated that the *optrA* genes of SS17 and SS20 located on the chromosome were associated with the Tn554 and araC genes. Tn554 carried the resistance genes *erm*(A) and *ant*(9). The *araC* gene was a transcriptional regulator gene, forming a core segment of 3453 bp with *optrA*. However, the *optrA* of *S. parasuis* H35 was flanked by IS1216E elements. The *optrA* of SS17 and SS20 had three SNPs (791, T→C; 1120, G→A; 1729, T→C) compared with *S. parasuis* H35 from the same host in the same country. BLASTn analysis revealed that the *optrA*-carrying fragment exhibited high similarity with the corresponding region in the chromosomal DNA of the *E. faecium* strain GJA5 (GenBank accession no. MK251151.1), *Staphylococcus* sp. MZ7 (GenBank accession no. CP076027.1), *Staphylococcus* sp. MZ1 (GenBank accession no. CP076025.1), and the plasmid pL15 of the *E. faecalis* strain L15 (GenBank accession no. CP042214.1) (Figure 1c).

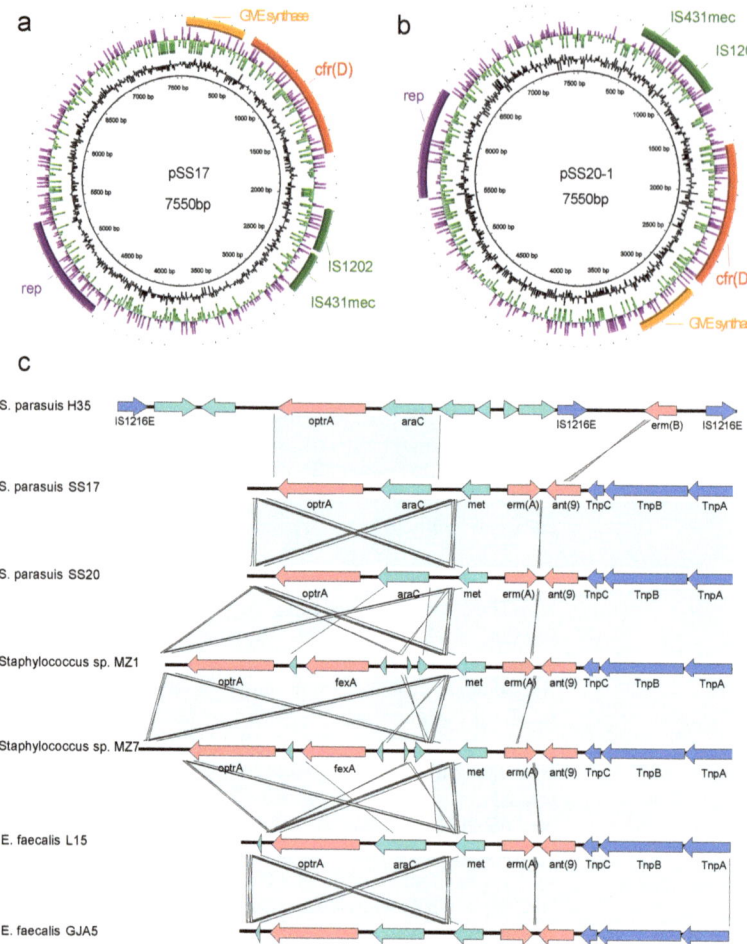

Figure 1. (**a**,**b**) are the structure and organization of the plasmids of pSS17 and pSS20-1, respectively. The circles (from the outside to inside) indicate the predicated coding sequences, GC-skew [(G + C)/(G + C)], GC content and scale in bp. The coding sequences with different functions are shown in different colors. Arrows indicate the direction of transcription of the genes. (**c**) Genetic environment of *optrA* in the chromosomal DNA of *S.parasuis* SS17 and SS20 compared to other plasmids and genomes. Resistance genes are indicated with pink arrows. Transposases are shown with blue arrows labeled by their name. Other elements are highlighted with green arrows. Shared regions with >99% identity are denoted by nattier blue shading.

The transposon Tn*554* containing *erm*(A) and *ant*(9) was detected upstream of araC–optrA of SS17 and SS20, sharing 100% nucleotide sequence identity with the *E. faecalis* strain L15 plasmid (GenBank accession no. CP042214.1), the *E. faecium* strain GJA5, *Staphylococcus* sp. MZ7, and *Staphylococcus* sp. MZ1 (Figure 1c). Tn*554* may play an important role in the horizontal transmission of optrA in Gram-positive bacteria [34,35]. The araC–optrA gene clusters in SS17 and SS20 had 100% nucleotide sequence identity with the E. faecium strain GJA5, the E. faecalis strain L15 plasmid, and the S. parasuis strain H35 (Figure 1c). The ability of the araC- optrA gene clusters in E. faecalis to form circular intermediates and spread horizontally has been confirmed [1]. The ability of the gene to form a covalent closure circle appeared to enhance its ability to excise and integrate into the chromosome or other mobile genetic elements, as previously characterized [36–38]. Therefore, here, we used inverse PCR to determine the ability of optrA to form circular intermediates by using genomes of SS17 and SS20 as templates with the primers designed at both ends of the optrA gene. The result revealed that optrA formed a circle with its flanking 269 base pairs among the two strains. However, no transconjugant harboring optrA was obtained in the transfer experiments. It is still necessary to confirm the optrA's transferability.

3.6. Phylogenetic Relatedness of Streptococcus parasuis Strains

A phylogenic tree was produced to analyze the evolution of *S. parasuis*. The phylogenic tree demonstrated that all *S. parasuis* strains were closely related. No SNPs were identified in SS17 and SS20. Therefore, it is clear that *S. parasuis* has not evolved significantly among different hosts or geographical locations. (Figure 2). These strains carried only a few ARGs, e.g., *ant(6)-la* and *erm*(B), and some did not contain any ARGs. At the same time, the distribution of ARGs explained the results of the antibiotic resistance testing.

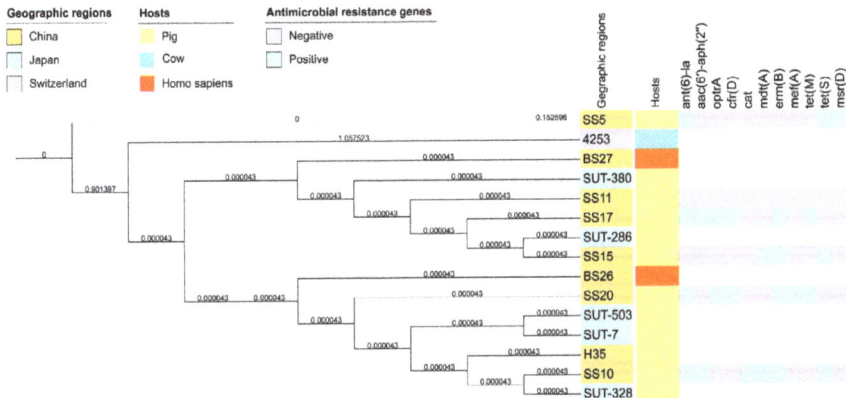

Figure 2. The phylogenetic analysis of *S. parasuis* isolates. The geographic regions of the sources of these isolates and the hosts are displayed in different colors. The antimicrobial resistance genes are indicated using a heatmap; light blue is positive, and purple is negative.

4. Discussion

A major factor in the prevalence of antibiotic resistance genes in the food chain is the presence of antibiotic-resistant bacteria in food animals, which poses a potential risk to public health and safety [39]. *Streptococcus suis* is an important zoonotic pathogen that can be transmitted to humans through contact with contaminated animal products or sick animals [40]. The ST25 and ST28 strains were dominant (9/30) among the isolates in this study. ST1 was identified as having a significantly higher virulence than ST25/28, and the remaining strains were ST242, ST27, ST1, ST7, and so on [41]. In addition to being extremely virulent, *S. suis* is recognized as a reservoir of ARGs, where transposons or integration and binding elements play a crucial role in the propagation of the organism [42]. *S. parasuis* is a close relative of *S. suis*, which may be an opportunistic pathogen, and it has been reported that it infects pigs, cattle, and humans [22]. The resistance of *S. parasuis* should also be taken into consideration. In this investigation, *S. suis* isolates only carried one to three ARGs, primarily *erm*(B) and *tet*(O), but *S. parasuis* isolates carried *ant(6)-la*, *aac(6′)-aph(2″)*, *mdt*(A), *lsa*(E), *cat*, *tet*(S) and other ARGs, which carry far more resistance genes. The detection rate of *tet*(O/M), *ant(6)-la*, and *erm*(B) in *S. parasuis* is higher, according to NCBI public data [43]. Based on these findings, *S. parasuis* is a potentially opportunistic zoonotic pathogen that may serve as a reservoir of resistance genes.

The spread of antibiotic resistance is significantly aided by both [44]. Since the *optrA* gene was discovered in China in 2015, it has been widely spread and detected in bacterial genera with diverse origins, including *Enterococcus* and *Staphylococcus*, in many different nations [45]. Platforms carrying the *optrA* gene can be categorized into three groups: those carrying *optrA* on chromosomally borne integration and conjugation elements (ICE), such as Tn*6674*, Tn*558*, and IS*1216E*; those on which the *optrA* gene is located on medium-sized plasmids (30–60 Kb) from the RepA_N, Inc18, and Rep_3 plasmid families to form *impB–fexA–optrA*; and those carrying *optrA–araC* on the chromosome or plasmids [46,47]. In this study, it was found that *optrA* was located in chromosomally borne Tn*554* carrying *erm*(A) and *ant*(9). The *cfr* gene was originally discovered on the multi-resistant pSCFS1 (16.5 kb) and pSCFS3 (35.7 kb) plasmids of *Staphylococcus sciuri* [48,49]. The *cfr*-carrying segment (IS*21-558-cfr*) was reported initially, which could form in tandem [50]. Mobile elements play an important role in the horizontal transfer of drug resistance genes. Subsequently, another multidrug-resistant plasmid (50 kb) carrying cfr was found in *Staphylococcus*, and a circular plasmid with five ORFs (*rep-Deltapre/mob-cfr-pre/mob-ermC*) was found in its transformants (7057 bp) [51]. Here, we found a new plasmid carrying the *cfr* gene in *S. parasuis*, 7550 bp, which is composed of 5 ORFs and *rep-IS431mec-IS1202-cfr-GME synthase*. Unfortunately, the transformants of *cfr* and *optrA* could not be obtained, and their transferability between different genera has yet to be confirmed. Interestingly, SS17 and SS20 remained sensitive to linezolid despite containing two oxazolidinone resistance mechanisms, *cfr*(D) and *optrA*. A study showed that *cfr*(D) did not produce any resistance when overexpressed in *E. faecalis* and *E. faecium*, but it was responsible for the phenicol resistance phenotype of *Escherichia coli* [52]. Meanwhile, the lack of *cfr* and *cfr*-like gene-mediated resistance to phenol and oxazolidinone in *E. faecalis* and *E. faecium* has been much reported [53,54]. Perhaps this phenomenon does not only occur in a single species. In contrast to the ubiquity of resistance in Gram-negative bacteria, Gram-positive bacteria still seem to preserve a defense against drug resistance genes. Since *optrA* was first identified, at least 69 variants have been identified; it is inferred that there are 1 to 20 amino acid differences. The different *optrA* variants may have an effect on the MIC of the oxazolidine of the corresponding isolates that show sensitivity/resistance [7].

In conclusion, this study reported the co-occurrence of *optrA* and *cfr*(D) operons in *S.parasuis*. The presence of Tn*554–optrA* in *Enterococcus* spp., *Staphylococcus* spp., and *Streptococcus* spp. with various genetic and source backgrounds demonstrated that the Tn*554* element plays an important role in the dissemination of *optrA*. Attention should be paid to the potential risks of plasmid-borne *cfr*(D) transference from streptococcus to other Gram-positive bacteria. Meanwhile, the existence of additional resistance genes, *erm*(A) and *ant*(9), and the use of various types of antibiotics may contribute to the prevalence of *optrA* and *cfr*(D). Therefore, it is urgently necessary to continuously monitor the spread of *optrA* and *cfr*(D) among Gram-positive bacteria, and monitor the prudent use of antibiotics in food animals.

Author Contributions: Conceptualization, N.H.; methodology, N.H. and J.L.; software, N.H. and Y.P.; validation, N.H., J.L. and P.W.; formal analysis, N.H.; resources, N.H. and P.W.; data curation, N.H.; writing—original draft preparation, N.H.; writing—review and editing, Z.Z., W.X. and T.X.; visualization, N.H.; supervision, Z.Z.; project administration, Z.Z.; funding acquisition, Z.Z. All authors have read and agreed to the published version of the manuscript.

Funding: This study was supported by the Local Innovative and Research Teams Project of Guangdong Pearl River Talents Program (2019BT02N054) and the Natural Science Foundation of Guangdong Province of China (2021A1515011159).

Data Availability Statement: The data presented in this study are available in article.

Acknowledgments: This study was supported by the Local Innovative and Research Teams Project of Guangdong Pearl River Talents Program (2019BT02N054) and the Natural Science Foundation of Guangdong Province of China (2021A1515011159).

Conflicts of Interest: The authors declare no conflict of interest.

References

1. Almeida, L.M.; Lebreton, F.; Gaca, A.; Bispo, P.M.; Saavedra, J.T.; Calumby, R.N.; Grillo, L.M.; Nascimento, T.G.; Filsner, P.H.; Moreno, A.M.; et al. Transferable Resistance Gene in Enterococcus faecalis from Swine in Brazil. *Antimicrob. Agents Chemother.* **2020**, *64*, e00142-20. [CrossRef] [PubMed]
2. Leach, K.L.; Brickner, S.J.; Noe, M.C.; Miller, P.F. Linezolid, the first oxazolidinone antibacterial agent. *Ann. N. Y. Acad. Sci.* **2011**, *1222*, 49–54. [CrossRef] [PubMed]
3. Klevens, R.M.; Morrison, M.A.; Nadle, J.; Petit, S.; Gershman, K.; Ray, S.; Harrison, L.H.; Lynfield, R.; Dumyati, G.; Townes, J.M.; et al. Invasive methicillin-resistant *Staphylococcus aureus* infections in the United States. *JAMA* **2007**, *298*, 1763–1771. [CrossRef]
4. Hoyert, D.L.; Xu, J. Deaths: Preliminary data for 2011. *Natl. Vital. Stat. Rep.* **2012**, *61*, 1–65. [PubMed]
5. Vehreschild, M.J.G.T.; Haverkamp, M.; Biehl, L.M.; Lemmen, S.; Fätkenheuer, G. Vancomycin-resistant enterococci (VRE): A reason to isolate? *Infection* **2019**, *47*, 7–11. [CrossRef]
6. Locke, J.B.; Hilgers, M.; Shaw, K.J. Novel ribosomal mutations in *Staphylococcus aureus* strains identified through selection with the oxazolidinones linezolid and torezolid (TR-700). *Antimicrob. Agents Chemother.* **2009**, *53*, 5265–5274. [CrossRef] [PubMed]
7. Schwarz, S.; Zhang, W.; Du, X.-D.; Krüger, H.; Feßler, A.T.; Ma, S.; Zhu, Y.; Wu, C.; Shen, J.; Wang, Y. Mobile Oxazolidinone Resistance Genes in Gram-Positive and Gram-Negative Bacteria. *Clin. Microbiol. Rev.* **2021**, *34*, e0018820. [CrossRef]
8. Jung, Y.-H.; Cha, M.-H.; Woo, G.-J.; Chi, Y.-M. Characterization of oxazolidinone and phenicol resistance genes in non-clinical enterococcal isolates from Korea. *J. Glob. Antimicrob. Resist.* **2021**, *24*, 363–369. [CrossRef]
9. Meka, V.G.; Gold, H.S. Antimicrobial resistance to linezolid. *Clin. Infect. Dis.* **2004**, *39*, 1010–1015. [CrossRef]
10. Aarestrup, F.M. The livestock reservoir for antimicrobial resistance: A personal view on changing patterns of risks, effects of interventions and the way forward. *Philos. Trans. R. Soc. Lond. B Biol. Sci.* **2015**, *370*, 20140085. [CrossRef]
11. Liu, B.G.; Yuan, X.L.; He, D.D.; Hu, G.Z.; Miao, M.S.; Xu, E.P. Research progress on the oxazolidinone drug linezolid resistance. *Eur. Rev. Med. Pharm. Sci.* **2020**, *24*, 9274–9281. [CrossRef]
12. Deshpande, L.M.; Castanheira, M.; Flamm, R.K.; Mendes, R.E. Evolving oxazolidinone resistance mechanisms in a worldwide collection of enterococcal clinical isolates: Results from the SENTRY Antimicrobial Surveillance Program. *J. Antimicrob. Chemother.* **2018**, *73*, 2314–2322. [CrossRef] [PubMed]
13. Wang, Y.; Gong, S.; Dong, X.; Li, J.; Grenier, D.; Yi, L. Mixed Biofilm of and Impacts Antibiotic Susceptibility and Modulates Virulence Factor Gene Expression. *Front. Microbiol.* **2020**, *11*, 507. [CrossRef] [PubMed]
14. Sharkey, L.K.R.; O'Neill, A.J. Antibiotic Resistance ABC-F Proteins: Bringing Target Protection into the Limelight. *ACS Infect. Dis.* **2018**, *4*, 239–246. [CrossRef]
15. Locke, J.B.; Finn, J.; Hilgers, M.; Morales, G.; Rahawi, S.; Kedar, G.C.; Picazo, J.J.; Im, W.; Shaw, K.J.; Stein, J.L. Structure-activity relationships of diverse oxazolidinones for linezolid-resistant *Staphylococcus aureus* strains possessing the cfr methyltransferase gene or ribosomal mutations. *Antimicrob. Agents Chemother.* **2010**, *54*, 5337–5343. [CrossRef]
16. Stojkovic, V.; Ulate, M.F.; Hidalgo-Villeda, F.; Aguilar, E.; Monge-Cascante, C.; Pizarro-Guajardo, M.; Tsai, K.; Tzoc, E.; Camorlinga, M.; Paredes-Sabja, D.; et al. cfr(B), cfr(C), and a New cfr-Like Gene, cfr(E), in *Clostridium difficile* Strains Recovered across Latin America. *Antimicrob. Agents Chemother.* **2019**, *64*, e01074-19. [CrossRef]
17. Huang, J.; Sun, J.; Wu, Y.; Chen, L.; Duan, D.; Lv, X.; Wang, L. Identification and pathogenicity of an XDR Streptococcus suis isolate that harbours the phenicol-oxazolidinone resistance genes optrA and cfr, and the bacitracin resistance locus bcrABDR. *Int. J. Antimicrob. Agents* **2019**, *54*, 43–48. [CrossRef]
18. Nomoto, R.; Maruyama, F.; Ishida, S.; Tohya, M.; Sekizaki, T.; Osawa, R. Reappraisal of the taxonomy of *Streptococcus suis* serotypes 20, 22 and 26: *Streptococcus parasuis* sp. nov. *Int. J. Syst. Evol. Microbiol.* **2015**, *65*, 438–443. [CrossRef]
19. Wang, J.; Yi, X.; Liang, P.; Tao, Y.; Wang, Y.; Jin, D.; Luo, B.; Yang, J.; Zheng, H. Investigation of the Genomic and Pathogenic Features of the Potentially Zoonotic. *Pathogens* **2021**, *10*, 834. [CrossRef]
20. Nomoto, R.; Ishida-Kuroki, K.; Nakagawa, I.; Sekizaki, T. Complete Genome Sequences of Four *Streptococcus parasuis* Strains Obtained from Saliva of Domestic Pigs in Japan. *Microbiol. Resour. Announc.* **2022**, *11*, e0124521. [CrossRef]
21. Zhu, Y.; Yang, Q.; Schwarz, S.; Yang, W.; Xu, Q.; Wang, L.; Liu, S.; Zhang, W. Identification of a Streptococcus parasuis isolate co-harbouring the oxazolidinone resistance genes cfr(D) and optrA. *J. Antimicrob. Chemother.* **2021**, *76*, 3059–3061. [CrossRef]
22. Yamada, R.; Tien, L.H.T.; Arai, S.; Tohya, M.; Ishida-Kuroki, K.; Nomoto, R.; Kim, H.; Suzuki, E.; Osawa, R.; Watanabe, T.; et al. Development of PCR for identifying *Streptococcus parasuis*, a close relative of *Streptococcus suis*. *J. Vet. Med. Sci.* **2018**, *80*, 1101–1107. [CrossRef] [PubMed]
23. Stevens, M.J.A.; Cernela, N.; Corti, S.; Stephan, R. Draft Genome Sequence of Streptococcus parasuis 4253, the First Available for the Species. *Microbiol. Resour. Announc.* **2019**, *8*, e00203-19. [CrossRef] [PubMed]
24. Clinical and Laboratory Standards Institute. *Performance Standards for an Timicrobial Susceptibility Testing*; Twenty-Sixth Informational Supplement M100-S26; CLSI: Wayne, PA, USA, 2016.
25. Clinical and laboratory Standards Institute. *Performance Standards for Antimi Crobial Disk and Diffusion Susceptibility Tests for Bacteria Isolated from Animals*; Second Informational Supplement VET01-S2; CLSI: Wayne, PA, USA, 2013.
26. Wang, Y.; Lv, Y.; Cai, J.; Schwarz, S.; Cui, L.; Hu, Z.; Zhang, R.; Li, J.; Zhao, Q.; He, T.; et al. A novel gene, optrA, that confers transferable resistance to oxazolidinones and phenicols and its presence in *Enterococcus faecalis* and *Enterococcus faecium* of human and animal origin. *J. Antimicrob. Chemother.* **2015**, *70*, 2182–2190. [CrossRef] [PubMed]

27. Wang, Y.; Zhang, W.; Wang, J.; Wu, C.; Shen, Z.; Fu, X.; Yan, Y.; Zhang, Q.; Schwarz, S.; Shen, J. Distribution of the multidrug resistance gene cfr in *Staphylococcus* species isolates from swine farms in China. *Antimicrob. Agents Chemother.* **2012**, *56*, 1485–1490. [CrossRef] [PubMed]
28. Chin, C.-S.; Alexander, D.H.; Marks, P.; Klammer, A.A.; Drake, J.; Heiner, C.; Clum, A.; Copeland, A.; Huddleston, J.; Eichler, E.E.; et al. Nonhybrid, finished microbial genome assemblies from long-read SMRT sequencing data. *Nat. Methods* **2013**, *10*, 563–569. [CrossRef]
29. Bitar, I.; Moussa, J.; Abboud, E.; Hrabak, J.; Tokajian, S. Integration of two pKPX-2-derived antibiotic resistance islands in the genome of an ESBL-producing Klebsiella pneumoniae ST3483 from Lebanon. *J. Glob. Antimicrob. Resist.* **2019**, *18*, 257–259. [CrossRef]
30. Zankari, E.; Hasman, H.; Cosentino, S.; Vestergaard, M.; Rasmussen, S.; Lund, O.; Aarestrup, F.M.; Larsen, M.V. Identification of acquired antimicrobial resistance genes. *J. Antimicrob. Chemother.* **2012**, *67*, 2640–2644. [CrossRef]
31. Stamatakis, A. RaxML version 8: A tool for phylogenetic analysis and post-analysis of large phylogenies. *Bioinformatics* **2014**, *30*, 1312–1313. [CrossRef]
32. Letunic, I.; Bork, P. Interactive Tree Of Life (iTOL) v5: An online tool for phylogenetic tree display and annotation. *Nucleic Acids Res.* **2021**, *49*, W293–W296. [CrossRef]
33. Yu, R.; Zhang, Y.; Xu, Y.; Schwarz, S.; Li, X.-S.; Shang, Y.-H.; Du, X.-D. Emergence of a (M) Variant Conferring Resistance to Tigecycline in. *Front. Vet. Sci.* **2021**, *8*, 709327. [CrossRef] [PubMed]
34. Li, D.; Li, X.Y.; Schwarz, S.; Yang, M.; Zhang, S.M.; Hao, W.; Du, X.D. Tn6674 Is a Novel Enterococcal optrA-Carrying Multiresistance Transposon of the Tn554 Family. *Antimicrob. Agents Chemother.* **2019**, *63*, e00142-20. [CrossRef]
35. Yao, T.G.; Li, B.Y.; Luan, R.D.; Wang, H.N.; Lei, C.W. Whole genome sequence of Enterococcus gallinarum EG81, a porcine strain harbouring the oxazolidinone-phenicol resistance gene optrA with chromosomal and plasmid location. *J. Glob. Antimicrob. Resist.* **2020**, *22*, 598–600. [CrossRef]
36. He, Y.Z.; Li, X.P.; Miao, Y.Y.; Lin, J.; Sun, R.Y.; Wang, X.P.; Guo, Y.Y.; Liao, X.P.; Liu, Y.H.; Feng, Y.; et al. The ISApl1 2 Dimer Circular Intermediate Participates in mcr-1 Transposition. *Front. Microbiol.* **2019**, *10*, 15. [CrossRef] [PubMed]
37. Lyras, D.; Rood, J.I. Transposition of Tn4451 and Tn4453 involves a circular intermediate that forms a promoter for the large resolvase, TnpX. *Mol. Microbiol.* **2000**, *38*, 588–601. [CrossRef]
38. Manganelli, R.; Romano, L.; Ricci, S.; Zazzi, M.; Pozzi, G. Dosage of Tn916 circular intermediates in *Enterococcus faecalis*. *Plasmid* **1995**, *34*, 48–57. [CrossRef]
39. García-Sánchez, L.; Melero, B.; Diez, A.M.; Jaime, I.; Rovira, J. Characterization of Campylobacter species in Spanish retail from different fresh chicken products and their antimicrobial resistance. *Food Microbiol.* **2018**, *76*, 457–465. [CrossRef]
40. Susilawathi, N.M.; Tarini, N.M.A.; Fatmawati, N.N.D.; Mayura, P.I.B.; Suryapraba, A.A.A.; Subrata, M.; Sudewi, A.A.R.; Mahardika, G.N. Streptococcus suis-Associated Meningitis, Bali, Indonesia, 2014–2017. *Emerg. Infect. Dis.* **2019**, *25*, 2235–2242. [CrossRef] [PubMed]
41. Segura, M.; Fittipaldi, N.; Calzas, C.; Gottschalk, M. Critical *Streptococcus suis* Virulence Factors: Are They All Really Critical? *Trends Microbiol.* **2017**, *25*, 585–599. [CrossRef]
42. Haenni, M.; Lupo, A.; Madec, J.-Y. Antimicrobial Resistance in spp. *Microbiol. Spectr.* **2018**, *6*, 585–599. [CrossRef] [PubMed]
43. Guo, G.; Wang, Z.; Li, Q.; Yu, Y.; Li, Y.; Tan, Z.; Zhang, W. Genomic characterization of Streptococcus parasuis, a close relative of *Streptococcus suis* and also a potential opportunistic zoonotic pathogen. *BMC Genom.* **2022**, *23*, 469. [CrossRef]
44. Mishra, S.; Klümper, U.; Voolaid, V.; Berendonk, T.U.; Kneis, D. Simultaneous estimation of parameters governing the vertical and horizontal transfer of antibiotic resistance genes. *Sci. Total Environ.* **2021**, *798*, 149174. [CrossRef]
45. Biggel, M.; Nüesch-Inderbinen, M.; Jans, C.; Stevens, M.J.A.; Stephan, R. Genetic Context of and in Florfenicol-Resistant Enterococci Isolated from Flowing Surface Water in Switzerland. *Antimicrob. Agents Chemother.* **2021**, *65*, e0108321. [CrossRef] [PubMed]
46. Freitas, A.R.; Tedim, A.P.; Novais, C.; Lanza, V.F.; Peixe, L. Comparative genomics of global optrA-carrying uncovers a common chromosomal hotspot for acquisition within a diversity of core and accessory genomes. *Microb. Genom.* **2020**, *6*, AAC0108321. [CrossRef] [PubMed]
47. Fan, R.; Li, D.; Feßler, A.T.; Wu, C.; Schwarz, S.; Wang, Y. Distribution of optrA and cfr in florfenicol-resistant *Staphylococcus sciuri* of pig origin. *Vet. Microbiol.* **2017**, *210*, 43–48. [CrossRef] [PubMed]
48. Schwarz, S.; Werckenthin, C.; Kehrenberg, C. Identification of a plasmid-borne chloramphenicol-florfenicol resistance gene in *Staphylococcus sciuri*. *Antimicrob. Agents Chemother.* **2000**, *44*, 2530–2533. [CrossRef]
49. Kehrenberg, C.; Ojo, K.K.; Schwarz, S. Nucleotide sequence and organization of the multiresistance plasmid pSCFS1 from *Staphylococcus sciuri*. *J. Antimicrob. Chemother.* **2004**, *54*, 936–939. [CrossRef]
50. Kehrenberg, C.; Aarestrup, F.M.; Schwarz, S. IS21-558 insertion sequences are involved in the mobility of the multiresistance gene cfr. *Antimicrob. Agents Chemother.* **2007**, *51*, 483–487. [CrossRef]
51. Li, S.-M.; Zhou, Y.-F.; Li, L.; Fang, L.-X.; Duan, J.-H.; Liu, F.-R.; Liang, H.-Q.; Wu, Y.-T.; Gu, W.-Q.; Liao, X.-P.; et al. Characterization of the Multi-Drug Resistance Gene in Methicillin-Resistant (MRSA) Strains Isolated from Animals and Humans in China. *Front. Microbiol.* **2018**, *9*, 2925. [CrossRef]

52. Guerin, F.; Sassi, M.; Dejoies, L.; Zouari, A.; Schutz, S.; Potrel, S.; Auzou, M.; Collet, A.; Lecointe, D.; Auger, G.; et al. Molecular and functional analysis of the novel cfr(D) linezolid resistance gene identified in *Enterococcus faecium*. *J. Antimicrob. Chemother.* **2020**, *75*, 1699–1703. [CrossRef]
53. Brenciani, A.; Morroni, G.; Vincenzi, C.; Manso, E.; Mingoia, M.; Giovanetti, E.; Varaldo, P.E. Detection in Italy of two clinical *Enterococcus faecium* isolates carrying both the oxazolidinone and phenicol resistance gene optrA and a silent multiresistance gene cfr. *J. Antimicrob. Chemother.* **2016**, *71*, 1118–1119. [CrossRef] [PubMed]
54. Fang, L.-X.; Duan, J.-H.; Chen, M.-Y.; Deng, H.; Liang, H.-Q.; Xiong, Y.Q.; Sun, J.; Liu, Y.-H.; Liao, X.-P. Prevalence of cfr in *Enterococcus faecalis* strains isolated from swine farms in China: Predominated cfr-carrying pCPPF5-like plasmids conferring "non-linezolid resistance" phenotype. *Infect. Genet. Evol.* **2018**, *62*, 188–192. [CrossRef] [PubMed]

Disclaimer/Publisher's Note: The statements, opinions and data contained in all publications are solely those of the individual author(s) and contributor(s) and not of MDPI and/or the editor(s). MDPI and/or the editor(s) disclaim responsibility for any injury to people or property resulting from any ideas, methods, instructions or products referred to in the content.

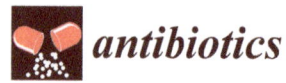

Article

Antimicrobial Resistant Pathogens Detected in Raw Pork and Poultry Meat in Retailing Outlets in Kenya

Patrick Muinde [1,*], John Maina [2], Kelvin Momanyi [1], Victor Yamo [1], John Mwaniki [2] and John Kiiru [2]

1. World Animal Protection, Westside Towers, 9th Floor, Suite 901, Along Lower Kabete Road, Westlands, P.O. Box 66580, Nairobi 00800, Kenya
2. Center for Microbiology Research, Kenya Medical Research Institute (KEMRI), P.O. Box 54840, Nairobi 00200, Kenya
* Correspondence: patrickmuinde@worldanimalprotection.org

Abstract: There is increasing proof of bacterial resistance to antibiotics all over the world, and this puts the effectiveness of antimicrobials that have been essential in decreasing disease mortality and morbidity at stake. The WHO has labeled some classes of antimicrobials as vitally important to human health. Bacteria from animals are thought to be reservoirs of resistance genes that can be transferred to humans through the food chain. This study aimed to identify the resistance patterns of bacteria from pork and poultry meat samples purchased from leading retail outlets in Kenya. Of the 393 samples collected, 98.4% of pork and 96.6% of poultry were contaminated with high levels of bacteria. Among the 611 bacterial isolates recovered, 38.5% were multi-drug resistant. This resistance was noted for critically essential antimicrobials (according to the WHO) such as rifampicin (96%), ampicillin (35%), cefotaxime (9%), cefepime (6%), and ciprofloxacin (6%). Moreover, there was high resistance to key antimicrobials for veterinary medicine such as tetracycline (39%), sulfamethoxazole (33%), and trimethoprim (30%). It is essential to spread awareness about the judicious use of antibiotics and take preventive measures to reduce disease burden.

Keywords: antibiotics; bacteria; isolates; antibiotic resistance; meat

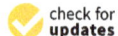

Citation: Muinde, P.; Maina, J.; Momanyi, K.; Yamo, V.; Mwaniki, J.; Kiiru, J. Antimicrobial Resistant Pathogens Detected in Raw Pork and Poultry Meat in Retailing Outlets in Kenya. *Antibiotics* **2023**, *12*, 613. https://doi.org/10.3390/antibiotics12030613

Academic Editors: Yongning Wu and Zhenling Zeng

Received: 9 February 2023
Revised: 2 March 2023
Accepted: 14 March 2023
Published: 20 March 2023

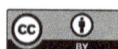

Copyright: © 2023 by the authors. Licensee MDPI, Basel, Switzerland. This article is an open access article distributed under the terms and conditions of the Creative Commons Attribution (CC BY) license (https://creativecommons.org/licenses/by/4.0/).

1. Introduction

Antimicrobial resistance (AMR) is a major global health concern, caused by the misuse and overuse of antimicrobials [1–4], which has led to microorganisms (including bacteria, fungi, viruses, and parasites) becoming resistant to the effects of these medications. The WHO defines AMR as the loss of susceptibility of these microorganisms to antimicrobials (such as antibiotics, antifungals, antivirals, and antiprotozoals). This imprudent use of antimicrobials in both the human and animal sector has resulted in the selection of pathogens resistant to multiple drugs.

It is now widely acknowledged that the rate of AMR development and spreading far outstrips the rate at which new antimicrobial drugs are being developed [5]. For instance, resistance to colistin, one of the last resort antibiotics used to treat multidrug-resistant Gram-negative infections, has been reported [6]. These multidrug-resistant (MDR) bacteria present a critical danger to public health. Such bacteria can survive the selective toxicity of antimicrobial use, enabling them to proliferate in clinical, on-farm, and environmental settings. For instance, patients infected with MDR bacteria tend to have a worse treatment outcome when compared to those infected with more susceptible organisms [7,8], in addition to being closely linked to the use of broad-spectrum antibiotics, both for empiric and definitive treatment [9].

AMR is a global issue that affects all nations including high, middle, and low-income countries, and it has increased the cost of health care and jeopardized gains made on goals set for Sustainable Development by 2030. A recent world bank report suggests AMR could cause low- and middle-income countries (LMICs) to lose more than 5% of their GDP and further push up to 28 million people, mostly in developing countries, into poverty by 2050 [10]. Globally, it is estimated that 1.27 million people die each year from drug resistant infections [11], which is projected to rise to 10 million deaths annually by 2050 [4]. By 2030, shocks due to antimicrobial resistance could cost the world up to USD 3.4 trillion a year [12], increasing to USD 100 trillion by 2050, with an overwhelming burden placed on LMICs [3].

Several antibiotic classes are used in both humans and animals, some of which are considered critically important to human health by the World Health Organization (WHO). Animal sectors chiefly use antimicrobials to prevent and treat infectious diseases [13] and promote growth in some countries [13]. Results from a recent analysis of global antibiotic sales data indicate that human antibiotic consumption is reported to have increased by 36% globally between 2000 and 2015, with most of the increase happening in LMICs where non-prescription use is still common [14].

In animals, antimicrobial use in animal production (especially in poultry and pigs) remains a key contributor to AMR [15]. The use is expected to increase exponentially due to the expansion of intensive production systems to meet the increasing demand for animal-sourced foods (ASFs), and the surge in disease burdens [16]. Over the next 20–40 years, the demand for ASFs will grow rapidly in Africa (meat consumption is forecast to grow by 30% by 2030) due to growth in the human population (from the current 1.2 billion to over 2.5 billion by 2050), increasing purchasing power and urbanization [17]. Across Africa, the current per capita annual consumption of meat and milk is about 14 kg and 30 L, respectively, and is projected to more than double to 26 kg and 64 L, respectively, by 2050 [18].

Of all antibiotics currently used in the world, approximately 73% are used within livestock [17], and a significant part is used for disease prevention (prophylaxis). The consumption is predicted to grow significantly by 2030 with the highest growth rates predicted within LMICs [19] because there will likely be a shift to more industrial livestock systems. The use of antimicrobials for growth promotion and routine disease prevention in groups of animals, without addressing the underlying animal welfare and husbandry practices that can prevent disease occurrences at farm levels, is contributing to the development and spread of AMR [20]. For instance, stressors have been documented to cause proliferation and colonization of pathogens such as *E. coli* O157:H7, *Campylobacter* and *Salmonella enterica*, which lead to fecal shedding as reported in pigs [21,22]. A review by Rostagno (2009) [23] reported how stress indirectly encourages the proliferation of enteric pathogens by suppressing the immune system and by physiological changes in the gastrointestinal tract via the action of the stress hormones.

Just like other countries, Kenya is already experiencing increasing levels of antimicrobial use and antimicrobial resistance. In 2013, it was estimated that 395 tons of antibiotics were used for food animal production in Kenya, of which 43% of them are classified as critically relevant by the WHO [16]. Notably, key antimicrobial-resistant foodborne pathogens such as *E. coli*, *Salmonella* and *Campylobacter* spp. have been documented in Kenya, with increasing frequency as causes of foodborne diseases of global public health significance [5,24]. Antimicrobial-resistant bacteria that originate in the gastrointestinal tract of animals can contaminate meat during animal slaughter and food processing or contaminate the environment with animal feces, and thus be transferred to humans through handling or consuming contaminated food or coming into contact with animal waste. This can lead to antimicrobial-resistant intestinal infections.

Studies have supported the hypothesis of the link between antimicrobial use in agricultural production systems and the emergence of AMR, especially the pronounced lack of biosecurity measures and low animal welfare practices. Since 1986, when the use of antimicrobials as growth promoters was banned in Sweden, the country has seen 65% considerable decrease in the utilization of antimicrobials in food animal production [25], resulting in a substantial reduction in the emergence and spread of AMR.

The demand for animal-based products has caused the intensification of production systems. As part of this intensification, antibiotics have been overused, both as growth promoters and as preventive measures. This has caused the emergence of pathogens that are resistant to antibiotics.

Antimicrobial-resistant bacteria have been reported in veterinary and food-related settings [26,27]. However, very few studies have assessed AMR in Kenya's pig and poultry meat products. Therefore, we conducted this study to determine the presence of foodborne bacteria in pork and chicken products and the resistance profiles of the isolates to selected clinically relevant antimicrobials.

2. Results

2.1. Sample Distribution across the Retailing Outlets

Table 1 shows that out of the 393 pork and poultry samples, 107 (27.2%) were obtained from an international outlet, followed by one regional outlet. The majority of the samples (53.4%: $n = 210$) were taken from the fridge/freezer and fresh meat section (44.8%: $n = 176$), while only seven (1.8%) samples were acquired from the supermarket shelves. Nairobi accounted for most of the samples collected (nearly 75% of the pork and 63% of the poultry). This is because most of the supermarkets are concentrated in Nairobi, with a few in other big towns in Kenya. For example, at the time of sampling, the publicly available information in their websites showed that 89% of international supermarket outlets were in Nairobi, while 37% of the regional supermarket outlets were found in Nairobi, with the rest situated in other big towns which include Mombasa, Kisumu, and Nakuru.

Table 1. Table showing the sample distribution across the selected retailing outlets in Kenya.

Type of Supermarket	Supermarket Name	No. of Poultry Samples Collected	No. of Pork Samples Collected	Total
International	A	31 (15.0%)	76 (40.6%)	107 (27.2%)
Regional	B	64 (31.1%)	33 (17.6%)	97 (24.7%)
Local	C	30 (14.6%)	32 (17.1%)	62 (15.8%)
	D	41 (19.9%)	15 (8.0%)	56 (14.2%)
	E	25 (12.2%)	26 (13.9%)	51 (13.0%)
	F	15 (7.3%)	5 (2.7%)	20 (5.1%)
Total		206 (100%)	187 (100%)	393 (100%)

The study anonymized the identities of the six retail outlets by assigning each an alphabetic designation from A to F (Table 1). Additionally, the outlets were classified into local, regional, or internationally based on criteria such as franchise status, ownership, and geographic reach.

2.2. Prevalence of Isolated Bacterial Contaminants

Nearly 98.4% (184/187) of pork and 96.6% (199/206) of poultry samples tested revealed the presence of at least one type of bacterium. In total, 611 bacterial isolates were recovered from the analysis of the 393 pork and poultry samples, but only 551 isolates were processed further depended on the resource availability. The majority (50.9%) of the isolates were detected in poultry samples but the difference was not found to be statistically significant ($p = 0.157$). Escherichia coli was the most common Gram-negative bacteria in both pork and poultry samples, at 47.7% and 49.2%, respectively. Meanwhile, *Staphylococcus* spp. (Gram-positive) was found in 28 (9.3%) of pork samples and 13 (4.2%) of poultry samples. However, it was difficult to identify *Staphylococcus aureus*, which is known to cause staphylococcal food poisoning, as the classical biochemical methods used were limited to identifying the genus level. Additional isolates included *Klebsiella* spp. (19.1%), *Salmonella* spp. (17.8%), *Shigella* (7.5%), and *Pseudomonas* spp. (0.3%), as seen in Figure 1.

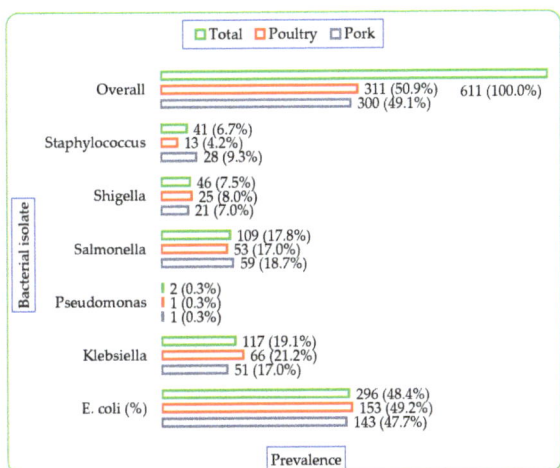

Figure 1. Figure showing the prevalence of bacterial contaminants that were isolated. The overall proportions for poultry and pork isolates were determined by analyzing the 611 total isolates recovered, which included 311 poultry and 300 pork.

2.3. The Overall Antimicrobial Resistance Profiles

Out of the 611 total isolates, 551 were chosen for analysis of antimicrobial resistance based on the sample type, retail store, and resources availability. The results, shown in Figure 2, revealed that rifampicin had the highest resistance rate of 96%. Ampicillin, sulfamethoxazole, trimethoprim, and tetracycline had resistance rates of 30–39%. The least resistance was seen with gentamicin (3%), cefepime (6%), ceftazidime (6%), and ciprofloxacin (7%).

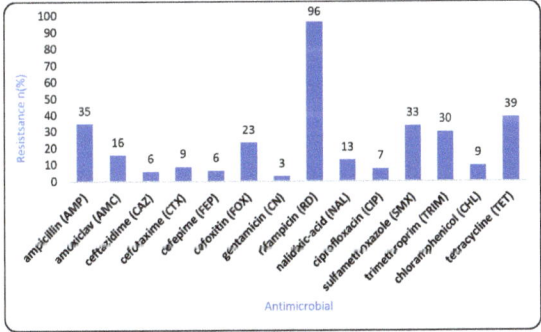

Figure 2. Figure showing the overall antimicrobial resistance profiles. The profiles of resistance were determined by examining 551 bacteria isolates taken from chicken and pork samples, comprising both Gram-positive and Gram-negative organisms. The percentage resistance was calculated by dividing the number of resistant isolates with the total number of test isolates.

As illustrated in Figure 3 below, isolates from chicken and pork samples exhibited the same resistance rate of 96% toward rifampicin. However, chicken isolates demonstrated higher resistance than those from pork against tetracycline (47% vs. 31%), sulfamethoxazole (41% vs. 26%), and trimethoprim (37% vs. 23%). Conversely, the resistance rates of pork isolate to ampicillin (35% vs. 34%), amoxicillin-clavulanic acid (19% vs. 12%), and cefoxitin (26% vs. 20%) were higher compared to that of chicken isolates.

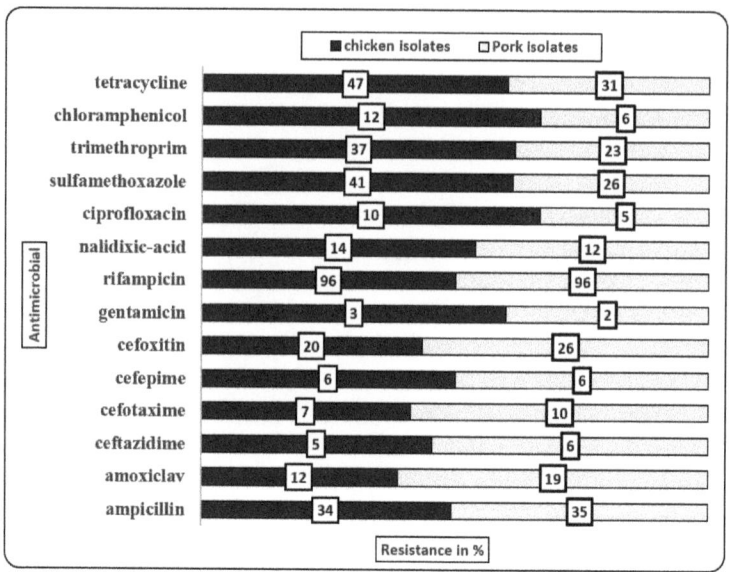

Figure 3. Figure showing the antimicrobial resistance profiles of chicken and pork isolates. The antimicrobial sensitivity testing is hinged on 268 chicken and 283 pork isolates.

2.4. The Antimicrobial Resistance Profiles of the Recovered Isolates

The comparative analysis of antimicrobial resistance (AMR) profiles was conducted using two *Pseudomonas aeruginosa* isolates, which had 100% resistance to eight antibiotics tested. Among the Gram-negatives, *Klebsiella* spp. had the highest level of resistance, particularly toward tetracycline (46%), sulfamethoxazole (43%), trimethoprim (37%), and cefoxitin (15%). Furthermore, this isolate also exhibited moderate resistance toward expanded spectrum antibiotics such as cefotaxime (5%), ceftazidime (3%), and cefepime (3%). As for *Staphylococcus* spp., its resistance profiles were higher than all other isolates for all antibiotics except rifampicin, which was higher in *Klebsiella* spp. (99%). *Salmonella* spp. was the least resistant, ranging from 1% to 31%, with the exception of rifampicin, which was at 97%. Table 2 shows the antimicrobial resistance profiles of the isolates mentioned above, *E. coli* and *Shigella* spp.

Table 2. Table showing the antimicrobial resistance profiles in recovered isolates.

Organism	N	AMP	AMC	CAZ	CTX	FEP	FOX	CN	RD	NAL	CIP	SMX	TRIM	CHL	TET
E. coli	275	71 (26)	41 (15)	5 (2)	11 (4)	6 (2)	70 (25)	11 (4)	269 (98)	33 (12)	26 (9)	95 (35)	78 (28)	28 (10)	100 (36)
Klebsiella spp.	95	53 (58)	11 (12)	3 (3)	5 (5)	3 (3)	14 (15)	1 (1)	94 (99)	9 (9)	8 (8)	41 (43)	35 (37)	8 (8)	44 (46)
P. aeruginosa	2	2 (100)	2 (100)	0	2 (100)	0	2 (100)	0	2 (100)	1 (50)	0	2 (100)	2 (100)	1 (50)	2 (100)
Salmonella spp.	101	18 (18)	7 (7)	1 (1)	4 (4)	3 (3)	15 (15)	0	98 (97)	10 (10)	5 (5)	20 (20)	24 (24)	6 (6)	31 (31)
Shigella spp.	36	7 (20)	4 (11)	1 (3)	4 (11)	1 (3)	6 (17)	0	34 (94)	3 (8)	2 (6)	10 (28)	10 (28)	2 (6)	11 (31)
Staph spp.	42	37 (88)	21 (50)	21 (50)	21 (50)	21 (50)	20 (48)	3 (7)	32 (76)	13 (32)	0	15 (36)	15 (36)	6 (14)	24 (57)

Out of the 551 isolates tested, 32.1% (177) were fully susceptible to the 14 antimicrobial agents in the 6 classes. *Shigella* had the highest number of fully susceptible isolates at 41.7% (15/36). The prevalence of multidrug resistance (MDR) was 16.2%, 6.9% of the isolates were resistant to 3 classes, 4.5% to 4 classes, 3.8% to 5 classes, and 0.9% to all 6 classes.

In addition, 100% of *P. aeruginosa* (2/2) isolates and 76.1% of *Staphylococcus* spp. (32/42) isolates had MDR, while 15.8% of *Klebsiella* spp. (15/95) isolates had MDR (Table 3).

Table 3. Table showing the isolation profiles based on antibiotics resistance class. The 14 antibiotics in this study were categorized into six classes based on CLSI 2021 guidelines. In addition, isolates resistant to three or more classes were considered MDR on the description of an earlier study by Basak et al. (2016) [28].

Organism		Number of Antibiotic Resistance Classes							Total
		0	1	2	3	4	5	6	
E. coli	Count	100 (36.4%)	96 (34.9%)	55 (20.0%)	17 (6.2%)	5 (1.8%)	1 (0.4%)	1 (0.4%)	275 (49.9%)
Klebsiella	Count	21 (22.1%)	39 (41.1%)	20 (21.1%)	8 (8.4%)	4 (4.2%)	2 (2.1%)	1 (1.1%)	95 (17.2%)
Pseudomonas	Count	0 (0.0%)	0 (0.0%)	0 (0.0%)	1 (50.0%)	1 (50.0%)	0 (0.0%)	0 (0.0%)	2 (0.4%)
Salmonella	Count	37 (36.6%)	30 (29.7%)	22 (21.8%)	7 (6.9%)	4 (4.0%)	0 (0.0%)	1 (1.0%)	101 (18.3%)
Shigella	Count	15 (41.7%)	11 (30.6%)	6 (16.7%)	2 (5.6%)	2 (5.6%)	0 (0.0%)	0 (0.0%)	36 (6.5%)
Staphylococcus	Count	4 (9.5%)	2 (4.8%)	4 (9.5%)	3 (7.1%)	9 (21.4%)	18 (42.9%)	2 (4.8%)	42 (7.6%)
	Count	177 (32.1%)	178 (32.3%)	107 (19.4%)	38 (6.9%)	25 (4.5%)	21 (3.8%)	5 (0.9%)	551 (100.0%)

3. Discussion

The results of this investigation give an excellent glimpse of the levels of bacterial carriage in chicken and poultry meat sold at major supermarkets across Kenya. This study noted a high prevalence of bacteria often considered commensals [29], such as *E. coli* (48.4%) and *Klebsiella* spp. (19.1%), and foodborne pathogens, such as *Salmonella* spp. (17.8%) and *Staphylococcus* spp. (6.7%). In addition, the study isolated *Shigella* spp. (7.5%) and *P. aeruginosa* (0.3%), bacteria associated with severe gastrointestinal infections such as chronic diarrhea and enterocolitis [30]; [31]. A similar study by Wardhana et al. (2021) [32] also reported a high prevalence of *S. aureus* (58.3%), *Salmonella* spp. (48.3%), and *E. coli* (40%) in retail chicken samples in Indonesia. Furthermore, a prevalence of 58.1% in *Salmonella* spp. [33], 18% in *E. coli* [34], 11.5% in *P. aeruginosa* [35], and 5.6% in *S. aureus* spp. [36] has been reported in pork sample from retail markets.

Though there was a potential of cross contamination in the fridge/freezer shelves through liquid drips from one food item to another, the likelihood of this happening was reduced because the samples were found to be shrink wrapped in polymer plastic film bags at the time of sampling. Therefore, the reported bacterial contamination of pork and chicken meat might have its origins at the farm level during the slaughtering process or packaging.

The extensive use of antibiotics for prevention and growth promotion in chickens and pigs has been a major factor in the development of antimicrobial resistance in bacteria with zoonotic potential, which is a serious public health issue [37]. For instance, according to a recent study by Ndukui et al. (2021), oxytetracycline (85%) and Amoxil (88%) are widely used antibiotics in commercial chicken raising in Kenya [38]. Our study findings of 39% and 35% frequencies against tetracycline and ampicillin are possibly a reflection of the implications of heavy antibiotics usage, as reported previously [38].

The development of antibiotic resistance to broad-spectrum medications such as ciprofloxacin, gentamicin, and cefepime, which are all on the WHO list of critically important antimicrobials for human medicine, is a growing concern. These medications provide limited alternatives, and it may be difficult to treat bacterial infections that do not respond to them with readily available drugs. The situation is further exacerbated by the increasing resistance to amoxiclav, ceftazidime, and gentamicin, which has risen to 16%, 6% and 3%, respectively, from levels of 2.6%, 0% and 0.6% reported in a similar study in Kenya less than 10 years ago [39]. The resistance to sulfamethoxazole and trimethoprim, two highly important antimicrobials used to treat bacterial and coccidial infections in humans and animals, has risen alarmingly. Furthermore, the resistance to tetracycline, ampicillin, amoxicillin-clavulanic, and ciprofloxacin, which are widely used to treat septicemia and respiratory infections in livestock, has reached 39%, 35%, 16% and 6%, respectively. These results could suggest that the bacteria in poultry and chicken farming sectors have developed resistance to antimicrobials due to heavy usage. Even though the use of rifampicin is prohibited or limited in many countries, it still remained the most resistant in all the isolates, which may indicate its use for prophylaxis purposes in the livestock sector. The reported high resistance towards rifampicin is expected considering the antibiotic is not recommended and is conventionally less active against infections caused by Gram-negative bacteria. Nonetheless, the resistance to antibiotics in chicken and pork isolates was found to be similarly high, which emphasizes the need for stewardship in chicken and pig farming and proper hygienic handling to avoid microbial contamination.

Though strains of *E. coli*, which was the most isolated bacteria in this study, are not harmful, some strains have acquired traits such as toxin production, making them pathogenic [40] and capable to cause serious foodborne pathogens. *Klebsiella* spp. and other known pathogens such as *Salmonella* and *Shigella* spp. were also found to be highly resistant to antibiotics commonly used to treat foodborne illnesses, for example ciprofloxacin (5% and 6%, respectively). Notably, *Pseudomonas aeruginosa*, which the WHO has identified as a critical pathogen due to its high resistance to antimicrobials, was among the most resistant to the antibiotics tested in chicken and pork samples.

In a similar study conducted in Kenya [41], in Vietnam, Salmonella isolates from chicken and pork samples exhibited a lower level of resistance to ampicillin (15%), tetracycline (36.7%), nalidixic acid (12.0%), and chloramphenicol (10%) than the corresponding rates seen in *E. coli* (85%, 66.7%, 24.1%, and 14.8%, respectively). Additionally, the resistance levels of ceftazidime, cefepime, ciprofloxacin, and tetracycline were reported to be 4.4%, 0.9%, 21%, and 66.4%, respectively [42]. It is alarming that 16.2% of the bacteria isolates studied were resistant to different antibiotics, as it jeopardizes the efficacy of antibiotic treatment for foodborne illnesses.

4. Materials and Methods

4.1. Sample Collection

For this cross-sectional study, we collected a total of uncooked 187 pork and 206 chicken samples between April and July 2020 from six leading supermarkets across five towns (Nairobi, Kisumu, Nakuru, Nanyuki and Eldoret) in Kenya. The leading supermarkets in Kenya are concentrated in cities (Nairobi, Kisumu, Mombasa, and Nakuru) and other big towns such as Eldoret and Naivasha. This is because urbanization has created easily accessible market for them in addition to improved infrastructure that facilitates transportation and storing of the perishable animal-sourced foods in their outlets. At the time of conducting this study, publicly available information showed that 89% of the international supermarket outlets and over a third of regional supermarket outlets were in Nairobi, the capital city of Kenya, with a population of over 4 million people as reported in 2019 [43]. All the samples were purchased either as wrapped/sealed by the supplier or repackaged by the outlet, within their expiry date, and the product branding was covered to blind the laboratory personnel. The samples were then transported in coolers to the Kenya Medical Research Institute within five hours, where processing began immediately. Moreover, data on the freshness of the sample, packaging method, storage temperature, and the type of PPE worn by the supermarket attendant was also collected.

4.2. Processing of the Samples in the Laboratory

Laboratory tests were carried out to detect foodborne bacteria in poultry meat and pork samples. Enrichment strategies and media were chosen carefully to enable the growth of non-fastidious bacteria.

To do this, 10 g of the meat sample was added into 90 mL of buffered peptone water (BPW) contained in a sterile stomacher bag and then homogenized with a stomacher machine (Stomacher® 400 Circulator). The resulting homogenate was transferred into as sterile 250 mL culture media bottle, loosely capped to allow growth of facultative bacteria, and incubated for 24 h at 37 °C. To grow Gram-negative (such as *E. coli*, *Shigella* and *Klebsiella* spp.) and *Staphylococcus* spp., a loopful (10 µL) of the BPW enrichment was streaked on MacConkey and Mannitol salt agar, respectively, and incubated overnight at 37 °C. Concurrently, 1 mL of the BPW pre-enrichment was added into 9 mL of Rappaport Vassiliadis (RV) enrichment media and incubated for 24 h at 37 °C to enhance enrichment of *Salmonella* spp. A loopful (10 µL) of RV enrichment was streaked on Xylose lysine deoxycholate (XLD), and incubated for 24 h at 37 °C, for isolation of *Salmonella* spp. Gram stain test was used to identify Gram-positive and negative isolates. Classical biochemistry methods were utilized to determine the species of the isolates. To identify Gram-negative bacteria, a pure colony was inoculated in triple sugar iron (TSI), lysin indole motility (LIM), methyl red voges Proskauer (MRVP), urea and citrate media and incubated overnight at 37 °C. To identify *Staphylococcus* species, we used the catalase test.

Antimicrobial susceptibility was then tested by the disc diffusion method with a selection of antimicrobials in line with the World Health Organization's recommendations for each species. In addition to the recommended antimicrobials, we also added nalidixic acid, chloramphenicol, and rifampicin to the antibiotics list because they are rarely tested drugs against enteric bacteria. A fresh, pure overnight culture was used to make a 0.5-equivalent MacFarland standard suspension in sterile normal saline. The suspension was evenly spread on Mueller–Hinton agar plates and antimicrobial discs (Oxoid) dispensed on the surface, after which the plates were incubated at 35 °C for 16–18 h. The *Escherichia coli* ATCC® 25,922 and *Staphylococcus aureus* ATCC® 25,923 were used for quality control. To analyze the antimicrobial resistance profiles and multidrug resistance, WHONET 2022 software (https://whonet.org/software.html, accessed on 2 November 2022) using the CLSI breakpoints interpretation guidelines were utilized.

4.3. Statistical Data Analysis

Data were gathered quantitatively and qualitatively using Epicollect5 mobile and web applications and were then exported to SPSS Statistics Software® (IBM Corp., Armonk, NY, USA, v.22) for statistical analysis. The chi-square test or Fisher's exact test was used to assess differences, and a p-value of less than 0.05 was considered as significant.

5. Conclusions

To sum up, this research suggests a high risk of food safety concerns, with chicken meat and pork from both local and international supermarkets in Kenya being found contaminated with bacterial contaminants, potentially spreading foodborne illnesses. It is essential to enforce high standards of food hygiene and sanitation throughout the supply chain, especially at the time of slaughter and packaging, in order to prevent the introduction of bacteria to the food and the subsequent spread of foodborne pathogens. Although we did not establish the source of microbial contamination, it is essential for retailing outlets to adhere to hygienic principles when handling and processing pork and chicken meat products to reduce the potential risk of microbial contamination. This study revealed that the resistance to essential classes of antibiotics, such as cephalosporins, aminoglycosides, and fluoroquinolones, is not high; however, an analysis of similar data showed that resistance might be increasing over time. Moreover, the analysis of our data showed worrying levels of resistance to tetracycline and penicillin, two of the most commonly used antibiotics in animal agriculture, demonstrating the necessity of responsible antibiotic use, improved and humane animal production methods, and increased biosecurity levels. It is particularly concerning that a few isolates were resistant to more than three types of antibiotics, which could make it more difficult to treat foodborne illnesses and other diseases. With new resistance mechanisms emerging and spreading globally, there is a need for a concerted effort to gain insights on how to better tackle AMR as well as raise awareness.

Author Contributions: Conceptualization, P.M., J.K., K.M. and V.Y.; methodology, P.M., J.K., K.M. and V.Y.; data curation, P.M., J.M. (John Maina) and K.M.; formal analysis, P.M., J.M. (John Maina). and J.K.; funding acquisition, P.M., V.Y. and J.K.; investigation, P.M., K.M. and V.Y.; project administration: P.M., V.Y. and J.K.; writing—original draft preparation, P.M. and J.M. (John Maina); writing—review and editing, P.M., J.M. (John Maina), K.M., V.Y., J.M. (John Mwaniki) and J.K. All authors have read and agreed to the published version of the manuscript.

Funding: This research was funded by World Animal Protection and Kenya Medical Research Institute (KEMRI).

Institutional Review Board Statement: This study was approved by the Institutional Review Board of the Kenya Medical Research Institute (KEMRI), under reference number EMRI/SERU/CMR/P00044/3487 (RESUBMISSION).

Informed Consent Statement: Not applicable.

Data Availability Statement: Data are available upon request from the corresponding author.

Acknowledgments: We are grateful to The National Research Fund (NRF) for partially supporting this study. We gratefully acknowledge the contributions and valuable support offered by Tennyson Williams and Patrick Kamunyo, and the KEMRI lab teams for the diagnostic support.

Conflicts of Interest: The authors declare no conflict of interest.

References

1. Davies, S.C.; Fowler, T.; Watson, J.; Livermore, D.M.; Walker, D. Annual Report of the Chief Medical Officer: Infection and the rise of antimicrobial resistance. *Lancet* **2013**, *381*, 1606–1609. [CrossRef] [PubMed]
2. WHO. *Global Action Plan on Antimicrobial Resistance*; World Health Organization: Geneva, Switzerland, 2017; pp. 1–28.
3. O'Neill, J. Tackling Drug-Resistant Infections Globally: Final Report and Recommendations. 2016. Available online: https://iiif.wellcomecollection.org/file/b28644797_160525_Final%20paper_with%20cover.pdf (accessed on 22 December 2022).
4. World Health Organization. Antimicrobial Resistance. 2022. Available online: https://www.who.int/westernpacific/health-topics/antimicrobial-resistance (accessed on 29 November 2022).
5. Government of Kenya. *Republic of Kenya National Policy on Prevention and Containment of Antimicrobial Resistance*; Ministry of Health of Kenya: Nairobi, Kenya, 2017; pp. 1–42. Available online: www.health.go.ke (accessed on 14 October 2022).
6. Xu, Y.; Zhong, L.-L.; Srinivas, S.; Sun, J.; Huang, M.; Paterson, D.L.; Lei, S.; Lin, J.; Li, X.; Tang, Z.; et al. Spread of MCR-3 Colistin Resistance in China: An Epidemiological, Genomic and Mechanistic Study. *Ebiomedicine* **2018**, *34*, 139–157. [CrossRef] [PubMed]
7. Vardakas, K.Z.; Rafailidis, P.I.; Konstantelias, A.A.; Falagas, M.E. Predictors of mortality in patients with infections due to multi-drug resistant Gram negative bacteria: The study, the patient, the bug or the drug? *J. Infect.* **2013**, *66*, 401–414. [CrossRef] [PubMed]
8. Bodi, M.; Ardanuy, C.; Rello, J. Impact of Gram-positive resistance on outcome of nosocomial pneumonia. *Crit. Care Med.* **2001**, *29*, N82–N86. [CrossRef]
9. Ena, J.; Dick, R.W.; Jones, R.N.; Wenzel, R.P. The Epidemiology of Intravenous Vancomycin Usage in a University Hospital: A 10-Year Study. *JAMA* **1993**, *269*, 598–602. [CrossRef]
10. World Bank. *Drug-Resistant Infections: A Threat to Our Economic Future*; World Bank: Washington, DC, USA, 2017; pp. 433–448. [CrossRef]
11. Murray, C.J.; Ikuta, K.S.; Sharara, F.; Swetschinski, L.; Aguilar, G.R.; Gray, A.; Han, C.; Bisignano, C.; Rao, P.; Wool, E.; et al. Global burden of bacterial antimicrobial resistance in 2019: A systematic analysis. *Lancet* **2022**, *399*, 629–655. [CrossRef]
12. International Livestock Research Institution. Managing Antimicrobial Use in Livestock Farming Promotes Human and Animal Health and Supports Livelihoods. 2021. Available online: https://hdl.handle.net/10568/113057 (accessed on 12 January 2023).
13. Page, S.; Gautier, P. Use of antimicrobial agents in livestock. *Rev. Sci. Tech.-OIE* **2012**, *31*, 145–188. [CrossRef]
14. Klein, E.Y.; Van Boeckel, T.P.; Martinez, E.M.; Pant, S.; Gandra, S.; Levin, S.A.; Goossens, H.; Laxminarayan, R. Global increase and geographic convergence in antibiotic consumption between 2000 and 2015. *Proc. Natl. Acad. Sci. USA* **2018**, *115*, E3463–E3470. [CrossRef]
15. Van Boeckel, T.P.; Pires, J.; Silvester, R.; Zhao, C.; Song, J.; Criscuolo, N.G.; Gilbert, M.; Bonhoeffer, S.; Laxminarayan, R. Global trends in antimicrobial resistance in animals in low- and middle-income countries. *Science* **2019**, *365*, eaaw1944. [CrossRef]

16. Van Boeckel, T.P.; Glennon, E.E.; Chen, D.; Gilbert, M.; Robinson, T.P.; Grenfell, B.T.; Levin, S.A.; Bonhoeffer, S.; Laxminarayan, R. Reducing antimicrobial use in food animals. *Science* **2017**, *357*, 1350–1352. [CrossRef]
17. FAO. *The Future of Food and Agriculture—Alternative Pathways to 2050 | Global Perspectives Studies | Food and Agriculture Organization of the United Nations*; Food and Agriculture Organization: Rome, Italy, 2018.
18. African Union—Interafrican Bureau for Animal Resources (AU–IBAR). Livestock Policy Landscape in Africa: A Review; Vet-Gov. 2016. Available online: https://www.au-ibar.org/sites/default/files/2020-11/doc_20160524_livestock_policy_lanscape_africa_en.pdf (accessed on 16 November 2022).
19. Van Boeckel, T.P.; Brower, C.; Gilbert, M.; Grenfell, B.T.; Levin, S.A.; Robinson, T.P.; Teillant, A.; Laxminarayan, R. Global trends in antimicrobial use in food animals. *Proc. Natl. Acad. Sci. USA* **2015**, *112*, 5649–5654. [CrossRef] [PubMed]
20. OIE. *OIE Annual Report on Antimicrobial Agents Intended for Use in Animals*; World Organisation for Animal Health: Paris, France, 2021; pp. 1–134. Available online: https://www.oie.int/en/document/fifth-oie-annual-report-on-antimicrobial-agents-intended-for-use-in-animals/ (accessed on 29 November 2022).
21. Jones, P.; Roe, J.; Miller, B. Effects of stressors on immune parameters and on the faecal shedding of enterotoxigenic Escherichia coli in piglets following experimental inoculation. *Res. Vet. Sci.* **2001**, *70*, 9–17. [CrossRef] [PubMed]
22. Callaway, T.R.; Morrow, J.L.; Edrington, T.S.; Genovese, K.J.; Dowd, S.; Carroll, J.; Dailey, J.W.; Harvey, R.B.; Poole, T.L.; Anderson, R.C.; et al. Social stress increases fecal shedding of Salmonella typhimurium by early weaned piglets. *Curr. Issues Intest. Microbiol.* **2006**, *7*, 65–72. [PubMed]
23. Rostagno, M.H. Can Stress in Farm Animals Increase Food Safety Risk? *Foodborne Pathog. Dis.* **2009**, *6*, 767–776. [CrossRef] [PubMed]
24. Carron, M.; Chang, Y.-M.; Momanyi, K.; Akoko, J.; Kiiru, J.; Bettridge, J.; Chaloner, G.; Rushton, J.; O'Brien, S.; Williams, N.; et al. Campylobacter, a zoonotic pathogen of global importance: Prevalence and risk factors in the fast-evolving chicken meat system of Nairobi, Kenya. *PLoS Negl. Trop. Dis.* **2018**, *12*, e0006658. [CrossRef] [PubMed]
25. Bengtsson, B.; Wierup, M. Antimicrobial resistance in Scandinavia after ban of antimicrobial growth promoters. *Anim. Biotechnol.* **2006**, *17*, 147–156. [CrossRef]
26. Oniciuc, E.-A.; Nicolau, A.I.; Hernández, M.; Rodríguez-Lázaro, D. Presence of methicillin-resistant *Staphylococcus aureus* in the food chain. *Trends Food Sci. Technol.* **2017**, *61*, 49–59. [CrossRef]
27. Manyi-Loh, C.; Mamphweli, S.; Meyer, E.; Okoh, A. Antibiotic Use in Agriculture and Its Consequential Resistance in Environmental Sources: Potential Public Health Implications. *Molecules* **2018**, *23*, 795. [CrossRef]
28. Basak, S.; Singh, P.; Rajurkar, M. Multidrug Resistant and Extensively Drug Resistant Bacteria: A Study. *J. Pathog.* **2016**, *2016*, 4065603. [CrossRef]
29. European Food Safety Authority; European Centre for Disease Prevention and Control. The European Union Summary Report on Antimicrobial Resistance in zoonotic and indicator bacteria from humans, animals and food in 2017/2018. *EFSA J.* **2020**, *18*, e06007. [CrossRef]
30. Hoff, R.T.; Patel, A.; Shapiro, A. Pseudomonas aeruginosa: An Uncommon Cause of Antibiotic-Associated Diarrhea in an Immunocompetent Ambulatory Adult. *Case Rep. Gastrointest. Med.* **2020**, *2020*, 6261748. [CrossRef] [PubMed]
31. McQuade, E.T.R.; Shaheen, F.; Kabir, F.; Rizvi, A.; Platts-Mills, J.A.; Aziz, F.; Kalam, A.; Qureshi, S.; Elwood, S.; Liu, J.; et al. Epidemiology of Shigella infections and diarrhea in the first two years of life using culture-independent diagnostics in 8 low-resource settings. *PLoS Negl. Trop. Dis.* **2020**, *14*, e0008536. [CrossRef]
32. Wardhana, D.K.; Haskito, A.E.P.; Purnama, M.T.E.; Safitri, D.A.; Annisa, S. Detection of microbial contamination in chicken meat from local markets in Surabaya, East Java, Indonesia. *Vet. World* **2021**, *14*, 3138–3143. [CrossRef]
33. Ngo, H.H.T.; Nguyen-Thanh, L.; Pham-Duc, P.; Dang-Xuan, S.; Le-Thi, H.; Denis-Robichaud, J.; Nguyen-Viet, H.; Le, T.T.; Grace, D.; Unger, F. Microbial contamination and associated risk factors in retailed pork from key value chains in Northern Vietnam. *Int. J. Food Microbiol.* **2021**, *346*, 109163. [CrossRef] [PubMed]
34. Scheinberg, J.A.; Dudley, E.G.; Campbell, J.; Roberts, B.; DiMarzio, M.; DebRoy, C.; Cutter, C.N. Prevalence and Phylogenetic Characterization of *Escherichia coli* and Hygiene Indicator Bacteria Isolated from Leafy Green Produce, Beef, and Pork Obtained from Farmers' Markets in Pennsylvania. *J. Food Prot.* **2017**, *80*, 237–244. [CrossRef] [PubMed]
35. McLellan, J.E.; Pitcher, J.I.; Ballard, S.A.; Grabsch, E.A.; Bell, J.M.; Barton, M.; Grayson, M.L. Superbugs in the supermarket? Assessing the rate of contamination with third-generation cephalosporin-resistant gram-negative bacteria in fresh Australian pork and chicken. *Antimicrob. Resist. Infect. Control* **2018**, *7*, 1–7. [CrossRef]
36. Rortana, C.; Nguyen-Viet, H.; Tum, S.; Unger, F.; Boqvist, S.; Dang-Xuan, S.; Koam, S.; Grace, D.; Osbjer, K.; Heng, T.; et al. Prevalence of *Salmonella* spp. and *Staphylococcus aureus* in Chicken Meat and Pork from Cambodian Markets. *Pathogens* **2021**, *10*, 556. [CrossRef]
37. Dafale, N.A.; Srivastava, S.; Purohit, H.J. Zoonosis: An Emerging Link to Antibiotic Resistance Under "One Health Approach". *Indian J. Microbiol.* **2020**, *60*, 139–152. [CrossRef]
38. Ndukui, J.G.; Gikunju, J.K.; Aboge, G.O.; Mbaria, J.M. Antimicrobial Use in Commercial Poultry Production Systems in Kiambu County, Kenya: A Cross-Sectional Survey on Knowledge, Attitudes and Practices. *Open J. Anim. Sci.* **2021**, *11*, 658–681. [CrossRef]
39. Odwar, J.A.; Kikuvi, G.; Kariuki, J.N.; Kariuki, S. A cross-sectional study on the microbiological quality and safety of raw chicken meats sold in Nairobi, Kenya. *BMC Res. Notes* **2014**, *7*, 1–8. [CrossRef]

40. García, A.; Fox, J.G.; Besser, T.E. Zoonotic Enterohemorrhagic *Escherichia coli*: A One Health Perspective. *ILAR J.* **2010**, *51*, 221–232. [CrossRef] [PubMed]
41. Deng, M.T.A.; Bebora, L.C.; Odongo, M.O.; Muchemi, G.M.; Kariuki, S.M.; Gathumbi, P.K. Antimicrobial resistance profiles of *E. coli* isolated from pooled samples of Sick, Farm and Market chickens in Nairobi County, Kenya. *Res. Sq.* **2022**, *5456*, 1–12. [CrossRef]
42. Nhung, N.T.; Van, N.T.B.; Van Cuong, N.; Duong, T.T.Q.; Nhat, T.T.; Hang, T.T.T.; Nhi, N.T.H.; Kiet, B.T.; Hien, V.B.; Ngoc, P.T.; et al. Antimicrobial residues and resistance against critically important antimicrobials in non-typhoidal Salmonella from meat sold at wet markets and supermarkets in Vietnam. *Int. J. Food Microbiol.* **2018**, *266*, 301–309. [CrossRef] [PubMed]
43. Kenya National Bureau of Statistics (KNBS). 2019 Kenya Population and Housing Census Results. Available online: https://www.knbs.or.ke/2019-kenya-population-and-housing-census-results/ (accessed on 27 February 2023).

Disclaimer/Publisher's Note: The statements, opinions and data contained in all publications are solely those of the individual author(s) and contributor(s) and not of MDPI and/or the editor(s). MDPI and/or the editor(s) disclaim responsibility for any injury to people or property resulting from any ideas, methods, instructions or products referred to in the content.

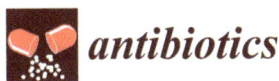

Article

Prevalence of Antibiotic Residues in Pork in Kenya and the Potential of Using Gross Pathological Lesions as a Risk-Based Approach to Predict Residues in Meat

Nicholas Bor [1,2], Alessandro Seguino [2], Derrick Noah Sentamu [1,3], Dorcas Chepyatich [1,3], James M. Akoko [1], Patrick Muinde [4] and Lian F. Thomas [1,5,*]

1. International Livestock Research Institute (ILRI), Nairobi P.O. Box 30709-00100, Kenya
2. The Royal (Dick) School of Veterinary Studies, University of Edinburgh, Easter Bush Campus, Midlothian EH25 9RG, UK
3. Faculty of Veterinary Medicine, University of Nairobi, Kangemi P.O. Box 29053-00625, Kenya
4. World Animal Protection, Nairobi P.O. Box 66580-00800, Kenya
5. Institute of Infection, Veterinary and Ecological Sciences, University of Liverpool, Leahurst Campus, Neston CH64 7TE, UK
* Correspondence: lian.thomas@liverpool.ac.uk

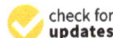

Citation: Bor, N.; Seguino, A.; Sentamu, D.N.; Chepyatich, D.; Akoko, J.M.; Muinde, P.; Thomas, L.F. Prevalence of Antibiotic Residues in Pork in Kenya and the Potential of Using Gross Pathological Lesions as a Risk-Based Approach to Predict Residues in Meat. *Antibiotics* 2023, 12, 492. https://doi.org/10.3390/antibiotics12030492

Academic Editors: Yongning Wu and Zhenling Zeng

Received: 13 January 2023
Revised: 24 February 2023
Accepted: 25 February 2023
Published: 1 March 2023

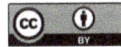

Copyright: © 2023 by the authors. Licensee MDPI, Basel, Switzerland. This article is an open access article distributed under the terms and conditions of the Creative Commons Attribution (CC BY) license (https://creativecommons.org/licenses/by/4.0/).

Abstract: The human population is growing and urbanising. These factors are driving the demand for animal-sourced proteins. The rising demand is favouring livestock intensification, a process that frequently relies on antibiotics for growth promotion, treatment and prevention of diseases. Antibiotic use in livestock production requires strict adherence to the recommended withdrawal periods. In Kenya, the risk of residues in meat is particularly high due to lack of legislation requiring testing for antibiotic residues in meat destined for the local market. We examined pig carcasses for gross pathological lesions and collected pork samples for antibiotic residue testing. Our aim was to determine if a risk-based approach to residue surveillance may be adopted by looking for an association between lesions and presence of residues. In total, 387 pork samples were tested for antibiotic residues using the Premi®Test micro-inhibition kit. The prevalence of antibiotic residues was 41.26% (95% CI, 34.53–48.45%). A logistic regression model found no significant associations between gross pathological lesions and the presence of antibiotic residues. We recommend that the regulating authorities strongly consider routine testing of carcasses for antibiotic residues to protect meat consumers. Future studies should research on farming practices contributing to the high prevalence of residues.

Keywords: antibiotic residues; food safety; gross pathological lesions; maximum residue limits; public health

1. Introduction

The global human population has been steadily rising, and estimates project an increase from the current 7 billion to 9.6 billion people by 2050. Most of the population growth is expected in Africa, which has an annual growth rate of 1.2% [1]. The ballooning population, urbanisation and improved incomes are likely to increase the demand for animal-sourced protein in low-income countries [2]. To cope with this increasing demand, livestock keepers are likely to use more antibiotics to prevent diseases and promote growth [3].

Globally, it was reported in 2017 that about 73% of all antimicrobials produced are used within food animal production [4] with pigs receiving the highest amount of antimicrobials at 172 mg/kg produced [5]. It is predicted that antibiotic use will rise by 67% between 2010 and 2030 [5] and usage is likely to be relatively higher in sub-Saharan Africa than other regions due to higher disease burden, limited diagnostic capacity, strained health facilities, limited personnel training on antibiotic use and unregulated access to antimicrobials [6]. Tetracyclines, sulphonamides, aminoglycosides and beta-lactams are the most commonly used classes of antibiotics for treatment and prevention of infections in food animals in Kenya with no current evidence of their use specifically for growth promotion [7].

Although antibiotics have the potential to improve production levels with regard to producer income and food security, when used inappropriately residues can be present in meat. These residues present public health risks such as allergenicity, toxicity, carcinogenicity and disruption of normal gastrointestinal flora therefore becoming a One Health issue. Residues may also promote the development of antibiotic-resistant microbes [8]. There have been concerted efforts by European Union (EU) member countries to reduce antimicrobial use in food animals by regulating veterinary antibiotic use and medicated feeds [9].

Failure to observe withdrawal periods has been cited as a major contributor to antibiotic residues in foods of animal origin [10]. Prior research has indicated that livestock farmers in Kenya have relatively unrestricted access to many antimicrobials without any prescription [11] despite having limited knowledge on withdrawal periods. A study in Busia County, Kenya, for example, showed that 12.9% of the interviewed farmers had no knowledge on withdrawal periods while 34.3% had scanty information on withdrawal periods, indicating a very high potential for antibiotic residues to be present in the meat produced by this group of farmers [12].

Ideally, food meant for human consumption should be free of antibiotic residues. Since a zero-residue level in meat may be impractical, the joint Food and Agriculture Organization of the United Nations and World Health Organization (FAO/WHO) Codex Alimentarius Commission has set maximum residue limits (MRL), above which meat is considered unsafe for human consumption [13]. This recommendation has led to routine national surveillance of antibiotic residues in meat products in most European countries. In Denmark for example, 0.1% of slaughtered pigs are routinely sampled and tested for antibiotic residues [14]. However, the situation is different in most African countries where financial constraints are widespread, and weak regulatory frameworks as is the case in Kenya [15]. As a result, national surveillance of residues remains a challenge [16].

In Switzerland, studies have established that risk-based sampling is 100% efficient in detecting tetracycline residues in calves [17]. Another risk-based surveillance study in Denmark found that chronic pleuritis may be used as a risk indicator for carcasses with antibiotic residues [18]. Although these risk-based approaches to monitoring and surveillance to antibiotic residues have the potential to be economically efficient, it is yet to be demonstrated in the Kenyan context [19].

To date, and to our knowledge, no study has investigated the prevalence of antibiotic residues in pork in Kenya. Therefore, this study aimed to establish the prevalence of antibiotic residues in pigs slaughtered and consumed in Nairobi and its environs. As a preliminary step to considering a risk-based surveillance system for Kenya, we also investigated the association between gross lesions detectable at slaughter and antibiotic residues in order to determine if gross lesions detectable at slaughter may be a suitable indicator to use in such a program. We hypothesized that animals with gross pathological lesions may have either been treated with antibiotics resulting in residues or may have originated from farms with generally poor husbandry practices, increasing the likelihood of both poor adherence to withdrawal times and presence of gross lesions in pigs presented for slaughter.

2. Results

A total of three hundred and eighty seven pork samples, each from an individual pig, were collected and tested for antibiotic residues. 126 of these 387 meat samples tested positive for the presence of antibiotics residues above the MRL. The apparent prevalence of antimicrobial residues above the MRL in the sampled population was 32.55% (95% CI 28.08–37.37%). Considering the reported sensitivity and specificity of the diagnostic assay, a true prevalence of 41.26% (95% CI 34.53–48.45%) was calculated. The prevalence of gross lesions in the full study population has been previously described [20] and only data from the 387 pigs with samples available for testing was analysed and reported in this paper. Table 1 shows the univariate analysis results for association of variables with presence of antibiotic residues at 5% significance level.

Table 1. Univariate analysis results showing the association between the presence of antibiotic residues over the recommended MRL and different predictor variables. The level of association is denoted by the *p* value in the last column.

Variables	N *	Variable Observation	Residue Result		p Value
			Negative	Positive	
Pleuropneumonia	266				0.727
		Absent	125	61	
		Present	52	28	
Tail bites	364				0.107
		Absent	233	116	
		Present	13	2	
Liver milk spots	348				0.612
		Absent	220	107	
		Present	13	8	
Loin bruising	364				0.423
		Absent	223	114	
		Present	13	4	
Hind limb bursitis	364				0.111
		Absent	241	112	
		Present	5	6	
Tether lesions	364				0.868
		Absent	239	115	
		Present	7	3	
Lung abscess	266				0.480
		Absent	175	87	
		Present	2	2	
Lacerations	364				0.961
		Absent	242	116	
		Present	4	2	
Cysts in the liver	362				0.480
		Absent	243	118	
		Present	1	0	
Pleurisy	266				0.593
		Absent	173	86	
		Present	4	3	
Husbandry type	381				0.558
		Housed	247	122	
		Outdoor	9	3	
Sex	384				0.084
		Female	143	58	
		Male	115	68	
Farm size	381				0.72
		<10	167	80	
		10 < 50	59	34	
		50 < 100	2	1	
		>100	28	10	
Lung score	266				0.642
		Mean (SD)	6.96 (13.40)	7.78 (14.21)	
		Range	0.00–55.00	0.00–48.00	

Table 1. Cont.

Variables	N *	Variable Observation	Residue Result		p Value
			Negative	Positive	
Live weight	366				0.199
		Mean (SD)	60.996 (28.308)	57.193 (22.257)	
		Range	13.0–230.0	27.0–157.0	
County of origin	383				0.558
		Homabay	1	0	
		Kajiado	6	3	
		Kiambu	200	103	
		Makueni	0	0	
		Murang'a	1	1	
		Nairobi	39	16	
		Nakuru	11	2	

* N varies based on the data that was successfully collected. Data was unavailable on all variables due to the rapid slaughter process and some traders being unwilling or unable to provide data, or to allow us to purchase the biological samples for closer inspection at the post-mortem room.

On univariate analysis, no statistically significant associations were found between gross pathological lesions and antibiotic residues in pork samples as seen in the last column in Table 1.

Sex, liveweight, tail bite lesions and hindlimb bursitis variables had p values of <0.2 and thus were included in the logistic regression model. Variable combination with the lowest Akaike Information Criterion (AIC) figure was picked as the best model. This model included sex, tail bites and hindlimb bursitis variables. The variance inflation factors output for sex, tail bites and hindlimb bursitis were 1.005, 1.008 and 1.01, respectively, indicating that these predictor variables were unrelated. No statistically significant associations were identified from the logistic regression model as shown in Table 2.

Table 2. Logistic regression output for the best model.

Variable	Estimate	Standard Error	Z Value	p Value
Intercept	−0.9020	0.1644	−5.487	4.1×10^{-8}
Sex male	0.3761	0.2276	1.652	0.0985
Presence of tail bite	−1.292	0.7806	−1.655	0.0979
Presence of hindlimb bursitis	1.0651	0.6278	1.697	0.0898

3. Discussion

We identified a high prevalence of antibiotic residues above the MRL in pork consumed in Nairobi and its environs. These findings indicate poor adherence to withdrawal periods by farmers and potential public health hazards to pork consumers through toxicity, allergic reactions and potential contribution to antimicrobial resistance development. Contrary to our hypothesis, we found no statistically significant associations between gross lesions and antibiotic residues in this population.

Due to resource limitations, we utilised Premi®Test (R-Biopharm AG, Pfungstadt, Germany) a broad-spectrum antibiotic screening method to detect the presence of residues above the MRL. Although the Premi®Test has been certified for use as a screening test based upon its comparability to current reference tests [21], the sensitivity and specificity are still suboptimal at 72.5% sensitivity and 95.3% specificity. Within statutory residue surveillance programs, positive screening results are generally followed by a confirmatory test to avoid false positives [22]. This indicates the potential for both false negatives and false positives when using the Premi®Test as a sole analytical technique, as was used in this study.

Although we adjusted the reported prevalence to account for the reported diagnostic performance, the sensitivity and specificity of the Premi®Test can vary among antibiotic classes. This means that there is a possibility that certain classes of antibiotic were not detected in this study. Sub-optimal detection of tetracyclines [23,24] and quinolones [25] in chicken by the Premi®Test have previously been reported, indicating that a parallel screening test sensitive for these classes of antibiotic in particular may be required to ensure all positive samples are accurately detected.

Freezing has been demonstrated to reduce the concentration of some antibiotics in meat [21] which may have resulted in an artificially reduced prevalence of samples with residues above the MRL in our study. The effect does, however, appear to be time related and we therefore expect that immediate freezing of the samples at $-80\ ^\circ$C for under six months with a single defrosting event will have reduced the impact of freezing to an acceptable level [26]. More research is required to quantify what impact this may have on residue collection and is highly relevant for the design of future studies or proposed surveillance activities.

Despite the possibility that some positive samples may have been incorrectly classified as negative through use of an imperfect screening test and freezing effects, there is a worryingly high prevalence of residues over MRL as indicated in this study. One possible explanation for the high prevalence of antibiotic residues in pork is that Kenyan authorities lack laws requiring testing of antibiotic residues for locally consumed meat [15].

The lack of current legislation in this area results in no financial or legal consequences for farmers and traders to present animals for slaughter where residues may still be present. Lack of legislation and current paucity of data on residues in food products may also lead to low level of awareness among farmers and consumers on the potential public health threats of these residues perpetuating a relaxed attitude to withdrawal periods.

It has been established that 100% of veterinary shops in Nairobi sell antibiotics without prescriptions with the buyer's/or farmer's preferences guiding purchasing decisions [11]. In rural areas of western Kenya, 60% of veterinary shop attendants have been reported to sell antibiotics to farmers without asking for a prescription [12]. This suggests that antibiotic accessibility is higher for pigs raised in urban areas than rural areas, which is potentially due to higher demand for animal-sourced proteins among urban residents with better incomes. Antibiotic residues have also been observed in Kenyan milk [27], indicating that the problem of antimicrobial residues should be addressed across different sectors for a safer food system.

The current legislative deficit can be rectified by regulatory bodies, such as the Kenya Veterinary Board (KVB) and the Veterinary Medicine Directorate (VMD). The two bodies should impose stricter regulations on sale of antibiotics by ensuring that antimicrobials are only accessible to licenced animal health practitioners. This should be combined with raising awareness among stakeholders regarding the negative health impacts of antibiotic residues in animal sourced proteins.

Kenya's National Action Plan on containment of antimicrobial resistance proposes residue testing as a strategic intervention [28]. The establishment of such a residue surveillance program would require investment in diagnostic technologies (e.g., mass spectrometry for confirmatory testing), training of staff in sample collection and testing and the creation and management of an appropriate data management system. In addition to fixed investments, there would also be additional per-sample costs like consumables and technician time. This would require an appropriate legislative framework and enforcement that is currently missing. If appropriately resourced, a surveillance program such as this would aid in generation of evidence and better adherence of withdrawal periods hence protecting the health of pork consumers from harmful effects of antibiotic residues.

In regulating antibiotic usage, regulatory authorities should encourage farmers to engage with cost-effective disease prevention alternatives. These include timely vaccinations, emphasis on biosecurity measures at the farm and appropriate stocking density. These alternatives will support animal health by reducing both the transmission and susceptibility to pathogens, thus reducing overreliance of antibiotics. These lessons should be taught using agricultural economic models that illustrate the benefits of disease prevention over treatment. Thereafter, legislation may be amended to require testing for residues in locally consumed meat. Such recommendations will supplement Kenya's National Action Plan of containing antimicrobial resistance and maintaining the efficacy of antimicrobials.

Very few willingness-to-pay studies have been performed for animal source products in Kenya, though one recent study indicates that antibiotic use had a negative impact on consumers' willingness-to-pay for chicken [29]. Similar results have been found in many other countries indicating that it is likely that consumers, particularly more affluent urban consumers, may be less willing to purchase meat with residues. This consumer pressure has the potential to drive future legislative development in Kenya and should be further explored.

At this stage, we have not identified any gross pathological lesions that may be used as predictors for the presence of antibiotic residues that could be utilised as an indicator in a risk-based surveillance program. Future studies should examine antimicrobial use at the farm level and may find other relevant factors which may be useful indicators for risk-based surveillance.

4. Materials and Methods

4.1. Ethical Approval

This study was approved by the International Livestock Research Institute, Institutional Animal Care and Use Committee (ILRI IACUC Ref no. 2019-36) and the Institutional Research Ethics Committee (ILRI-IREC 2020-14). An additional permit was obtained from the National Commission for Science, Technology, and Innovation permit (NACOSTI/P/20/4847). Both the national and county Directorate of Veterinary Services granted permission to conduct the study at the local abattoir.

4.2. Study Site and Data Collection Procedure

This cross-sectional study was conducted between 5 January and 5 March 2021 in a medium-sized, non-integrated abattoir, which slaughters an average of 215 pigs per week for sale. Consumption occurs in Nairobi and its environs [30]. A minimum sample size for estimation of antibiotic residue prevalence was calculated as 384 based upon a 5% level of precision, 95% confidence interval and an assumed prevalence of 50% due to lack of previous data in Kenya [31].

This antibiotic residue study was embedded in a larger study, researching food safety and animal welfare themes that required 529 pigs to be sampled. The study site and sampling strategy have previously been described in detail [20]. All pigs brought to the abattoir were eligible for sampling. A systematic sampling method was used where the first person presenting a pig to slaughter after 6 a.m. was the first to be recruited on each sampling day. After that, every second pig presented to slaughter was recruited into the study. If a presented pig had originated from the same farm as the previously recruited pig (i.e., belonged to the same batch), this pig would be skipped and the next pig from a separate batch would be recruited to reduce the impact of clustering on our prevalence results.

We had a team of 7 members and for ease of data collection the abattoir was divided into 3 stations, i.e., recruitment, evisceration area and dispatch point with each member assigned different roles.

At the recruitment station, the person presenting the pig for slaughter was approached and study objectives explained to him or her. If they agreed to participate, an informed consent form would be filled in, and data collection begun. Data on the pig's origin, farm size, husbandry type, sex and live weights were collected and recorded. We did not consider breed since the majority of the pigs presented to the slaughterhouse were of 'European origin or European mix' with previous studies on pig breeds in Kenya showing a heterogeneous control [32]. Therefore, identifying the breed that matches the pig's phenotype and genotype would have been difficult or even impossible. All recruited pigs were stunned and exsanguinated by the slaughterhouse workers. An ear tag was applied on each recruited pig for ease of follow-up along the slaughter line.

At the evisceration area, carcasses were visually examined for any gross pathological lesions. Two members of the research team, both qualified veterinarians, were responsible for inspecting the carcasses and collecting biological samples. One member examined the carcass for external lesions including ear marks (lacerations made on the ears of pigs with a sharp object to identify their pigs), tail bites, loin bruising, tether wounds, hindlimb bursitis and lacerations. The presence and absence and severity of each lesion was recorded as 1 and 0, respectively. The second team member examined thoracic and abdominal cavities and associated visceral organs namely lungs, heart and liver for cysts, abscesses, pleurisy, pneumonia, and milk spots in the liver. The lungs, liver and heart were collected, labelled and put in Ziploc bags for further examination at ILRI post-mortem room for gross pathological lesions. Finally, at the dispatch point, a 9 cm by 7 cm by 2 cm sample was collected from the left-side of *Biceps femoris* muscle [20]. These samples were placed in prelabelled Ziplock bags and kept in a cool box (at approximately 4 °C) for transport to ILRI laboratories within 2 h after sampling. Meat samples were taken from every available carcass until the sample size for the antimicrobial residue prevalence study was obtained. In the laboratory, the samples were frozen at -80 °C for later testing for antibiotic residues. The samples were stored for three months and tested between 11 June and 24 June 2021 once consumables had been delivered to Kenya.

In the post-mortem room, lungs, heart and liver samples were inspected for lesions that may have been missed due to the rapid slaughter process at the abattoir. The 7 lung lobes were scored according to the BPEX Pig Health Scheme [33]. The cranial and caudal lobes on the left and right side were scored between 0 and 10 while the accessory lobe and the two middle lobes were scored between 0–5 depending on their health condition. The maximum score was 55 and the minimum score was 0 denoting a healthy lung [33].

All collected data were entered into an Open Data Kit (ODK) form on a mobile phone (https://opendatakit.org/) and later uploaded to the ILRI server. Data was cleaned and checked for consistency on a weekly basis. Each sampling day took an average of 4 h.

4.3. Antibiotic Residue Testing

Pork samples were tested for antibiotic residues using the Premi®Test kit (R-Biopharm AG, Germany). This kit is a micro-inhibition screening test containing *Bacillus stearothermophilus* spores in an agar medium and a bromocresol purple indicator. In the absence of inhibitory substances, antibiotics in this case, the spores germinate and multiply to form an acid. This causes the bromocresol indicator to change colour from purple to yellow. If antibiotics are present above the MRL, the colour of the indicator remains purple and was recorded as a positive result [34]. Premi®Test is one of the most commonly used screening test for β-lactams, macrolides, tetracyclines and sulphonamides in meat in the EU with confirmatory tests generally utilised to confirm positive samples [22].

Before testing the 387 pork samples, we ran positive and negative controls. The negative meat sample was obtained from Farmers Choice. This a model firm and food processing plant that adheres to best farming practices, withdrawal periods and food safety standards. Its design and operations have been certified under ISO 22000:2005 on Food Safety Management Systems. The facility is licensed by the Director of Veterinary Services to exports their meat products and we are confident that residues would not be present. We bought 500 g of pork from Farmers Choice and obtained 100 µL of meat juice using a meat juice extractor. Further, 20 µL of meat juice was added to 2 ampoules. In addition, 2 mL of Betamox® (Norbrook, UK), which contains Penicillin as its active ingredient, was spiked into the positive control ampoule. Nothing was added to the negative control ampoule. The Premi®Test incubator was pre-heated to 64 °C. The 2 control ampoules were placed in the incubator, covered with foil, and incubated for approximately three hours. After this period, the negative control turned yellow while the positive control retained it purple colour as shown in Figure 1.

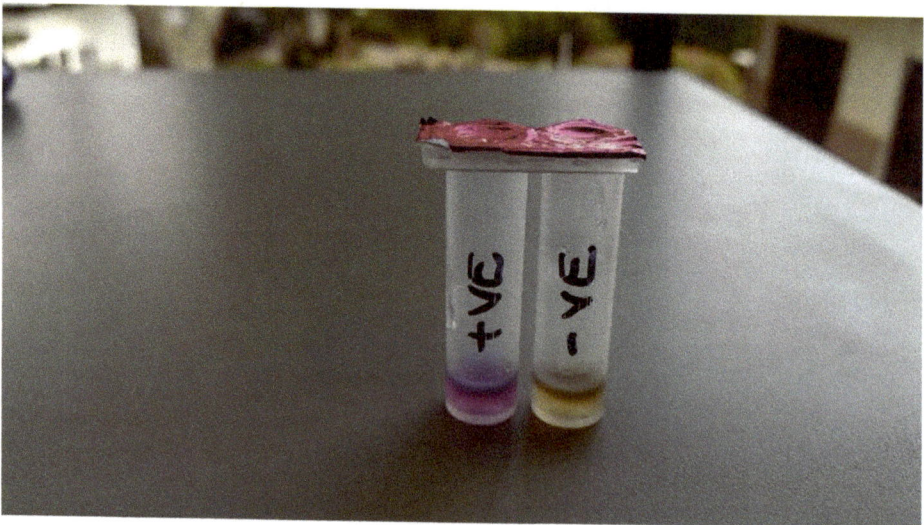

Figure 1. Images of positive and negative controls after incubation.

The frozen pork samples were defrosted on the bench, and a meat juice extractor was used to extract 100 µL of meat juice from each of the defrosted pork sample. The juice was vortexed to obtain a homogenous sample. Further, 20 µL of the vortexed juice was added to a pre-labelled ampoule corresponding to the pig ID and incubated at room temperature for 20 min. The ampoules were turned upside down to pour out meat juices and flushed with deionised water. They were then placed on a rack in an upside down position for 5 min to allow them to dry completely.

The ampoules were then placed in the incubator that had been preheated to 64 °C, as seen in Figure 2. The ampoules were covered with foil and incubated for approximately 3 h until the negative control turned yellow. The resultant colour for each ampoule was read against the provided colour chart and the result recorded in the ODK tool for later analysis. A negative control was always included in every batch of tested samples. This served as a guide to when to stop the incubation.

4.4. Data Analysis

All the uploaded data were downloaded as .csv files (comma-separated values files) from the ILRI server, cleaned and loaded into R version 4.2.2 for analysis (https://www.R-project.org/). Prevalence of antibiotic residues at 95% confidence interval was calculated using the epi.prev function under the epiR package [35]. This package accounted for the diagnostic performance of the test kit which has a reported 72.5% sensitivity and 95.5% specificity [36]. Univariate analysis was performed to explore the association between each potential predictor variable and the presence of antibiotic residues using the arsenal package in R [37].

A logistic regression model was then built utilising the generalised linear model function in the MASS package, utilising the binomial family since the outcome was binary [38]. An initial model was built with variables demonstrating potential association in univariate analysis with $p < 0.2$ as shown in Table 1. The best model was determined by looking at the variable combinations with the lowest AIC using the dredge function from MuMin package [38]. We tested for multicollinearity among independent variables by regressing these variables against each other. From the R^2 output, we calculated the variance inflation factor using the formula $VIF_j = 1/(1 − R^2)$. Since they were all below 2, they were all retained in the model.

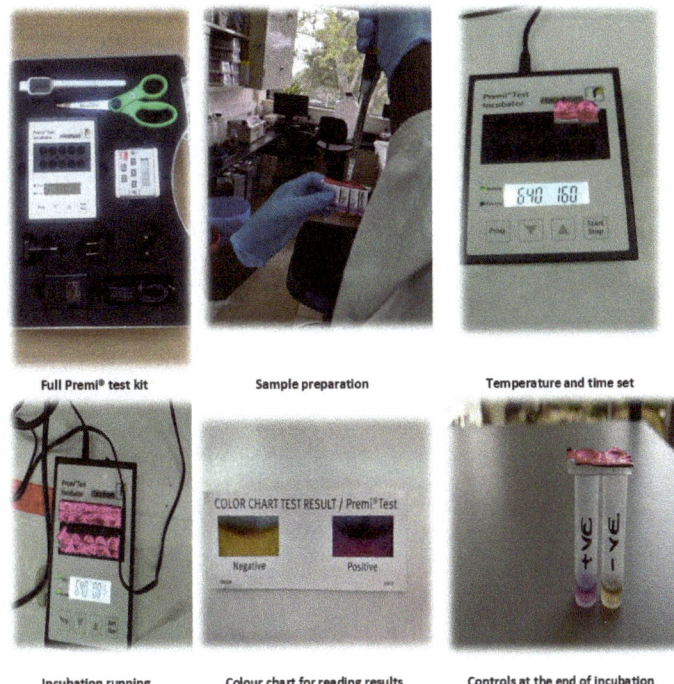

Figure 2. Premi®Test kit and summary of incubation process.

5. Conclusions

Close to half of the pork destined for consumption in Nairobi and its environs contained antibiotic residues above the recommended maximum residue limit. This poses potential public health risks to pork consumers. Action is urgently needed to address the underlying antibiotic misuse that has resulted in such a high prevalence of residues in pork. We recommend that regulating authorities strongly consider routine testing of carcasses for antibiotic residues for the protection of public health. We acknowledge that the establishment of a residue surveillance program would require huge investment in diagnostic technologies, e.g., high-performance liquid chromatography mass spectrometry for confirmatory testing, training of staff in sample collection and testing and the creation and management of an appropriate data management system. In addition to the fixed investments, there would be additional per-sample costs (e.g., consumables, technician time). To reduce the cost of residue surveillance, a sampling plan would be required, which could be based upon random or risk-based sampling.

The lack of a significant association between gross pathological lesions and the presence of antibiotic residues suggests that, for the time being, we cannot recommend a risk-based surveillance system based on gross lesions as predictors of residues in this population until antibiotic access enforcement is addressed. Future studies should research farming practices and antimicrobial use contributing to the high prevalence of residues.

To ensure better practices in the sale and use of antibiotics, appropriate legislation must be developed and enforced. There needs to be random testing of meat samples for residues and condemning of carcasses that test positive for residues. Meanwhile, producers should be sensitized on the judicious use of antibiotics and importance of adhering to recommended withdrawal times. Antibiotic stewardship, food safety and improved health outcomes will be ensured through this multifaceted approach.

Author Contributions: Conceptualization, N.B., A.S. and L.F.T.; data curation, N.B.; formal analysis, N.B., D.N.S. and L.F.T.; funding acquisition, J.M.A. and L.F.T.; investigation, N.B., D.N.S. and D.C.; methodology, N.B., A.S., P.M. and L.F.T.; project administration, N.B. and L.F.T.; writing—original draft, N.B.; writing—review and editing, all authors. All authors have read and agreed to the published version of the manuscript.

Funding: The fieldwork for this study was supported by the University of Liverpool Welcome Trust Institutional Strategic Support Fund (Grant number 204822/Z/16/Z), the Soulsby Foundation, the University of Liverpool Early Career Research Fund, World Animal Protection and the German Federal Ministry for Economic Cooperation and Development through the One Health Research, Education and Outreach Centre in Africa (OHRECA), RSMH. D.N.S. and D.C. are supported through ILRI Graduate Fellowships, funded by OHRECA and the CGIAR Research Program on Agriculture for Nutrition and Health (A4NH), led by the International Food Policy Research Institute (IFPRI). We also acknowledge the CGIAR Fund Donors (http://www.cgiar.org/funders).

Data Availability Statement: All data is freely available at: https://doi.org/10.17638/datacat.liverpool.ac.uk/1441.

Acknowledgments: We are indebted to the slaughterhouse workers and the management for their time and cooperation during data collection at the abattoir. Special thank you to Mary Nduati, Margaret Kemboi, Nelly Bargoiyet and Dennis Kigano for collecting data and processing biological samples. We are grateful to Dishon Muloi, Robert Ofwete and Luke Korir for their guidance in using R for data analysis and to William Pass and Paul Karimu for proofreading the paper.

Conflicts of Interest: The authors declare no conflict of interest.

References

1. Gerland, P.; Raftery, A.E.; Ševčíková, H.; Li, N.; Gu, D.; Spoorenberg, T.; Alkema, L.; Fosdick, B.K.; Chunn, J.; Lalic, N.; et al. World Population Stabilization Unlikely This Century. *Science* **2014**, *346*, 234–237. [CrossRef]
2. Gilbert, W.; Thomas, L.; Coyne, L.; Rushton, J. Review: Mitigating the risks posed by intensification in livestock production: The examples of antimicrobial resistance and zoonoses. *Animal* **2021**, *15*, 100123. [CrossRef]
3. Aidara-Kane, A.; the WHO Guideline Development Group; Angulo, F.J.; Conly, J.M.; Minato, Y.; Silbergeld, E.K.; McEwen, S.A.; Collignon, P.J. World Health Organization (WHO) guidelines on use of medically important antimicrobials in food-producing animals. *Antimicrob. Resist. Infect. Control* **2018**, *7*, 234–237. [CrossRef]
4. Van Boeckel, T.P.; Glennon, E.E.; Chen, D.; Gilbert, M.; Robinson, T.P.; Grenfell, B.T.; Levin, S.A.; Bonhoeffer, S.; Laxminarayan, R. Reducing antimicrobial use in food animals. *Science* **2017**, *357*, 1350–1352. [CrossRef]
5. Van Boeckel, T.P.; Brower, C.; Gilbert, M.; Grenfell, B.T.; Levin, S.A.; Robinson, T.P.; Teillant, A.; Laxminarayan, R. Global trends in antimicrobial use in food animals. *Proc. Natl. Acad. Sci. USA* **2015**, *112*, 5649–5654. [CrossRef]
6. Ayukekbong, J.A.; Ntemgwa, M.; Atabe, A.N. Atabe The threat of antimicrobial resistance in developing countries: Causes and control strategies. *Antimicrob. Resist. Infect. Control* **2017**, *6*, 100123. [CrossRef]
7. Mitema, E.S.; Kikuvi, G.M.; Wegener, H.C.; Stohr, K. An assessment of antimicrobial consumption in food producing animals in Kenya. *J. Vet. Pharmacol. Ther.* **2001**, *24*, 385–390. Available online: http://journal.um-surabaya.ac.id/index.php/JKM/article/view/2203 (accessed on 12 January 2023). [CrossRef]
8. Agmas, B.; Adugna, M. Antimicrobial residue occurrence and its public health risk of beef meat in Debre Tabor and Bahir Dar, Northwest Ethiopia. *Vet. World* **2018**, *11*, 902–908. [CrossRef]
9. More, S.J. European perspectives on efforts to reduce antimicrobial usage in food animal production. *Ir. Vet. J.* **2020**, *73*, 2. [CrossRef]
10. Nisha, A.R. Antibiotic residues—A global health hazard. *Vet. World* **2008**, *1*, 375–377. [CrossRef]
11. Muloi, D.; Fèvre, E.M.; Bettridge, J.; Rono, R.; Ong'Are, D.; Hassell, J.M.; Karani, M.K.; Muinde, P.; van Bunnik, B.; Street, A.; et al. A cross-sectional survey of practices and knowledge among antibiotic retailers in Nairobi, Kenya. *J. Glob. Health* **2019**, *9*, 010412. [CrossRef]
12. Kemp, S.A.; Pinchbeck, G.L.; Fèvre, E.M.; Williams, N.J. A Cross-Sectional Survey of the Knowledge, Attitudes & Practices of Antimicrobial Users and Providers in an Area of High-Density Livestock-Human Population in Western Kenya Abstract Background. *Front. Vet. Sci.* **2021**, *8*, 1070. [CrossRef]
13. FAO, OMS, and CODEX. Maximun Residue Limits (MRLs) and Risk Management Recommendations (RMRs) for residues of veterinary drugs in foods CAC/MRL 2-2015. 2015. Available online: https://www.fao.org/input/download/standards/45/MRL2_2015e (accessed on 12 January 2023).

14. Alban, L.; Rugbjerg, H.; Petersen, J.V.; Nielsen, L.R. Nielsen Comparison of risk-based versus random sampling in the monitoring of antimicrobial residues in Danish finishing pigs. *Prev. Vet. Med.* **2016**, *128*, 87–94. [CrossRef]
15. Government of Kenya Meat Control Act. *Natl. Counc. Law Report.* **2016**, *356*, 1–83. Available online: http://kenyalaw.org:8181/exist/kenyalex/actview.xql?actid=CAP (accessed on 12 January 2023).
16. Kimera, Z.I.; Mshana, S.E.; Rweyemamu, M.M.; Mboera, L.E.G.; Matee, M.I.N. Matee Antimicrobial use and resistance in food-producing animals and the environment: An African perspective. *Antimicrob. Resist. Infect. Control* **2020**, *9*, 37. [CrossRef]
17. Presi, P.; Stärk, K.D.C.; Knopf, L.; Breidenbach, E.; Sanaa, M.; Frey, J.; Regula, G. Efficiency of risk-based vs. random sampling for the monitoring of tetracycline residues in slaughtered calves in Switzerland. *Food Addit. Contam.—Part A Chem. Anal. Control Expo. Risk Assess* **2008**, *25*, 566–573. [CrossRef]
18. Alban, L.; Pacheco, G.; Petersen, J.V. Petersen Risk-based surveillance of antimicrobial residues in pigs—Identification of potential risk indicators. *Prev. Vet. Med.* **2014**, *114*, 88–95. [CrossRef]
19. Hoinville, L.J.; Alban, L.; Drewe, J.; Gibbens, J.; Gustafson, L.; Häsler, B.; Saegerman, C.; Salman, M.; Stärk, K. Proposed terms and concepts for describing and evaluating animal-health surveillance systems. *Prev. Vet. Med.* **2013**, *112*, 1–12. [CrossRef]
20. Sentamu, D.N.; Onono, J.O.; Muinde, P.; Bor, N.; Chepyatich, D.; Thomas, L.F. Thomas Prevalence of gross lesions and handling practices in pigs and their association with pork quality, Kiambu, Kenya. *PLoS ONE* **2022**, *17*, e0272951. [CrossRef]
21. Shaltout, F. Impacts of Different Types of Cooking and Freezing on Antibiotic Residues in Chicken Meat. *Food Sci. Nutr.* **2019**, *5*, 45. [CrossRef]
22. Kožárová, I.; Juščáková, D.; Šimková, J.; Milkovičová, M.; Kožár, M. Effective screening of antibiotic and coccidiostat residues in food of animal origin by reliable broad-spectrum residue screening tests. *Ital. J. Anim. Sci.* **2020**, *19*, 487–501. [CrossRef]
23. Okerman, L.; Croubels, S.; Cherlet, M.; De Wasch, K.; De Backer, P.; Van Hoof, J. Evaluation and establishing the performance of different screening tests for tetracycline residues in animal tissues. *Food Addit. Contam.* **2004**, *21*, 145–153. [CrossRef]
24. Pikkemaat, M.G.; Rapallini, M.L.; Dijk, S.O.-V.; Elferink, J.A. Comparison of three microbial screening methods for antibiotics using routine monitoring samples. *Anal. Chim. Acta* **2009**, *637*, 298–304. [CrossRef]
25. Pikkemaat, M.G.; Mulder, P.P.J.; Elferink, J.W.A.; De Cocq, A.; Nielen, M.W.F.; Van Egmond, H.J. Improved microbial screening assay for the detection of quinolone residues in poultry and eggs. *Food Addit. Contam.* **2007**, *24*, 842–850. [CrossRef]
26. Monir, H.H.; Fayez, Y.M.; Nessim, C.K.; Michael, A.M. When is it safe to eat different broiler chicken tissues after administration of doxycycline and tylosin mixture? *J. Food Sci.* **2021**, *86*, 1162–1171. [CrossRef] [PubMed]
27. Brown, K.; Mugoh, M.; Call, D.R.; Omulo, S. Antibiotic residues and antibiotic-resistant bacteria detected in milk marketed for human consumption in Kibera, Nairobi. *PLoS ONE* **2020**, *15*, e0233413. [CrossRef]
28. Ministry of Health of Kenya. *Government of Kenya National Policy for the Prevention and Containment of Antimicrobial Resistance, Nairobi, Kenya*; Ministry of Health of Kenya: Nairobi, Kenya, 2017; pp. 1–42. Available online: www.health.go.ke (accessed on 12 January 2023).
29. Otieno, D.J.; Ogutu, S.O. Consumer willingness to pay for chicken welfare attributes in Kenya. *J. Int. Food Agribus. Mark.* **2020**, *32*, 379–402. [CrossRef]
30. Murungi, M.K.; Muloi, D.M.; Muinde, P.; Githigia, S.M.; Akoko, J.; Fèvre, E.M.; Rushton, J.; Alarcon, P. The Nairobi Pork Value Chain: Mapping and Assessment of Governance, Challenges, and Food Safety Issues. *Front. Vet. Sci.* **2021**, *8*, 581376. [CrossRef]
31. Charan, J.; Biswas, T. How to calculate sample size for different study designs in medical research? *Indian J. Psychol. Med.* **2013**, *35*, 121–126. [CrossRef]
32. Mujibi, F.D.; Okoth, E.; Cheruiyot, E.K.; Onzere, C.; Bishop, R.P.; Fevre, E.; Thomas, L.; Masembe, C.; Plastow, G.; Rothschild, M. Genetic diversity, breed composition and admixture of Kenyan domestic pigs. *PLoS ONE* **2018**, *13*, e0190080. [CrossRef]
33. Holt, H.R.; Alarcon, P.; Velasova, M.; Pfeiffer, D.U.; Wieland, B. Wieland BPEX Pig Health Scheme: A useful monitoring system for respiratory disease control in pig farms? *BMC Vet. Res.* **2011**, *7*, 2005. [CrossRef]
34. Rakotoharinome, M.; Pognon, D.; Randriamparany, T.; Ming, J.C.; Idoumbin, J.-P.; Cardinale, E.; Porphyre, V. Prevalence of antimicrobial residues in pork meat in Madagascar. *Trop. Anim. Health Prod.* **2014**, *46*, 49–55. [CrossRef]
35. Chongsuvivatwong, V. *Analysis of Epidemiological Data Using R and Epicalc*; Epidemiology Unit Prince of Songkla University: Songkhla, Thailand, 2008.
36. Gaudin, V.; Juhel-Gaugain, M.; Morétain, J.-P.; Sanders, P. AFNOR validation of Premi®Test, a microbiological-based screening tube-test for the detection of antimicrobial residues in animal muscle tissue. *Food Addit. Contam.—Part A Chem. Anal. Control Expo. Risk Assess* **2008**, *25*, 1451–1464. [CrossRef]
37. Heinze, E.; Sinnwell, J.; Atkinson, E.; Tina Gunderson, T.; Dougherty, G.; Votruba, P.; Lennon, R.; Hanson, A.; Goergen, K.; Lundt, E.; et al. Package 'arsenal' R topics documented: 2022. Available online: https://cran.r-project.org/web/packages/arsenal/arsenal.pdf (accessed on 12 January 2023).
38. Bartoń, K. Package "MuMIn": Multi-Model Inference, version 1.47.1. 2022. Available online: https://cran.r-project.org/web/packages/MuMIn/MuMIn.pdf (accessed on 12 January 2023).

Disclaimer/Publisher's Note: The statements, opinions and data contained in all publications are solely those of the individual author(s) and contributor(s) and not of MDPI and/or the editor(s). MDPI and/or the editor(s) disclaim responsibility for any injury to people or property resulting from any ideas, methods, instructions or products referred to in the content.

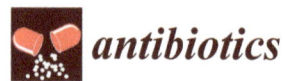

Brief Report

Synergistic Effects of Capric Acid and Colistin against Colistin-Susceptible and Colistin-Resistant *Enterobacterales*

Yi-Yun Liu [1,2,†], Zong-Hua Qin [3,†], Hui-Ying Yue [1], Phillip J. Bergen [4], Li-Min Deng [1], Wan-Yun He [1], Zhen-Ling Zeng [1], Xian-Feng Peng [3,*] and Jian-Hua Liu [1,2,*]

[1] National Risk Assessment Laboratory for Antimicrobial Resistance of Animal Original Bacteria, Guangdong Provincial Key Laboratory of Veterinary Pharmaceutics Development and Safety Evaluation, South China Agricultural University, Guangzhou 510642, China
[2] Guangdong Laboratory for Lingnan Modern Agriculture, Guangzhou 510642, China
[3] Guangzhou Insighter Biotechnology Co., Ltd., Guangzhou 510642, China
[4] Biomedicine Discovery Institute, Department of Microbiology, School of Biomedical Sciences, Monash University, Clayton, VIC 3800, Australia
* Correspondence: istpeng@hotmail.com (X.-F.P.); jhliu@scau.edu.cn (J.-H.L.)
† These authors contributed equally to this work.

Abstract: Colistin is a last-line antibiotic against Gram-negative pathogens. However, the emergence of colistin resistance has substantially reduced the clinical effectiveness of colistin. In this study, synergy between colistin and capric acid was examined against twenty-one Gram-negative bacterial isolates (four colistin-susceptible and seventeen colistin-resistant). Checkerboard assays showed a synergistic effect against all colistin-resistant strains [(FICI, fractional inhibitory concentration index) = 0.02–0.38] and two colistin-susceptible strains. Time–kill assays confirmed the combination was synergistic. We suggest that the combination of colistin and capric acid is a promising therapeutic strategy against Gram-negative colistin-resistant strains.

Keywords: colistin resistance; combination therapy; capric acid; synergy

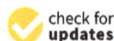

Citation: Liu, Y.-Y.; Qin, Z.-H.; Yue, H.-Y.; Bergen, P.J.; Deng, L.-M.; He, W.-Y.; Zeng, Z.-L.; Peng, X.-F.; Liu, J.-H. Synergistic Effects of Capric Acid and Colistin against Colistin-Susceptible and Colistin-Resistant *Enterobacterales*. *Antibiotics* **2023**, *12*, 36. https://doi.org/10.3390/antibiotics12010036

Academic Editor: Manuel Simões

Received: 29 November 2022
Revised: 20 December 2022
Accepted: 23 December 2022
Published: 26 December 2022

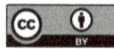

Copyright: © 2022 by the authors. Licensee MDPI, Basel, Switzerland. This article is an open access article distributed under the terms and conditions of the Creative Commons Attribution (CC BY) license (https://creativecommons.org/licenses/by/4.0/).

Global antimicrobial resistance poses a serious threat to human health. Over the last decade, there has been a rapid increase in the number of multidrug-resistant (MDR) and extensively drug-resistant (XDR) Gram-negative bacteria [1,2]. Of particular concern is the emergence of carbapenem-resistant Gram-negative pathogenic bacteria such as *Acinetobacter baumannii*, *Escherichia coli*, *Pseudomonas aeruginosa* and *Klebsiella pneumoniae* which represent a special clinical challenge [3,4]. This situation has only been made worse by the slow development of new antibiotics and the rapid spread of drug-resistant genes, which have led to a decline in the number of effective antibiotics available to treat infections caused by MDR bacteria. Thus, the emergence of such pathogens including carbapenemase-producing *Enterobacterales* has resulted in the reintroduction of colistin as a last-resort antibiotic treatment [5]. Colistin, a polymyxin antibiotic discovered in the 1950s, is a cationic polypeptide antibiotic produced by *Bacillus polymyxa* which acts as a bactericidal agent by targeting the polyanionic lipid A of lipopolysaccharide (LPS) in the outer membrane of Gram-negative bacteria [6]. However, widespread use of this agent has given rise to a remarkable increase in colistin-resistant strains [7]. Polymyxin resistance was previously thought to be due solely to mutations in chromosomal genes which led to the modification of lipid A with phosphoethanolamine (pEtN) and/or 4-amino-4-deoxy-L-arabinose (L-Ara4N), thereby reducing the interaction of lipid A with polymyxins [7]. This paradigm changed when we reported for the first time plasmid-mediated colistin resistance via the *mcr-1* gene in an isolate from China [8]. Subsequently, more than 60 countries and regions have demonstrated the presence of *mcr-1*-harboring strains [9], with other *mcr* family genes (*mcr-2* to *mcr-10*) having since been reported worldwide [10]. The *mcr* genes encode a pEtN transferase that modifies lipid A with pEtN residues [10]. These reports have led to global concern regarding the efficacy of colistin, raising an urgent need for the identification of new antimicrobial compounds to address these challenges.

Synergy with colistin has been investigated for a variety of traditional antimicrobial agents including rifampicin, rifabutin, carbapenems, clarithromycin, novobiocin, macrolides, minocycline, tigecycline, and glycopeptides [11]. MacNair, C. R et al., demonstrated that when used in combination with colistin, the best synergistic killing activity was achieved with rifampicin, novobiocin, rifabutin, minocycline, and clarithromycin [11]. Synergy with polymyxins has also been shown with several FDA-approved non-antibiotic drugs, representing another promising alternative treatment pathway that is currently underexplored [12–14]. Of these, particularly noteworthy are recent studies that have described synergy against a variety of MDR Gram-negative bacteria with colistin in combination with the signal peptidase inhibitor MD3, the antiretroviral HIV drugs zidovudine and azidothymidine, as well as curcumin, netropsin, and auranofin [15–18]. For example, Martinez-Guitian et al., confirmed that not only did the combination of MD3 and colistin increase the susceptibility of colistin-susceptible clinical isolates of *A. baumannii*, but that potent synergy with this combination was also observed against colistin-resistant strains with mutations in *pmrB* and phosphoethanolamine modification of lipid A [15]. Similarly, Feng et al., reported potent synergy when colistin was combined with auranofin against problematic colistin-resistant Gram-negative bacteria both in vitro (*K. pneumoniae*, *A. baumannii*, *E. coli* and *Pseudomonas aeruginosa*) and in vivo (*K. pneumoniae*, *A. baumannii*) [18]. Altogether, these results suggest that the use of colistin in combination with such compounds has the potential to enhance bacterial killing of MDR pathogens and prolong the utility of this increasingly important last-line antibiotic. Accordingly, the aim of this study was to find an agent with potential synergistic activity with colistin and assess the in vitro activity of the combination against colistin-susceptible and -resistant Gram-negative bacterial isolates.

We initially screened over 200 compounds for antimicrobial activity against a colistin-resistant *E. coli* strain, with capric acid identified as a candidate compound. Capric acid is a saturated free fatty acid (FFA) with 10 carbon atoms in the carbon chain and a carboxyl group (–COOH) at one end and a methyl group (–CH$_3$) at the other [19]. FFAs are found in marine organisms and plants and have been reported to show antimicrobial activity by targeting the cell membrane and causing damage to cellular energy production and enzyme activity [20,21]. Although capric acid has been shown to have killing activity against the Gram-positive organism *Cutibacterium acnes* [22] and the fungus *Candida albicans* cells [23], activity against Gram-negative organisms has not been investigated. We examined the synergistic potential of capric acid in combination with colistin in vitro against 21 Gram-negative bacterial isolates.

Four colistin-susceptible and seventeen colistin-resistant strains were tested (Table 1), comprising *K. pneumoniae* (n = 7), *E. coli* (n = 7), *Salmonella* (n = 5), and *Pseudomonas aeruginosa* (n = 2). Of the colistin-resistant strains, twelve carried the *mcr-1* gene, three the *mcr-8* gene, while two harbored mutations in chromosomal genes associated with colistin-resistance. The minimum inhibitory concentrations (MICs) of colistin and capric acid determined for all strains using broth dilution as per the Clinical Laboratory Standards Institute (CLSI) guidelines (M07-A11) are shown in Table 1. The colistin MICs of the colistin-resistant strains were ≥4 mg/L, while the colistin MICs of susceptible strains ranged from 0.5 to 1 mg/L. The MICs of capric acid were all ≥3200 mg/L, suggesting capric acid had no antimicrobial activity against the tested strains when used as monotherapy.

Synergy between colistin and capric acid was then evaluated by checkerboard assay in a 96-well microtiter plate as previously described [24]. In brief, serial 2-fold dilutions of colistin and capric acid were undertaken with the final concentrations ranging from 0.06 to 32 mg/L for colistin and from 25 to 3200 mg/L for capric acid. Each test organism was added to a density of 5×10^6 CFU/mL, with the final volume in each well being 200 µL. The 96-well plate was then incubated at 37 °C for 18 h. The fractional inhibitory concentration index (FICI) for the interaction of the combination was calculated as follows:

FICI = FIC of drug A + FIC of drug B = [(MIC of drug A in combination/MIC of drug A alone) + (MIC of drug B in combination/MIC of drug B alone)]. The FICI was interpreted as follows: FICI $\leq$ 0.5, synergy; FICI > 0.5–4, indifference; FICI > 4, antagonism. The antibacterial activity of colistin increased when used in combination with capric acid, with synergy observed against 19 of the 21 strains, including against all four bacterial species examined (FICI values ranged from 0.02 to 0.38; Table 1). Importantly, the combination of colistin and capric acid was synergistic against all colistin-resistant strains. The only two strains for which synergy was not observed were Salmonella SH47 (FICI, 0.51) and P. aeruginosa 10104 (FICI, 2) (Table 1).

Table 1. FICI and MIC (mg/L) values for the strains tested in this study.

Strain	Origin	PCR for mcr-1 [a]	MIC (mg/L)				FICI [b]
			Single Drug		Combination		
			Colistin	Capric Acid	Colistin	Capric Acid	
K. pneumoniae P11	Human	-	1	>3200	0.13	400	0.26
K. pneumoniae P11+ pHNSHP45	Transformant	+	8	>3200	0.5	200	0.13
K. pneumoniae 117	Pig	+	16	>3200	2	400	0.26
K. pneumoniae 281	Pig	+	16	>3200	1	200	0.13
K. pneumoniae SDQ8C53R [c]	Chicken	-	>512	3200	1	50	0.02
K. pneumoniae HNJ9C285 [c]	Chicken	-	>512	3200	4	200	0.07
K. pneumoniae HNJ9C245 [c]	Chicken	-	>512	3200	2	100	0.04
E. coli C600	-	-	0.5	>3200	0.125	200	0.26
E. coli C600 + pHNSHP45	Transformant	+	8	>3200	0.5	200	0.13
E. coli 2D-8 [d]	Pig	-	8	>3200	0.5	200	0.13
E. coli SHP7	Pig	+	8	>3200	2	200	0.31
E. coli SHP8	Pig	+	8	>3200	1	200	0.19
E. coli SHP50	Pig	+	8	>3200	0.5	200	0.13
E. coli GDF36	Fish	+	8	3200	1	800	0.38
Salmonella SA316	Pig	+	8	>3200	1	400	0.26
Salmonella SH271	Pig	+	4	3200	1	50	0.27
Salmonella SH138	Pig	+	8	>3200	1	400	0.26
Salmonella SH47	Pig	-	1	>3200	0.25	800	0.51
Salmonella SH17	Pig	+	4	3200	1	50	0.27
P. aeruginosa 10104	CVCC [f]	-	1	>3200	1	>3200	2.00
P. aeruginosa 10104 (R) [e]	Induced	-	8	>3200	1	400	0.26

[a] + and - indicate positive and negative for mcr-1. [b] FICI—Fractional Inhibitory Concentration Index. [c] K. pneumoniae strains harboring colistin resistance gene mcr-8. [d] E. coli 2D-8 harbors mutations in phoP (Y114I), phoQ (E232D), and pmrA (L3S). [e] P. aeruginosa 10104 (R) harbors mutations in phoQ (K151R), parS (T222R), colR (L1M), and cprR (T171P). [f] CVCC—China Veterinary Culture Collection Center.

To further examine the potential for synergy with capric acid combined with an antibiotic, we repeated the checkerboard study above using two E. coli isolates (2D-8 and SHP50) and ciprofloxacin, cefotaxime, neomycin, tetracycline, and ampicillin. As shown in Table 2, synergy between capric acid and other antimicrobials was not observed (FICI range, 1–2).

Table 2. MIC (mg/L) values of capric acid and various antibiotics and FICI values of capric acid when combined with each antibiotic against two colistin-resistant E. coli strains.

Strain		Antibiotic					
		Colistin	Ciprofloxacin	Cefotaxime	Neomycin	Tetracycline	Ampicillin
E. coli 2D-8	MIC [a]	8	0.5	0.06	256	32	128
	FICI [b]	0.13	2	2	1	1	1
E. coli SHP50	MIC [a]	8	32	0.5	0.25	128	8
	FICI [b]	0.19	1	2	1	1	1

[a] MIC of the single drug. [b] FICI—Fractional Inhibitory Concentration Index.

Based on the checkerboard study results, the potential for enhanced bacterial killing with the combination of colistin (0.5× MIC) and capric acid (800 mg/L) was examined using time-kill studies against a colistin-susceptible reference strain (*E. coil* C600) and *mcr-1*-positive colistin-resistant strain (*E. coli* C600 + pHNSHP45) according to a previously reported method [25]. The starting inoculum was ~10^6 CFU/mL and experiments were conducted for 36 h. Antibiotic-free Mueller-Hinton broth served as the control. Synergy was considered to be a $\geq$2-$\log_{10}$ reduction in CFU/mL with the combination when compared to the most active monotherapy at the specified time [26]. Bacterial cultures (5 mL) were incubated with shaking (180 rpm) at 37 °C and samples (5 mL) collected at 0, 2, 4, 8, 24, 28, 32 and 36 h for viable counting. The results of time–kill studies are shown in Figure 1. For both strains, no bacterial killing was observed with capric acid monotherapy and growth mirrored that of the growth control. For the colistin-susceptible reference strain (*E. coli* C600), initial bacterial killing of ~4 $\log_{10}$ CFU/mL with colistin monotherapy at 4 h was followed by rapid regrowth that had returned to control values by 28 h (Figure 1A). Amplification of colistin-resistant subpopulations in heteroresistant isolates, namely susceptible isolates based upon their MICs but which contain resistant subpopulations, is known to contribute to regrowth following polymyxin monotherapy [27]. However, synergy was observed with combination therapy from 4 h onwards such that no viable bacteria were observed across 4–8 h, with subsequent regrowth remaining at ~5 $\log_{10}$ CFU/mL below that of the control and monotherapies. Synergistic killing was also observed from 8 h onwards with the *mcr-1*-positive colistin-resistant strain (*E. coli* C600 + pHNSHP45), although the enhancement of bacterial killing with the combination was less than that observed with *E. coli* C600 (Figure 1B). Altogether, the time-kill experiments showed good bactericidal activity ($\geq$3 $\log_{10}$ CFU/mL) and synergy with combination therapy against both strains (Figure 1).

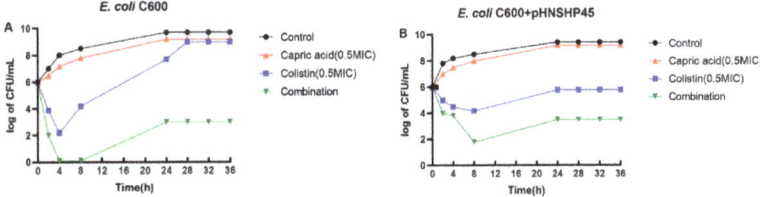

Figure 1. Time-kill study performed with *E. coli* C600 (**A**) and *E. coli* C600 + pHNSHP45 (**B**) with colistin monotherapy (0.5× MIC), capric acid monotherapy (800 mg/L), and their combination (equivalent concentrations).

Resistance genes are often associated with various mobile genetic structures, facilitating their dissemination among different *Enterobacterales* species. The plasmid-mediated transmission of the colistin resistance gene *mcr-1* has raised serious concerns for the efficacy of colistin, pointing to the urgent need for new agents to effectively treat clinical infections caused by colistin-resistant isolates [8]. Here, we demonstrated synergistic bacterial killing with the combination of colistin and capric acid against a variety of *mcr-1*-positive Gram-negative bacterial strains (Table 1 and Figure 1). While the specific mechanism(s) for the observed synergy with this combination is not yet known, one possible explanation is that capric acid disturbs the stability and activity of the bacterial membrane, enabling more colistin to target lipid A. Like other FFAs, capric acid can cross the cell membrane and disrupt the electron transport chain, resulting in a reduction of ATP production [19]. It has previously been shown that capric acid has anti-adhesion activity and inhibits the adhesion of *C. albicans* cells to abiotic surfaces [23]. A recent study by Jakub et al., showed that capric acid combined with either fluconazole or amphotericin B achieved synergistic killing of *C. albicans* by causing the MDR transporter Cdr1p to relocalize from the plasma membrane to the interior of the cell, leading to reduced efflux activity of Cdr1p [28]. These findings raise the possibility that capric acid may have an impact on the function/integrity of bacterial membranes, thereby enabling more colistin to bind lipid A and thus increasing bacterial susceptibility to colistin.

Another possible mechanism for the synergy between colistin and capric acid involves the prevention of lipid A modifications by capric acid. The bactericidal activity of colistin begins when it binds to the lipid A component of LPS. The LPS structure can be altered via two-component regulatory systems (TCSs, e.g., PmrAB, ParRS, CprRS, PhoPQ and CrrAB) [7]. The TCSs are sensitive to environmental stimuli including exposure to exogenous compounds or metal ions such as Mg^{2+} and Fe^{2+}, which usually results in the modification of the lipid A phosphate groups via the addition of cationic L-Ara4N and/or pEtN moieties [7]. MCR-1 is phosphoethanolamine (pEtN) transferase that leads to the addition of pEtN to lipid A. It is possible that exogenous capric acid prevents such modifications of lipid A, thereby retaining sensitivity to colistin. However, further studies specifically examining the mechanism(s) of synergy are required.

In conclusion, we have demonstrated that capric acid can enhance bacterial killing of colistin-resistant Gram-negative bacteria when combined with colistin. Although the underlying mechanism(s) of synergy with this combination remains to be elucidated, our results suggest that further exploration of this combination against MDR pathogens is warranted.

Author Contributions: Conceptualization, Y.-Y.L. and X.-F.P.; methodology, Y.-Y.L., H.-Y.Y. and L.-M.D.; software, H.-Y.Y. and Z.-L.Z.; validation, H.-Y.Y. and W.-Y.H.; formal analysis, Y.-Y.L.; investigation, Y.-Y.L.; resources, Z.-L.Z., Z.-H.Q. and X.-F.P.; data curation, Y.-Y.L. and P.J.B.; writing—original draft preparation, Y.-Y.L.; writing—review and editing, Y.-Y.L., P.J.B. and J.-H.L.; visualization, Y.-Y.L. and H.-Y.Y.; supervision, X.-F.P. and J.-H.L.; project administration, X.-F.P. and J.-H.L.; funding acquisition, J.-H.L. All authors have read and agreed to the published version of the manuscript.

Funding: This research was funded by the National Natural Science Foundation of China (No. 31830099), Science and Technology Program of Guangzhou (No. 202201010300), Project of Educational Commission of Guangdong Province of China (2021KQNCX006), Science and Technology Program of Guangzhou, China (202201010300), the Innovation Team Project of Guangdong University (No. 2019KCXTD001), and the 111 Project (No. D20008). The APC was funded by National Natural Science Foundation of China (No. 31830099).

Institutional Review Board Statement: Not applicable.

Informed Consent Statement: Not applicable.

Data Availability Statement: Not applicable.

Conflicts of Interest: The authors declare no conflict of interest.

References

1. De Oliveira, D.; Forde, B.M.; Kidd, T.J.; Harris, P.; Schembri, M.A.; Beatson, S.A.; Paterson, D.L.; Walker, M.J. Antimicrobial Resistance in ESKAPE Pathogens. *Clin. Microbiol. Rev.* **2020**, *33*, e00181-19. [CrossRef]
2. Du, H.; Chen, L.; Tang, Y.W.; Kreiswirth, B.N. Emergence of the *mcr-1* colistin resistance gene in carbapenem-resistant Enterobacteriaceae. *Lancet Infect. Dis.* **2016**, *16*, 287–288. [CrossRef]
3. Dortet, L.; Cuzon, G.; Ponties, V.; Nordmann, P. Trends in carbapenemase-producing *Enterobacteriaceae*, France, 2012 to 2014. *Eurosurveillance* **2017**, *22*, 30461. [CrossRef]
4. Schuelter-Trevisol, F.; Schmitt, G.J.; Araujo, J.M.; Souza, L.B.; Nazario, J.G.; Januario, R.L.; Mello, R.S.; Trevisol, D.J. New Delhi metallo-beta-lactamase-1-producing *Acinetobacter* spp. infection: Report of a survivor. *Rev. Soc. Bras. Med. Trop.* **2016**, *49*, 130–134. [CrossRef]
5. Livermore, D.M.; Warner, M.; Mushtaq, S.; Doumith, M.; Zhang, J.; Woodford, N. What remains against carbapenem-resistant Enterobacteriaceae? Evaluation of chloramphenicol, ciprofloxacin, colistin, fosfomycin, minocycline, nitrofurantoin, temocillin and tigecycline. *Int. J. Antimicrob. Agents* **2011**, *37*, 415–419. [CrossRef]
6. Abdul, R.N.; Cheah, S.E.; Johnson, M.D.; Yu, H.; Sidjabat, H.E.; Boyce, J.; Butler, M.S.; Cooper, M.A.; Fu, J.; Paterson, D.L.; et al. Synergistic killing of NDM-producing MDR *Klebsiella pneumoniae* by two 'old' antibiotics-polymyxin B and chloramphenicol. *J. Antimicrob. Chemother.* **2015**, *70*, 2589–2597. [CrossRef]
7. Poirel, L.; Jayol, A.; Nordmann, P. Polymyxins: Antibacterial Activity, Susceptibility Testing, and Resistance Mechanisms Encoded by Plasmids or Chromosomes. *Clin. Microbiol. Rev.* **2017**, *30*, 557–596. [CrossRef]

8. Liu, Y.Y.; Wang, Y.; Walsh, T.R.; Yi, L.X.; Zhang, R.; Spencer, J.; Doi, Y.; Tian, G.; Dong, B.; Huang, X.; et al. Emergence of plasmid-mediated colistin resistance mechanism MCR-1 in animals and human beings in China: A microbiological and molecular biological study. *Lancet Infect. Dis.* **2016**, *16*, 161–168. [CrossRef]
9. Nang, S.C.; Li, J.; Velkov, T. The rise and spread of *mcr* plasmid-mediated polymyxin resistance. *Crit. Rev. Microbiol.* **2019**, *45*, 131–161. [CrossRef]
10. Hussein, N.H.; Al-Kadmy, I.; Taha, B.M.; Hussein, J.D. Mobilized colistin resistance (*mcr*) genes from 1 to 10: A comprehensive review. *Mol. Biol. Rep.* **2021**, *48*, 2897–2907. [CrossRef]
11. Macnair, C.R.; Stokes, J.M.; Carfrae, L.A.; Fiebig-Comyn, A.A.; Coombes, B.K.; Mulvey, M.R.; Brown, E.D. Overcoming *mcr-1* mediated colistin resistance with colistin in combination with other antibiotics. *Nat. Commun.* **2018**, *9*, 458. [CrossRef]
12. Hussein, M.; Schneider-Futschik, E.K.; Paulin, O.; Allobawi, R.; Crawford, S.; Zhou, Q.T.; Hanif, A.; Baker, M.; Zhu, Y.; Li, J.; et al. Effective Strategy Targeting Polymyxin-Resistant Gram-Negative Pathogens: Polymyxin B in Combination with the Selective Serotonin Reuptake Inhibitor Sertraline. *ACS Infect. Dis.* **2020**, *6*, 1436–1450. [CrossRef]
13. Falagas, M.E.; Voulgaris, G.L.; Tryfinopoulou, K.; Giakkoupi, P.; Kyriakidou, M.; Vatopoulos, A.; Coates, A.; Hu, Y. Synergistic activity of colistin with azidothymidine against colistin-resistant *Klebsiella pneumoniae* clinical isolates collected from inpatients in Greek hospitals. *Int. J. Antimicrob. Agents* **2019**, *53*, 855–858. [CrossRef]
14. Zhou, Y.F.; Liu, P.; Dai, S.H.; Sun, J.; Liu, Y.H.; Liao, X.P. Activity of Tigecycline or Colistin in Combination with Zidovudine against *Escherichia coli* Harboring *tet(X)* and *mcr-1*. *Antimicrob. Agents Chemother.* **2020**, *65*, e01172-20. [CrossRef]
15. Martinez-Guitian, M.; Vazquez-Ucha, J.C.; Odingo, J.; Parish, T.; Poza, M.; Waite, R.D.; Bou, G.; Wareham, D.W.; Beceiro, A. Synergy between Colistin and the Signal Peptidase Inhibitor MD3 Is Dependent on the Mechanism of Colistin Resistance in *Acinetobacter baumannii*. *Antimicrob. Agents Chemother.* **2016**, *60*, 4375–4379. [CrossRef]
16. Chung, J.H.; Bhat, A.; Kim, C.J.; Yong, D.; Ryu, C.M. Combination therapy with polymyxin B and netropsin against clinical isolates of multidrug-resistant *Acinetobacter baumannii*. *Sci. Rep.* **2016**, *6*, 28168. [CrossRef]
17. Dai, C.; Wang, Y.; Sharma, G.; Shen, J.; Velkov, T.; Xiao, X. Polymyxins-Curcumin Combination Antimicrobial Therapy: Safety Implications and Efficacy for Infection Treatment. *Antioxidants* **2020**, *9*, 506. [CrossRef]
18. Feng, X.; Liu, S.; Wang, Y.; Zhang, Y.; Sun, L.; Li, H.; Wang, C.; Liu, Y.; Cao, B. Synergistic Activity of Colistin Combined With Auranofin Against Colistin-Resistant Gram-Negative Bacteria. *Front. Microbiol.* **2021**, *12*, 676414. [CrossRef]
19. Desbois, A.P.; Smith, V.J. Antibacterial free fatty acids: Activities, mechanisms of action and biotechnological potential. *Appl. Microbiol. Biotechnol.* **2010**, *85*, 1629–1642. [CrossRef]
20. McGaw, L.J.; Jäger, A.K.; Van Staden, J.; Houghton, P.J. Antibacterial effects of fatty acids and related compounds from plants. *South Afr. J. Bot.* **2002**, *68*, 417–423. [CrossRef]
21. Li, L.; Chen, H.; Liu, Y.; Xu, S.; Wu, M.; Liu, Z.; Qi, C.; Zhang, G.; Li, J.; Huang, X. Synergistic effect of linezolid with fosfomycin against *Staphylococcus aureus* in vitro and in an experimental *Galleria mellonella* model. *J. Microbiol. Immunol. Infect.* **2020**, *53*, 731–738. [CrossRef]
22. Huang, W.C.; Tsai, T.H.; Chuang, L.T.; Li, Y.Y.; Zouboulis, C.C.; Tsai, P.J. Anti-bacterial and anti-inflammatory properties of capric acid against *Propionibacterium acnes*: A comparative study with lauric acid. *J. Dermatol. Sci.* **2014**, *73*, 232–240. [CrossRef]
23. Murzyn, A.; Krasowska, A.; Stefanowicz, P.; Dziadkowiec, D.; Bukaszewicz, M. Capric acid secreted by *S. boulardii* inhibits *C. albicans filamentous* growth, adhesion and biofilm formation. *PLoS ONE* **2010**, *5*, e12050. [CrossRef]
24. Vidaillac, C.; Benichou, L.; Duval, R.E. In vitro synergy of colistin combinations against colistin-resistant *Acinetobacter baumannii*, *Pseudomonas aeruginosa*, and *Klebsiella pneumoniae* isolates. *Antimicrob. Agents Chemother.* **2012**, *56*, 4856–4861. [CrossRef]
25. Betts, J.W.; Sharili, A.S.; La Ragione, R.M.; Wareham, D.W. In Vitro Antibacterial Activity of Curcumin-Polymyxin B Combinations against Multidrug-Resistant Bacteria Associated with Traumatic Wound Infections. *J. Nat. Prod.* **2016**, *79*, 1702–1706. [CrossRef]
26. Pillai, S.K.; Moellering, R.C.; Eliopoulos, G.M. Antimicrobial combinations. In *Antibiotics in Laboratory Medicine*, 5th ed.; Lorian, V., Ed.; The Lippincott Williams & Wilkins Co.: Philadelphia, PA, USA, 2005; pp. 365–440.
27. Bergen, P.J.; Smith, N.M.; Bedard, T.B.; Bulman, Z.P.; Cha, R.; Tsuji, B.T. Rational Combinations of Polymyxins with Other Antibiotics. *Adv. Exp. Med. Biol.* **2019**, *1145*, 251–288. [CrossRef]
28. Suchodolski, J.; Derkacz, D.; Bernat, P.; Krasowska, A. Capric acid secreted by *Saccharomyces boulardii* influences the susceptibility of *Candida albicans* to fluconazole and amphotericin B. *Sci. Rep.* **2021**, *11*, 6519. [CrossRef]

Disclaimer/Publisher's Note: The statements, opinions and data contained in all publications are solely those of the individual author(s) and contributor(s) and not of MDPI and/or the editor(s). MDPI and/or the editor(s) disclaim responsibility for any injury to people or property resulting from any ideas, methods, instructions or products referred to in the content.

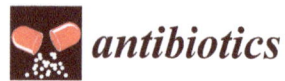

Article

Characterization of the Composition Variation of Healthy Human Gut Microbiome in Correlation with Antibiotic Usage and Yogurt Consumption

Shaofei Yan [1,†], Xiaofan Zhang [2,†], Xiaofang Jia [2], Jiguo Zhang [2], Xiaomin Han [1], Chang Su [2], Jianyun Zhao [1], Wanglong Gou [3], Jin Xu [1,*] and Bing Zhang [2,*]

1. NHC Key Laboratory of Food Safety Risk Assessment, China National Center for Food Safety Risk Assessment, Beijing 100021, China
2. National Institute for Nutrition and Health, Chinese Center for Disease Control and Prevention, Key Laboratory of Trace Element Nutrition, National Health Commission of the People's Republic of China, Beijing 100050, China
3. Key Laboratory of Growth Regulation and Translational Research of Zhejiang Province, School of Life Sciences, Westlake University, Hangzhou 310024, China
* Correspondence: xujin@cfsa.net.cn (J.X.); zhangbing@chinacdc.cn (B.Z.)
† These authors contributed equally to this work.

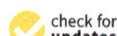

Citation: Yan, S.; Zhang, X.; Jia, X.; Zhang, J.; Han, X.; Su, C.; Zhao, J.; Gou, W.; Xu, J.; Zhang, B. Characterization of the Composition Variation of Healthy Human Gut Microbiome in Correlation with Antibiotic Usage and Yogurt Consumption. *Antibiotics* 2022, *11*, 1827. https://doi.org/10.3390/antibiotics11121827

Academic Editor: Carlos M. Franco

Received: 31 October 2022
Accepted: 15 November 2022
Published: 16 December 2022

Publisher's Note: MDPI stays neutral with regard to jurisdictional claims in published maps and institutional affiliations.

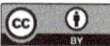

Copyright: © 2022 by the authors. Licensee MDPI, Basel, Switzerland. This article is an open access article distributed under the terms and conditions of the Creative Commons Attribution (CC BY) license (https://creativecommons.org/licenses/by/4.0/).

Abstract: Antibiotic usage and yogurt consumption are the major interventions for gut microbiota, yet their shared characteristics and disparities in healthy human gut microbiome remain unclear. This study aimed to decipher the composition changes among healthy humans, comparing antibiotic usage and yogurt consumption. The relative bacterial abundances of 1113 fecal samples were collected from an ongoing, population-based longitudinal cohort study in China that covered lifestyle, diet, disease status and physical measurements, and biological indicators of participants were obtained by the sequencing of 16S rRNA. The samples were divided into three groups, which were antibiotic users (122), yogurt consumers (497) and controls (494), where data visualization, alpha diversity, beta diversity and LEfSe analysis were conducted. At the family level, the relative abundances of *Streptococcaceae*, *Enterobacteriaceae* and *Enterococcaceae* families in antibiotic users increased almost 50%, 70% and 200%, respectively, while yogurt consumption also increased relative abundances of *Streptococcaceae* and *Enterococcaceae*, but not *Enterobacteriaceae*. Alpha diversity analyses suggested that the microbiome of the antibiotic usage and yogurt consumption groups exhibited an alpha diversity lower than that of the control. LEfSe analysis showed that, at the family level, the number of biomarkers in the yogurt consumption and antibiotic usage group were respectively 5 and 7, lower than that of the control (13). This study demonstrated the importance in considering the potential assistance of yogurt consumption on ARG gene transfer from commensal bacteria to pathogens in the human gut, which may pose a risk for human health. Antibiotic usage and yogurt consumption share more identical changes on healthy human gut flora than disparities. Therefore, in order to understand the potential risks of antibiotic usage and yogurt consumption on antibiotic resistance transmission in human gut microbiota, further research needs to be undertaken.

Keywords: gut microbiota; antibiotic usage; yogurt consumption; metagenomics

1. Introduction

The human gut microbiota comprises the microorganisms that live in the human gut, including bacteria, archaea, fungi, and viruses, from which bacteria are dominant [1]. The functions of gut microbiota are resisting pathogens, maintaining the intestinal epithelium, metabolizing dietary and pharmaceutical compounds, controlling immune function, and so on [2,3]. There are four dominant bacterial phyla in the composition of human gut microbiota: *Bacillota*, *Bacteroidota*, *Actinomycetota*, and *Pseudomonadota* [4]. *Bacteroides*,

Clostridium, Faecalibacterium, Eubacterium, Ruminococcus, Peptococcus, Peptostreptococcus, and *Bifidobacterium* are the dominant genera that are found to inhabit the human gut [1]. The composition of human gut microbiota responds to a variety of factors and changes all the time [5]. It has been reported by a human-cohort-based analysis that dynamic change in the gut ecosystem correlates strongly with complex interactions such as host lifestyle, dietary, ecological and other factors [4,6].

Antibiotic resistance is a global concern. Some bacteria in the gut are naturally resistant to certain antibiotics, while other commensal bacteria may acquire resistance genes from fellow resistant bacteria through horizontal gene transfer (HGT), including conjugation, transduction and transformation [7]. The human gut micobiota is directly affected by the clinical use of antibiotics [8]. Antibiotic usage can disrupt the ability of gut micobiota to inhibit pathogen growth, due to the reduction of native bacterial species, therefore causing antibiotic diarrhea [9]. Antibiotic usage may also enhance horizontal AMR gene transfer from commensal bacteria to pathogens in gut microbiota, through which antibiotic resistant pathogens that are difficult to treat with common antibiotics are created [10,11]. Probiotics are microorganisms that are beneficial to health when supplemented as part of the human diet [12]. It has been reported that the consumption of probiotics containing *Lactobacillus* species might help prevent antibiotic-associated diarrhea [13].

Diet may influence gut resistome in healthy humans. Researchers found that subjects with a diverse, fiber-rich diet had a lower abundance of ARGs in their gut, through changing the composition of gut microbiota to harbor more antibiotic resistance genes [14]. As a food type in the human diet that contains probiotics *Lactobacillus delbrueckii* subsp. *bulgaricus* and *Streptococcus thermophilus* bacteria, yogurt consumption is gradually increasing around the world. However, although yogurt consumption is good for human health, as reported [15], does the influence of the yogurt consumption on human gut microbiome also go against gut resistome? This study therefore focuses on deciphering the composition changes among healthy humans in comparison with antibiotic usage and yogurt consumption.

2. Results

2.1. Baseline Characteristics among Study Groups

The average age of the three groups ranged from 48.0 to 54.7 years, with a slightly higher proportion of women than men. The yogurt group had higher levels of education and lower rates of smoking than the other two groups. Other basic characteristics, such as body mass index (BMI), waist circumference (WC), physical activity (PA), and total energy were presented as means in Table 1.

Table 1. Baseline characteristics of adults in different groups.

Characteristics	Control Group (n = 494)	Yogurt Group (n = 497)	Antibiotic Group (n = 122)
Gender (n, %)			
Male	202 (40.9)	202 (40.6)	58 (47.5)
Female	292 (59.1)	295 (59.4)	64 (52.5)
Age (year)	48.5	48.0	54.7
BMI (kg/m^2)	25.0	23.9	24.5
WC (cm)	86.3	83.4	85.7
Smoke (n, %)			
No	372 (75.6)	402 (81.1)	87 (71.9)
Yes	120 (24.4)	94 (18.9)	34 (28.1)
PA (METs/week)	148.6	117.0	140.7
Education (n, %)			
Primary and below	104 (23.5)	36 (7.7)	21 (21.6)
Junior high	175 (39.6)	136 (29.0)	42 (43.3)
Senior high and above	163 (36.9)	297 (63.3)	34 (35.1)
Total energy (kcal/d)	2000.0	2043.1	1931.9

2.2. Composition of the Gut Microbiota in groups of Antibiotic Usage and Yogurt Consumption

In our study, bacterial 16S rRNA sequences from 1113 healthy human fecal samples were identified. The composition of gut microbiota was shown in phylum and family levels, respectively (Figure 1A,B). The relative abundances of the *Bacteroidetes* phyla in feces from the antibiotic usage and yogurt group were both lower than those of the control group, with the yogurt group being the lowest among them. The relative abundances of *Actinobacteria* and *Proteobacteria* phyla showed opposite results while comparing with the control group, with *Actinobacteria* higher in the yogurt group, *Proteobacteria* higher in the antibiotic group, and control in the middle. At the order level, the relative abundances of *Bacillales* order in the antibiotic usage group increased notably. Both antibiotic and yogurt brought about observable increases in *Lactobacillales* order (Figure 1C). At the family level, the relative abundances of *Streptococcaceae*, *Enterobacteriaceae* and *Enterococcaceae* families in antibiotic users increased almost 50%, 70% and 200%, respectively, when compared with the control. Interestingly, the yogurt consumption group was also composed of increased relative abundances of *Streptococcaceae* and *Enterococcaceae* family, but not the *Enterobacteriaceae* family, compared with control (Figure 1B).

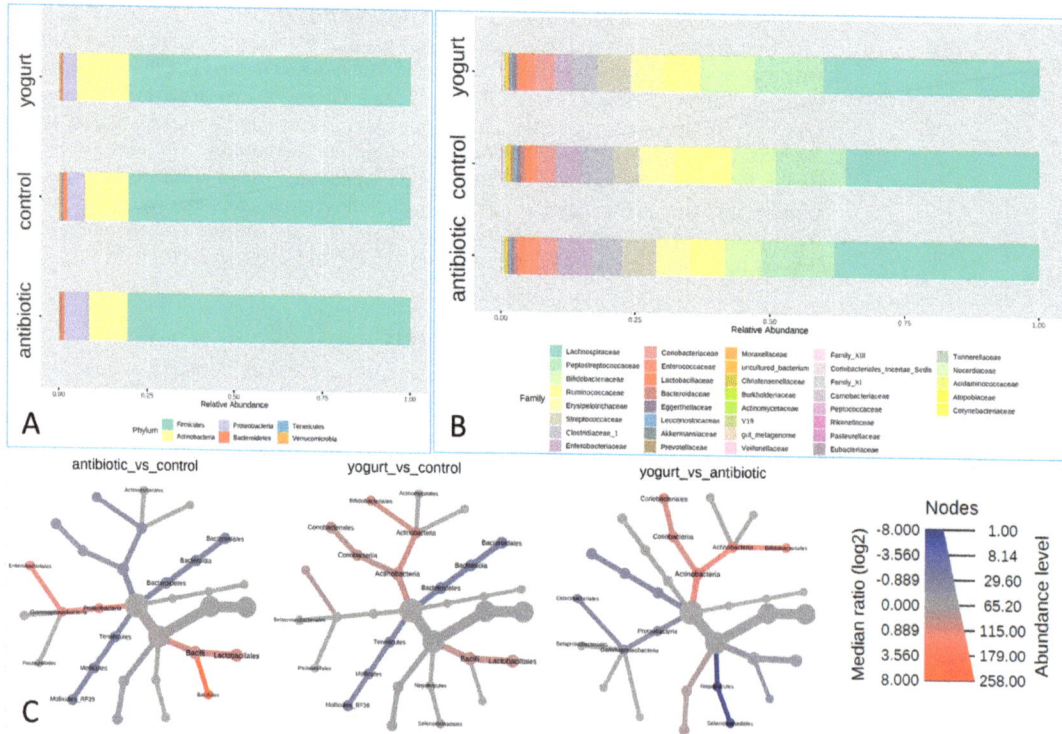

Figure 1. Composition of the Gut Microbiota of control, antibiotic usage and Yogurt consumption groups. (**A**) Gut microbiome composition at the phylum level; (**B**) Gut microbiome composition at the family level; (**C**) Heat tree demonstration of gut microbiome composition at the order level.

2.3. Alpha and Beta Diversity in the Gut Microbiome among Antibiotic Usage, Yogurt Consumption and Control

After operational taxonomic units (OTUs) were obtained and analyzed using QIIME 2 work flow, alpha and beta diversity analyses were carried out. Chao1, Shannon, Simpson and observed indexes were calculated to evaluate the alpha diversity in the human gut microbiome. The microbiomes of the antibiotic usage and yogurt consumption groups exhibited a lower alpha diversity than that of the control (Figure 2A). There was a significant difference in the Chao1, observed OTUs, and Shannon indices ($p = 1.0796 \times 10^{-10}$, $p = 1.7389 \times 10^{-12}$, and $p = 0.0001$, respectively). Principal coordinates analysis (PCoA) was performed to visualize the beta diversity based on the PERMANOVA statistic method in the microbial community structure, where antibiotic usage and yogurt consumption groups were shown in the Bray–Curtis Index analysis (Figure 2B, F-value: 8.3963; R-squared: 0.014916; p-value: 0.001).

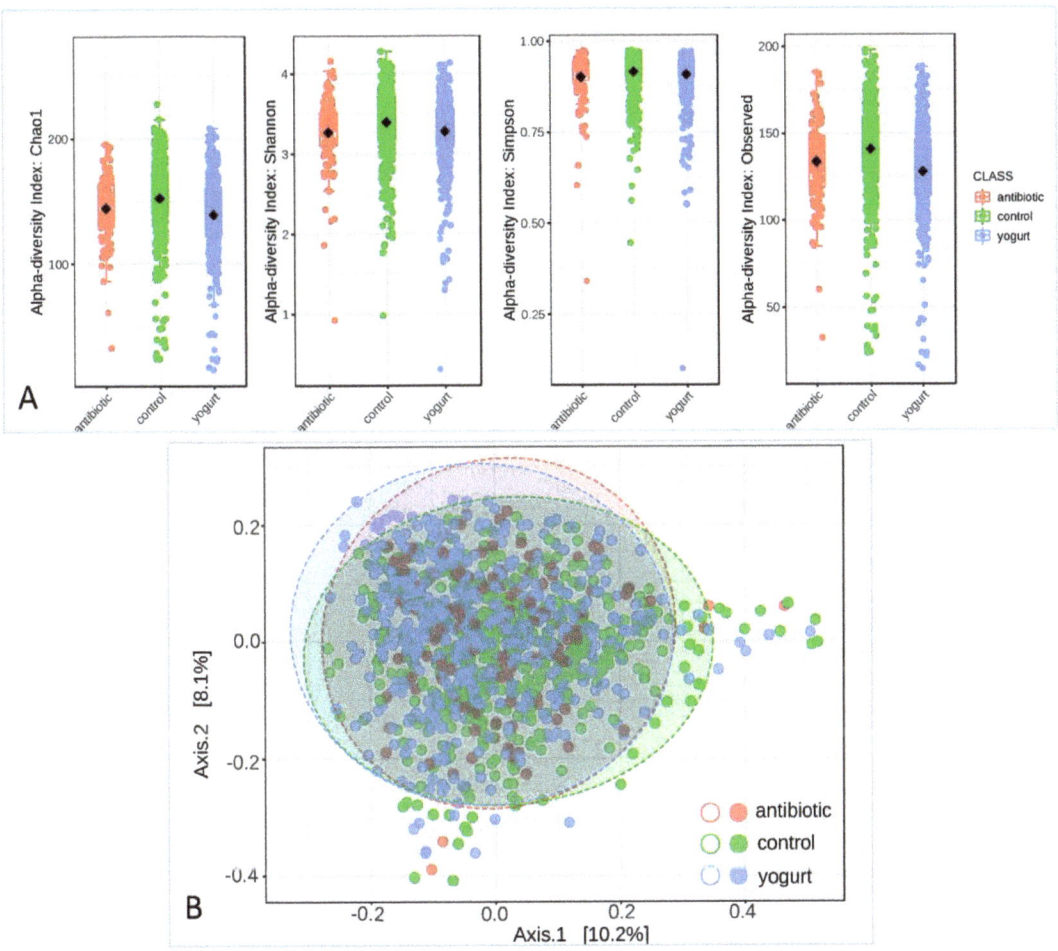

Figure 2. Alpha and Beta Diversity of the Gut Microbiome. (**A**) Alpha diversity evaluation at Chao1, Shannon, Simpson and observed indexes; (**B**) Beta diversity based on the PERMANOVA statistic method.

2.4. Biomarker Differences among Antibiotic Usage, Yogurt Consumption and Control

In this study, we carried out the linear discriminant analysis (LDA) effect size (LEfSe analysis) to investigate the differences in different taxa levels between groups using the Microbiome Analyst online platform [16,17]. At phylum level, *Proteobacteria* was the biomarker of the antibiotic usage group, and *Actinobacteria* the yogurt consumption group, where they were all four times higher than those in the control group. At Order level, *Enterobacteriales*, *Lactobacillales*, and *Actinomycetales* in the antibiotic usage group were three times higher than those in the control group. At family level, the number of biomarkers in the yogurt consumption and antibiotic usage group were respectively 5 and 7, lower than that of the control (13), as shown in Figure 3.

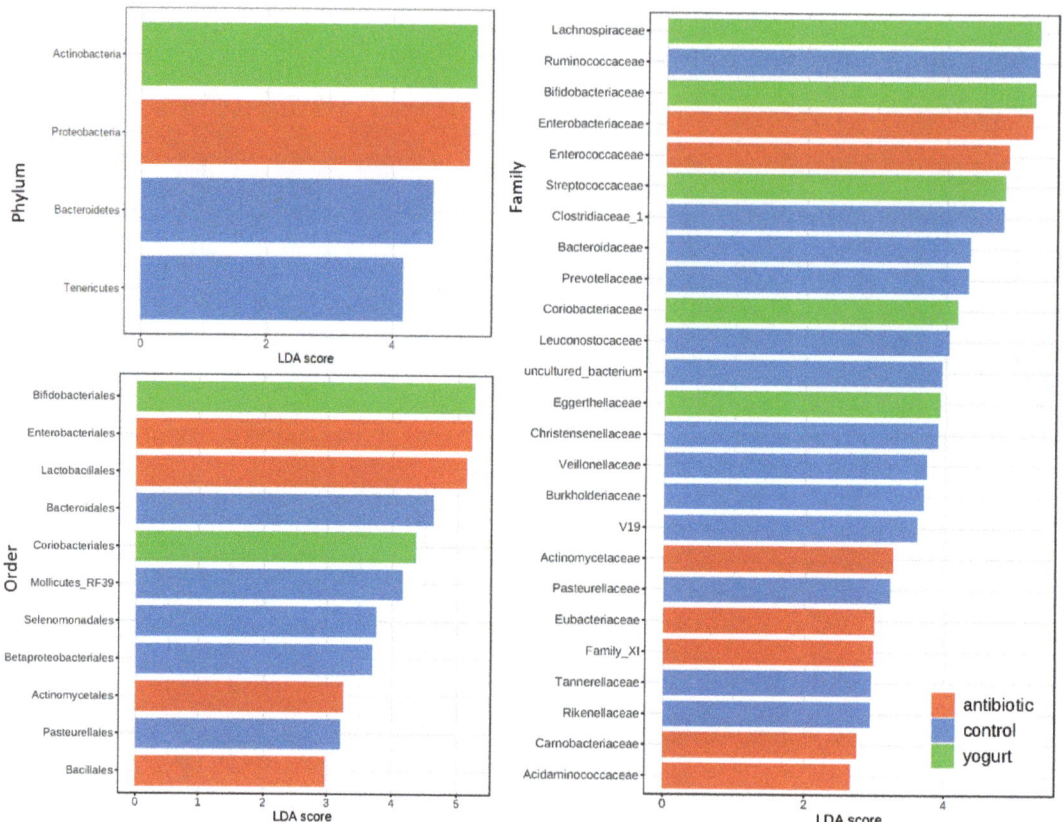

Figure 3. Biomarkers of different taxa level of the Gut Microbiome among antibiotic usage, Yogurt consumption and control (LEfSe analysis).

3. Discussion

Self-use of antibiotics in healthy humans is becoming a health concern, especially in low-income groups of people. Although clinical use of antibiotics has been proved to reduce diversity in the gut microbiome [8], the situation for antibiotic usage in healthy humans is unclear. As an important part of healthy human diet, how yogurt consumption influences human gut microbiome is under researched. Therefore, in order to better understand the effects of antibiotic usage and yogurt consumption on human gut, it is important to understand the similarities and differences between antibiotic usage and yogurt consumption among healthy humans.

Both the antibiotic usage and yogurt consumption groups exhibited a decrease in the richness and evenness of diversity compared with the control group. The insignificant result of the Simpson index showed that the dominance indices of gut flora remained stable in a large scale of healthy human gut microbiome. Alpha analysis indicated that antibiotic usage and yogurt consumption were making significant changes in healthy human gut microbiome. However, the overall diversity of the microbiome among these groups was not obvious enough, possibly due to attenuation of the potential effects on the physiology of the host organisms. This may also possibly be due to the limitation of the sample sets, and the deviation caused by other variables such as age, smoking state, and the evolutionary outcomes that keep getting the human gut microbiome back to a stable state should also be considered.

Yogurt is produced by adding a combination of probiotics to ferment milk, which are mostly *Lactobacillus delbrueckii subspecies bulgaricus* and *Streptococcus salivarius subspecies thermophiles, Lactobacilli* or *Bifidobacteria* [18]. The lactic-acid-secreting bacteria that are added to milk may modify the intestinal environment in two ways: (1) increasing tight junctions in the gut epithelium; (2) decreasing potentially harmful enzymes produced by the residential bacteria [19,20]. In our study, the relative abundances of the *Bacteroidetes* phyla in feces from the antibiotic usage and yogurt groups were both lower than those of the control group, with the yogurt group being the lowest among them. It is consistent with Odamaki's reports that the consumption of yogurt containing *Bifidobacterium longum* BB536 significantly decreases enterotoxigenic *Bacteroides fragilis* in the gut microbiota [21].

Yogurt consumption was reported to be good for human health, and is especially deemed beneficial to the human gut [22]. Yogurts made with *Bifidobacterium lactis* and other probiotics are considered to help maintain gut flora by providing organisms that are usually inhabited in the human gut [23]. However, we need to be careful when antimicrobial resistance is taken into consideration. It has been reported that antibiotic usage would assist AMR genes' horizontal transfer in patients [10]. However, the mechanisms of antibiotic resistance transmission during microbiome modification remain unclear. At the family level of the relative abundances in this study, *Streptococcaceae, Enterobacteriaceae* and *Enterococcaceae*, which are closely correlated with AMR, increased almost 50%, 70% and 200% in the antibiotic usage group, as expected. It has been suggested that probiotic supplementation may decrease the total load of ARGs within the gut [24,25]. However, in our study, interestingly, the yogurt consumption group was also composed of increased relative abundances of *Streptococcaceae* and *Enterococcaceae* family, the same as antibiotic usage group. Therefore, it is not negligible that we should consider the potentiality of yogurt consumption on bacterial ecosystems that will potentially increase the stress and/or selection pressure and, therefore, could induce an intensification of ARG gene transfer processes from commensal bacteria to pathogens in the human gut, posing a possible risk for human health.

Through LEfSe analysis, we can see that the number of biomarkers in the yogurt consumption and antibiotic usage group was much lower than that of control. This probably means that the yogurt consumption and antibiotic usage decreased gut micobiome diversity in healthy human. Antibiotic usage was more influential than yogurt consumption on healthy human gut microbiome. However, antibiotic usage and yogurt consumption do share more identical changes in healthy human gut microbiome than disparities. Therefore, in order to reduce the health and AMR transmitting risk, functional research based on an in-depth study from a meta-interactomics perspective and the use of advanced computing equipment under different metabolic states needs to be carried out to decipher the correlation between antibiotic usage and yogurt consumption on human gut microbiota.

4. Materials and Methods

4.1. Study Design and Participants

The present study was based on data from the China Health and Nutrition Survey (CHNS), an ongoing, population-based longitudinal cohort in China that covers lifestyle, diet and disease status, physical measurements and biological indicators. A total of 15 provinces/megacities in China participated. An overview of the CHNS study design has been published previously [26]. During the 2015 survey, stool samples were collected as well as dietary information. In the study, 16S rRNA analysis from stool samples was used to construct gut microbiota profiles (n = 3248). Participants were excluded if they had no FFQ information during 2015 (n = 9), or drank more than 150 g of yogurt more than once a week and took antibiotics within 6 months at the same time (n = 25). Participants were included if they drank yogurt more than once a week and consumed more than 150 g (n = 497, yogurt group), or had not drunk yogurt (n = 1987) in the past year, or had taken antibiotics within 6 months (n = 122, antibiotic group). The non-yogurt-drinkers were matched with the yogurt group 1:1 for gender and age (no more than 2 years' difference), and 494 people were finally matched as the control group (n = 494, control group). A total of 1113 participants from the 2015 survey were included in the present study (age 48.9 ± 13.5 years, mean ± SD).

4.2. Sample Collection

Adult participants collected stool samples themselves after receiving adequate instruction for the collection process during a home visit prior to collection, and samples were frozen immediately at $-20\ ^\circ$C. Stool samples were transported within 48 h by cold chain to the central laboratory and stored at $-20\ ^\circ$C to ensure proper processing.

4.3. Genomic DNA Extraction

The methods for DNA extraction, amplification and sequencing have been described previously [27]. A bead-beating procedure was used to extract bacterial DNA (TIANGEN Biotech, Beijing, China) following the manufacturer's instructions. For 16s ribosomal RNA (rRNA) genes, we adjusted the DNA concentration of each sample to 50 ng/L.

4.4. PCR Amplification of the V3-V4 Region of 16S rRNA Gene

The V3-V4 region of 16s rRNA gene with a 6-bp barcode unique to each sample was amplified with primers 515F/806R (5′-GTGCCAGCMGCCGCGGTAA-3′/ 5′-GGACTACHVGGGTWTCTAAT-3′) to characterize the taxonomic profile of gut microbiota. In an equimolar ratio, PCR products were combined. An Illumina HiSeq PE-250 platform was used to sequence the libraries, constructed with TruSeq DNA PCR-Free Library Preparation Kit (Illumina, CA, USA).

4.5. Microbial Data Analyses

The comparisons between groups were analyzed using parametric (chi-square test, analysis of variance) or non-parametric tests (Kruskal–Wallis test); a p-value was assessed as significant when <0.05.

An analysis of the 16S rRNA gene sequences was performed using the QIIME 2 bioinformatics pipeline [28]. The filtering and normalization, visualization of the data, alpha diversity, beta diversity, heat tree and LEfSe analysis were all produced using a web-based platform Microbiome Analyst [16,17]. The parameters for data filtering were minimum count = 4, prevalence in samples = 20%, percentage to remove based on interquantile range = 10%, sample size = 5000.

5. Conclusions

Antibiotic usage and yogurt consumption demonstrated significant changes in specific bacterial groups (*Streptococcaceae*, *Enterococcaceae* and so on) in healthy human gut microbiomes in this study. Antibiotic usage and yogurt consumption shared more identical changes in healthy human gut microbiome than disparities, especially ARG gene related bacteria groups that could induce an intensification of ARG gene transfer processes from commensal bacteria to pathogens in human gut. However, in order to understand the potential risks of antibiotic usage and yogurt consumption on antibiotic resistance transmission in human gut microbiota, further researches need to be carried out.

Author Contributions: Conceptualization, S.Y. and X.J.; formal analysis, S.Y., X.J. and W.G.; funding acquisition, B.Z.; investigation, X.Z., X.J., J.Z. (Jiguo Zhang) and C.S.; methodology, S.Y., X.Z. and W.G.; project administration, B.Z.; supervision, J.X.; visualization, S.Y.; writing—original draft, S.Y. and X.Z.; writing—review and editing, S.Y., J.Z. (Jiguo Zhang), X.H. and J.Z. (Jianyun Zhao). All authors have read and agreed to the published version of the manuscript.

Funding: This study was funded by Study of Diet and Nutrition Assessment and Intervention Technology (No.2020YFC2006300) from Active Health and Aging Technologic Solutions Major Project of National Key R&D Program. This research used data from CHNS, CHNS received funding from the National Institutes of Health (NIH) (R01HD30880, R01AG065357, P30DK056350, and R01HD38700) from 1989 to 2019, and was supported by the National Institutes of Health and National Institute of Diabetes and Digestive and Kidney Diseases (R01DK104371) and the Carolina Population Center P2CHD050924, P30AG066615.

Institutional Review Board Statement: The study met the standards for the ethical treatment of participants and was approved by the Institutional Review Board of the University of North Carolina at Chapel Hill, Chapel Hill, North Carolina, United States (NO. 07-1963). The National Institute for Nutrition and Health, Chinese Center for Disease Control and Prevention, approved the survey (No. 201524).

Informed Consent Statement: Informed consent was obtained from all participants involved in the study.

Data Availability Statement: Data are available upon reasonable request.

Acknowledgments: We are grateful to all subjects and investigators who participated in this study.

Conflicts of Interest: The authors declare no conflict of interest.

References

1. Thursby, E.; Juge, N. Introduction to the human gut microbiota. *Biochem. J.* **2017**, *474*, 1823–1836. [CrossRef]
2. Moszak, M.; Szulińska, M.; Bogdański, P. You Are What You Eat-The Relationship between Diet, Microbiota, and Metabolic Disorders-A Review. *Nutrients* **2020**, *12*, 1096. [CrossRef] [PubMed]
3. Bäumler, A.J.; Sperandio, V. Interactions between the microbiota and pathogenic bacteria in the gut. *Nature* **2016**, *535*, 85–93. [CrossRef]
4. Bresser, L.R.F.; de Goffau, M.C. Gut Microbiota in Nutrition and Health with a Special Focus on Specific Bacterial Clusters. *Cells* **2022**, *11*, 3091. [CrossRef]
5. Cook, J.; Prinz, M. Regulation of microglial physiology by the microbiota. *Gut Microbes* **2022**, *14*, 2125739. [CrossRef] [PubMed]
6. Nash, A.K.; Auchtung, T.A.; Wong, M.C.; Smith, D.P.; Gesell, J.R.; Ross, M.C.; Stewart, C.J.; Metcalf, G.A.; Muzny, D.M.; Gibbs, R.A.; et al. The gut mycobiome of the Human Microbiome Project healthy cohort. *Microbiome* **2017**, *5*, 153. [CrossRef] [PubMed]
7. Lamberte, L.E.; van Schaik, W. Antibiotic resistance in the commensal human gut microbiota. *Curr. Opin. Microbiol.* **2022**, *68*, 102150. [CrossRef]
8. Kwon, Y.; Cho, Y.S.; Lee, Y.M.; Kim, S.J.; Bae, J.; Jeong, S.J. Changes to Gut Microbiota Following Systemic Antibiotic Administration in Infants. *Antibiotics* **2022**, *11*, 470. [CrossRef] [PubMed]
9. Gu, X.; Sim, J.X.Y.; Lee, W.L.; Cui, L.; Chan, Y.F.Z.; Chang, E.D.; Teh, Y.E.; Zhang, A.N.; Armas, F.; Chandra, F.; et al. Gut Ruminococcaceae levels at baseline correlate with risk of antibiotic-associated diarrhea. *iScience* **2022**, *25*, 103644. [CrossRef] [PubMed]
10. Crits-Christoph, A.; Hallowell, H.A.; Koutouvalis, K.; Suez, J. Good microbes, bad genes? The dissemination of antimicrobial resistance in the human microbiome. *Gut Microbes* **2022**, *14*, 2055944. [CrossRef]
11. Khanna, S.; Tosh, P.K. A clinician's primer on the role of the microbiome in human health and disease. *Mayo Clin. Proc.* **2014**, *89*, 107–114. [CrossRef]
12. Kamińska, K.; Stenclik, D.; Błażejewska, W.; Bogdański, P.; Moszak, M. Probiotics in the Prevention and Treatment of Gestational Diabetes Mellitus (GDM): A Review. *Nutrients* **2022**, *14*, 4303. [CrossRef]
13. Kopacz, K.; Phadtare, S. Probiotics for the Prevention of Antibiotic-Associated Diarrhea. *Healthcare* **2022**, *10*, 1450. [CrossRef]
14. Oliver, A.; Xue, Z.; Villanueva, Y.T.; Durbin-Johnson, B.; Alkan, Z.; Taft, D.H.; Liu, J.; Korf, I.; Laugero, K.D.; Stephensen, C.B.; et al. Association of Diet and Antimicrobial Resistance in Healthy U.S. Adults. *mBio* **2022**, *13*, e0010122. [CrossRef]
15. Fernandez, M.A.; Panahi, S.; Daniel, N.; Tremblay, A.; Marette, A. Yogurt and Cardiometabolic Diseases: A Critical Review of Potential Mechanisms. *Adv. Nutr.* **2017**, *8*, 812–829. [CrossRef]
16. Dhariwal, A.; Chong, J.; Habib, S.; King, I.L.; Agellon, L.B.; Xia, J. MicrobiomeAnalyst: A web-based tool for comprehensive statistical, visual and meta-analysis of microbiome data. *Nucleic Acids Res.* **2017**, *45*, W180–W188. [CrossRef]
17. Chong, J.; Liu, P.; Zhou, G.; Xia, J. Using MicrobiomeAnalyst for comprehensive statistical, functional, and meta-analysis of microbiome data. *Nat. Protoc.* **2020**, *15*, 799–821. [CrossRef]
18. Kok, C.R.; Hutkins, R. Yogurt and other fermented foods as sources of health-promoting bacteria. *Nutr. Rev.* **2018**, *76* (Suppl. S1), 4–15. [CrossRef]
19. Alvaro, E.; Andrieux, C.; Rochet, V.; Rigottier-Gois, L.; Lepercq, P.; Sutren, M.; Galan, P.; Duval, Y.; Juste, C.; Doré, J. Composition and metabolism of the intestinal microbiota in consumers and non-consumers of yogurt. *Br. J. Nutr.* **2007**, *97*, 126–133. [CrossRef]

20. Lim, S.M.; Jeong, J.J.; Woo, K.H.; Han, M.J.; Kim, D.H. Lactobacillus sakei OK67 ameliorates high-fat diet-induced blood glucose intolerance and obesity in mice by inhibiting gut microbiota lipopolysaccharide production and inducing colon tight junction protein expression. *Nutr. Res.* **2016**, *36*, 337–348. [CrossRef]
21. Odamaki, T.; Sugahara, H.; Yonezawa, S.; Yaeshima, T.; Iwatsuki, K.; Tanabe, S.; Tominaga, T.; Togashi, H.; Benno, Y.; Xiao, J.Z. Effect of the oral intake of yogurt containing Bifidobacterium longum BB536 on the cell numbers of enterotoxigenic Bacteroides fragilis in microbiota. *Anaerobe* **2012**, *18*, 14–18. [CrossRef] [PubMed]
22. Gómez-Gallego, C.; Gueimonde, M.; Salminen, S. The role of yogurt in food-based dietary guidelines. *Nutr. Rev.* **2018**, *76* (Suppl. S1), 29–39. [CrossRef] [PubMed]
23. Tutunchi, H.; Naghshi, S.; Naemi, M.; Naeini, F.; Esmaillzadeh, A. Yogurt consumption and risk of mortality from all causes, cardiovascular disease, and cancer: A comprehensive systematic review and dose-response meta-analysis of cohort studies. *Public Health Nutr.* **2022**, 1–29, *online ahead of print*. [CrossRef]
24. Tsigalou, C.; Konstantinidis, T.; Stavropoulou, E.; Bezirtzoglou, E.E.; Tsakris, A. Potential Elimination of Human Gut Resistome by Exploiting the Benefits of Functional Foods. *Front. Microbiol.* **2020**, *11*, 50. [CrossRef] [PubMed]
25. Rosenberg, K. Multispecies Probiotic Can Prevent Antibiotic-Associated Diarrhea in Children. *Am. J. Nurs.* **2022**, *122*, 58. [CrossRef]
26. Popkin, B.M.; Du, S.; Zhai, F.; Zhang, B. Cohort Profile: The China Health and Nutrition Survey–monitoring and understanding socio-economic and health change in China, 1989-2011. *Int. J. Epidemiol.* **2010**, *39*, 1435–1440. [CrossRef]
27. Sun, S.; Wang, H.; Tsilimigras, M.C.; Howard, A.G.; Sha, W.; Zhang, J.; Su, C.; Wang, Z.; Du, S.; Sioda, M.; et al. Does geographical variation confound the relationship between host factors and the human gut microbiota: A population-based study in China. *Bmj Open* **2020**, *10*, e038163. [CrossRef]
28. Bolyen, E.; Rideout, J.R.; Dillon, M.R.; Bokulich, N.A.; Abnet, C.C.; Al-Ghalith, G.A.; Alexander, H.; Alm, E.J.; Arumugam, M.; Asnicar, F.; et al. Reproducible, interactive, scalable and extensible microbiome data science using QIIME 2. *Nat. Biotechnol.* **2019**, *37*, 852–857. [CrossRef]

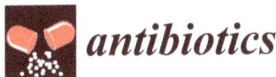

Article

Occurrence and Genomic Characterization of *mcr-1*-Harboring *Escherichia coli* Isolates from Chicken and Pig Farms in Lima, Peru

Dennis Carhuaricra [1,2,†], Carla G. Duran Gonzales [1,†], Carmen L. Rodríguez Cueva [1], Yennifer Ignacion León [1], Thalia Silvestre Espejo [1], Geraldine Marcelo Monge [1], Raúl H. Rosadio Alcántara [1], Nilton Lincopan [3,4], Luis Luna Espinoza [1] and Lenin Maturrano Hernández [1,*]

1. Research Group in Biotechnology Applied to Animal Health, Production and Conservation [SANIGEN], Laboratory of Biology and Molecular Genetics, Faculty of Veterinary Medicine, Universidad Nacional Mayor de San Marcos, Lima 15021, Peru
2. Programa de Pós-Graduação Interunidades em Bioinformática, Instituto de Matemática e Estatística, Universidade de São Paulo, Rua do Matão 1010, São Paulo 05508-090, Brazil
3. Department of Clinical Analysis, School of Pharmacy, University of São Paulo, São Paulo 05508-000, Brazil
4. Department of Microbiology, Institute of Biomedical Sciences, University of São Paulo, São Paulo 05508-000, Brazil
* Correspondence: amaturranoh@unmsm.edu.pe
† These authors contributed equally to this work.

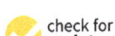

Citation: Carhuaricra, D.; Duran Gonzales, C.G.; Rodríguez Cueva, C.L.; Ignacion León, Y.; Silvestre Espejo, T.; Marcelo Monge, G.; Rosadio Alcántara, R.H.; Lincopan, N.; Espinoza, L.L.; Maturrano Hernández, L. Occurrence and Genomic Characterization of *mcr-1*-Harboring *Escherichia coli* Isolates from Chicken and Pig Farms in Lima, Peru. *Antibiotics* **2022**, *11*, 1781. https://doi.org/10.3390/antibiotics11121781

Academic Editors: Yongning Wu and Zhenling Zeng

Received: 24 October 2022
Accepted: 5 December 2022
Published: 8 December 2022

Publisher's Note: MDPI stays neutral with regard to jurisdictional claims in published maps and institutional affiliations.

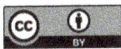

Copyright: © 2022 by the authors. Licensee MDPI, Basel, Switzerland. This article is an open access article distributed under the terms and conditions of the Creative Commons Attribution (CC BY) license (https://creativecommons.org/licenses/by/4.0/).

Abstract: Resistance to colistin generated by the *mcr-1* gene in *Enterobacteriaceae* is of great concern due to its efficient worldwide spread. Despite the fact that the Lima region has a third of the Peruvian population and more than half of the national pig and poultry production, there are no reports of the occurrence of the *mcr-1* gene in *Escherichia coli* isolated from livestock. In the present work, we studied the occurrence of *E. coli* carrying the *mcr-1* gene in chicken and pig farms in Lima between 2019 and 2020 and described the genomic context of the *mcr-1* gene. We collected fecal samples from 15 farms in 4 provinces of Lima including the capital Lima Metropolitana and recovered 341 *E. coli* isolates. We found that 21.3% (42/197) and 12.5% (18/144) of the chicken and pig strains were *mcr-1*-positive by PCR, respectively. The whole genome sequencing of 14 *mcr-1*-positive isolates revealed diverse sequence types (e.g., ST48 and ST602) and the presence of other 38 genes that confer resistance to 10 different classes of antibiotics, including beta-lactamase $bla_{CTX-M-55}$. The *mcr-1* gene was located on diverse plasmids belonging to the IncI2 and IncHI1A:IncHI1B replicon types. A comparative analysis of the plasmids showed that they contained the *mcr-1* gene within varied structures (*mikB*–*mcr1*–*pap2*, IS*Apl1*–*mcr1*–*pap2*, and Tn*6330*). To the best of our knowledge, this is the first attempt to study the prevalence of the *mcr-1* gene in livestock in Peru, revealing its high occurrence in pig and chicken farms. The genetic diversity of *mcr-1*-positive strains suggests a complex local epidemiology calling for a coordinated surveillance under the One-Health approach that includes animals, retail meat, farmers, hospitals and the environment to effectively detect and limit the spread of colistin-resistant bacteria.

Keywords: *mcr-1* gene; colistin; chicken farm; pig farm; *Escherichia coli*

1. Introduction

Antimicrobial resistance (AMR) represents a growing threat to global health, principally in developing countries, where the high population density, poor medical care and unregulated use of antibiotics provide a favorable environment for the emergence and dissemination of multidrug-resistant bacteria (MDR) [1]. The increased prevalence of bacterial pathogens resistant to last-line antibiotics (carbapenems, colistin and tigecycline) raises serious concerns about our ability to treat infectious diseases in humans and animals [2]. Colistin is one of the last-resort treatments against multidrug-resistant strains of *Enterobacterales*, but its unregulated overuse as a therapeutic drug and growth promoter in pig and poultry farming has favored the emergence of colistin-resistant strains [3,4]. Since the discovery of the plasmid-encoded colistin resistance gene named *mcr-1* in China in 2015 [5], this gene has been described in human, animal and environmental samples around the world [6]. The rapid spread of the *mcr-1* gene by efficient horizontal transfer is driven by the IncI2, IncHI2 and IncX4 plasmids [4].

Escherichia coli is a commensal bacterium that inhabits the gastrointestinal tract of humans and animals and represents a major reservoir of antimicrobial resistance genes (ARGs), mostly acquired through horizontal gene transfer [7,8]. As a result of this capacity, *E. coli* has been commonly used as an indicator to monitor AMR in livestock, food and humans [9,10]. Even though they are normally commensal, certain strains of *E. coli* are associated with infections. For example, pathogenic *E. coli* may cause neonatal and post-weaning diarrhea and edema in swine, while it may cause infections of the respiratory tract and soft tissues, resulting in colibacillosis, air sacculitis and cellulitis in chickens [11]. *E. coli* and *Klebsiella pneumoniae* carrying the *mcr-1* gene have recently been reported in isolates from Peruvian hospitals [12–15], as well as in isolates from slaughtered chickens destined for human consumption [16]. Due to the recurrent detection of resistant enterobacteria in hospitals, the Peruvian government decreed in late 2019 the prohibition of the manufacture, sale and import of veterinary products containing the active compound of colistin (Polymyxin E).

The Lima region has a third of the Peruvian population and concentrates the largest animal production in the country. In fact, by 2020, 53% and 43% of the national poultry and pig production were concentrated in Lima, mainly in farms located on the outskirts of the capital Lima Metropolitana. Reporting the growing colistin resistance and *mcr-1* prevalence in poultry and pig farms in low- and middle-income countries (LMIC) could be of high importance, but until now has been neglected in Peru [17]. Indeed, there is no information about the occurrence of *mcr* genes in livestock in Peru due to the absence of a systematic surveillance. In the present work, we investigated the occurrence of *E. coli* carrying the *mcr-1* gene isolated from chicken and pig farms in Lima, Peru, from 2019 to 2020 and performed a genomic analysis of the isolates carrying *mcr-1* to determine the genetic diversity and phylogenetic relationships of these isolates. Additionally, we characterized the virulence and ARGs profiles and explored the genomic context of the *mcr-1* gene.

2. Methods

2.1. Sample Collection and Bacterial Culture

We collected 348 fecal samples from 8 chicken farms and 300 samples from 7 pig farms in 4 provinces of Lima, including the Peruvian capital, Lima Metropolitana, between 2019 and 2020 (Supplementary Table S1). All samples were later organized in pools. One pool was prepared for each chicken shed or pigpen combining 2 g of feces in a 50 mL tube; at least 5 pools per farm were obtained. Each fecal pool was diluted in buffered saline solution (0.9%) and thereafter plated onto MacConkey agar (BD Difco) and incubated overnight at 37 °C. At least five suspected colonies of *E. coli* (lactose-fermenting colonies, convex morphology and pinkish color appearance) were selected from each pool, inoculated on eosin methylene blue agar (EMBA) and incubated for 24 h at 37 °C, observing the growth of typical metallic green colonies. Finally, a 7-parameter biochemical test including Simmon's citrate agar, lysine iron agar, triple sugar iron, motility–indole–lysine medium, sulfur indole motility medium, urea medium, red methyl and Voges Proskauer medium were used to confirm *E. coli*.

2.2. mcr-1 Gene Screening by PCR

All isolates were screened for the *mcr-1* gene using the procedures described by Rebelo et al. (2018) [18]. Shortly, we used forward 5′-AGTCCGTTTGTTCTTGTGGC-3′ and reverse 5′-AGATCCTTGGTCTCGGCTTG-3′ primers with 2 μL of 10X PCR Buffer (100 mM

KCl, 100 mM Tris-HCl, 20 mM MgCl$_2$), 1.6 µL of deoxynucleotide triphosphate (dNTPs) 10 mM, 0.2 µL of DreamTaq 5 U/µL (Thermo Fisher Scientific, Waltham, MA, USA) and 2 µL of DNA in a final volume of 20 µL. The following condition were used: 1 cycle of initial denaturation at 94 °C for 15 min, followed by 25 cycles of denaturation at 94 °C for 30 s, annealing at 58 °C for 90 s and elongation at 72 °C for 60 s, with a final extension step of 72 °C for 10 min. We used the *mcr-1*-harboring *E. coli* CDC-AR-0346A reference strain (https://www.microbiologics.com/01259P) (accessed on 27 November 2022) as a positive control for all PCR runs.

2.3. Whole-Genome Sequencing and Assembly

From all *mcr-1*-positive *E. coli*, we selected 14 isolates for whole-genome sequencing (accession numbers and sequencing statistics are provided in Supplementary Table S2). The DNA was extracted from pure colonies using the PureLink™ Genomic DNA Kit (Invitrogen', Cat. No K1820-02). DNA concentration was measured using the Qubit dsDNA HS assay (Invitrogen, Cat. No Q33230). Then 1 ng of DNA was used for Nextera XT library preparation and subsequent sequencing using 2 × 250 bp reads on the Illumina Miseq platform (Illumina, San Diego, CA, USA). The quality of the fastq files was evaluated with FastQC v0.11.9 [19], and the trimming of low-quality reads was performed with Trimmomatic v0.39 [20]. Finally, the assembly was performed with SPAdes v3.14.1 [21], and Prokka v1.14.6 [22] was used for genome annotation.

2.4. Sequence Analysis

We used the mlst v2.19.0 tool (https://github.com/tseemann/mlst) (accessed on 16 August 2022) and EzClermont v0.6.3 [23] to determine the multilocus sequence type (MLST) and phylogroup type, respectively. ARGs, virulence genes and plasmid replicon types were annotated using the Resfinder, VirulenceFinder and PlasmidFinder databases from the Center for Genomic Epidemiology with the ABRICATE v. 1.0.1 tool (https://github.com/tseemann/abricate) (accessed on 16 August 2022) using the following settings: a nucleotide identity of 80% and minimum coverage of 80%.

For the phylogenetic reconstruction, we used the following pipeline: Snippy v 4.6.0 (https://github.com/tseemann/snippy) (accessed on 15 July 2022) to generate the core-genome alignment of 14 *E. coli* genomes including the reference genome sequence *E. coli* K-12 (Genbank accession: NC_000913.3); given that recombination is widespread in bacteria genomes, Gubbins v3.2 [24] was used to detect and mask recombinant regions, and IQ-TREE v2.0 [25] to construct a maximum-likelihood tree based on a general time-reversible (GTR) nucleotide substitution model with 1000 bootstrap replicates. Tree visualization and annotation were created using the ggtree v3.0.4 [26] package in R 4.2. The genetic context of the *mcr-1*-encoding plasmid sequences was represented using Easyfig v2.2.2 [27].

We used a bioinformatics approach to identify the plasmid sequences. First, we used plasmidSPAdes [28] for plasmid assembly from raw data. Second, after checking if these sequences contained the *mcr-1* cassette, we used plasmidfinder [29] to check if the predicted plasmid has a replicon and then we used oriTfinder [30] to identify the origin of the transfer site (oriT) and conjugative elements. Finally, we performed a search in the PLSDB database [31] to identify similar plasmid sequences. Highly similar sequences were compared with the predicted plasmids to generate a circular view using Blast Ring Image generation (BRIG) software [32].

3. Results

3.1. Prevalence of the mcr-1 Gene in Poultry and Pig Farms

A total of 15 farms located in Lima were investigated in this study. We collected 648 fecal samples and recovered 197 *E. coli* isolates from 8 chicken farms and 144 *E. coli* isolates from 7 pig farms. The *mcr-1* gene was identified in four of eight chicken farms in three Lima provinces, and in five of seven pig farms located in three Lima provinces (Figure 1). The occurrence of the *mcr-1* gene was variable: 81% of the isolates were *mcr-1*-

positive in the AV8 farm (26/32 isolates), while 52.2% (12/23) were positive in the AV4 farm, and just 10.7% (3/28) were positive in the AV5 farm (see Supplementary Table S1). Overall, the *mcr-1*-specific PCR identified the gene in 21.3% (42/197) of the isolates from poultry and in 12.5% (18/144) of the isolates from pigs.

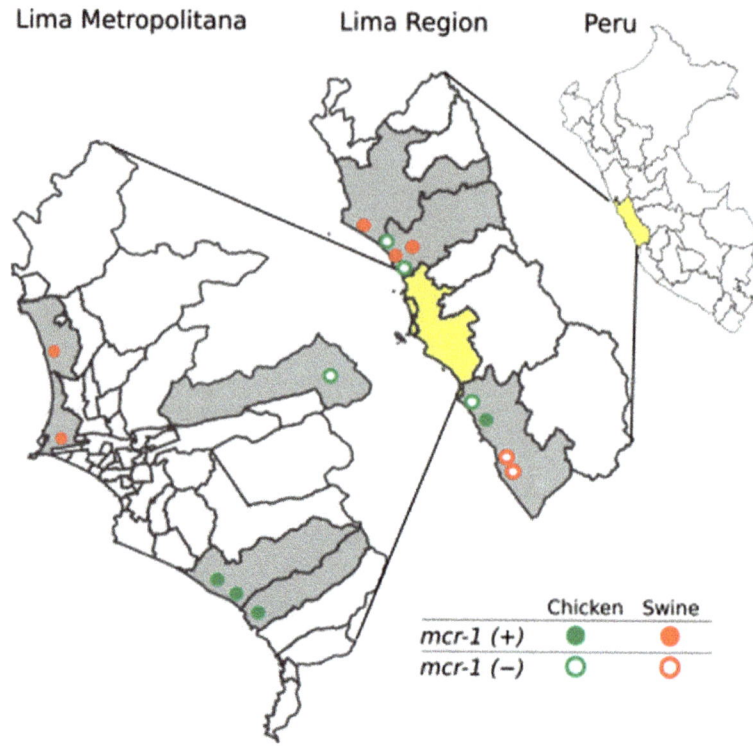

Figure 1. Geographical distribution of pig and poultry farms sampled in Lima, Peru. The location of the farms with the presence of *mcr-1*-positive *E. coli* isolates from chicken and swine is represented by circles filled in green and red, respectively. The location of the farms without the presence of *mcr-1*-positive *E. coli* isolates from chicken and swine is represented by green and red circles, respectively.

3.2. Genetic Characterization of E. coli Harboring mcr-1 and Resistome

The whole genome of 14 *mcr-1*-positive *E. coli* was sequenced (7 genomes from pigs and 7 from chicken). The sequence size varied from 4.75 to 5.90 Mb. A total of 10 different MLSTs were identified in 11 isolates, while 3 were not determined (Supplementary Table S2). Most isolates were identified as phylogenetic groups A ($n = 7$) and B1 ($n = 6$), while one isolate was typed as an unknown phylogroup (U). There was no differential clustering between the isolates from poultry and porcine sources (Figure 2).

Interestingly, the genome sequence analysis showed a high number of resistance genes. We detected 39 different genes that confer resistance to 10 different classes of antibiotics, including *mcr-1* (Table 1 and Figure 2). Five isolates contained the $bla_{CTX-M-55}$ gene for resistance to extended-spectrum beta-lactamase (ESBL). At least 70% of the isolates contained a gene for resistance to ampicillin, chloramphenicol, kanamycin and trimethoprim, and at least 90% of the isolates contained a gene for resistance to streptomycin, sulfisoxazole and tetracycline.

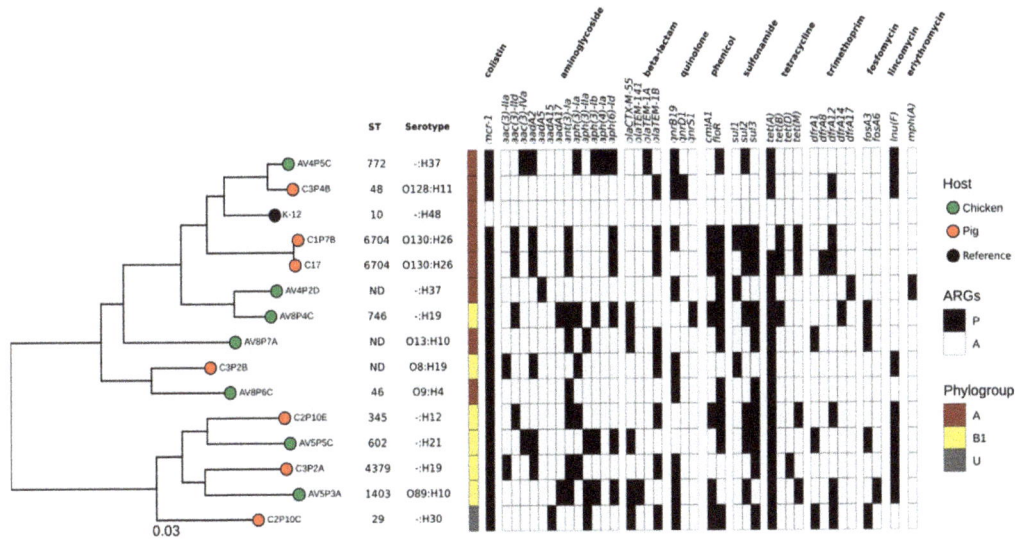

Figure 2. Resistome of 14 *mcr-1*-harboring *E. coli* isolated from pig and poultry farms in Lima, Peru. From left to right: phylogenomic tree based on SNPs of 14 *E. coli* genomes from chicken (circle filled with green) and pig (circle filled with red) farms. The *E. coli* K-12 strain was used as the reference. First column indicates the phylogroups A (red), B (yellow) or U (gray). The heatmap shows the presence/absence (P/A) of ARGs detected in *mcr-1*-positive *E. coli* genomes.

Table 1. ARGs profile of 14 *E. coli* genomes carrying *mcr-1*.

Class	Antibiotics	Number of *mcr-1* + *E. coli* (%)	Gene Name (n)
Aminoglycoside	gentamicin	8 (57)	aac(3)-IIa (2), aac(3)-IId (4), aac(3)-IVa (1), aac(3)-VIa (1)
	hygromycin B	1 (7)	aph(4)-Ia (1)
	kanamycin	11 (79)	aph(3′)-Ia (5), aph(3′)-IIa (4), aph(6)-Id (6)
	streptomycin	13 (93)	aadA2 (6), aadA5 (1), aadA15 (1), aadA17 (2), ant(3″)-Ia (8), aph(3″)-Ib (4)
Beta lactam	ampicillin	10 (71)	blaTEM-1A (1), blaTEM-1B (8), blaTEM-141 (1)
	ceftriaxone	5 (36)	blaCTX-M-55 (5)
Quinolone	ciprofloxacin	10 (71)	qnrB19 (9), qnrD1 (1), qnrS2 (1)
Folate pathway antagonist	trimethoprim	10 (71)	dfrA1 (3), dfrA8 (1), dfrA12 (6), dfrA14 (1), dfrA17 (1)
Fosfomycin	fosfomycin	5 (36)	fosA3 (4), fosA6 (1)
Glycylcycline	tetracycline	14 (100)	tet(A) (13), tet(B) (3), tet(D) (1), tet(M) (4)
	lincomycin	7 (50)	lnu(F) (7)
Macrolide	erythromycin	1 (7)	mph(A) (1)
Phenicol	chloramphenicol	11 (79)	cmlA1 (6), floR (10)
Sulphonamide	sulfamethoxazole	13 (93)	sul1 (3), sul2 (7), sul3 (9)

Forty-two genes encoding virulence factors were detected in all *E. coli* genomes using the VirulenceFinder tool v2.0 (see Supplementary Figure S1 and Table S3), including genes related to evasion/invasion (*capU, kpsE, kpsMII_K5, gad, iss, ompT, sepA, traT*), toxins (*astA, cea, cib, hlyF, stb, toxB*), secretion system (*cif, espABFJ, nleABC, terC, tir*), adherence (*eae, lpfA, perA, tsh*) and iron uptake (*fyuA, ireA, irp2, iucC, iutA, sitA*). The AV5P5C isolate from chicken was classified as APEC because it presented genes encoding outer membrane protein (*ompT*), hemolysin (*hlyF*), increased serum survival (*iss*), aerobactin siderophore receptor (*iutA*), temperature-sensitive hemagglutinin (*tsh*) and siderophores (*IucC, sitA*) [33,34].

Additionally, 33 types of plasmid replicons were identified in the analyzed genomes; the most overrepresented was IncFIB, followed by IncX1, ColRNAI, IncFIC(FII) and IncFII(pHN7A8) (Supplementary Figure S1 and Table S3).

3.3. Characterization of the Genetic Context of the mcr-1 Gene

The *mcr-1* sequence of all *E. coli* genomes was 100% identical to the *mcr-1* sequence from the Resfinder database. The exploration of the genetic context of *mcr-1* allowed us to identify three different types of *mcr-1*-containing cassettes suggesting a diverse genetic context of *mcr-1*-harboring *E. coli* in the farms of Lima (Figure 3). Two different context structures were identified in chicken farms. The IS*Apl1–mcr1–pap2*–IS*Apl1* was identified in the AV4P5C isolate, which belongs to ST48. This cassette shows a structure called Tn*6330* inserted into an IncHI1A:IncHI1B hybrid plasmid. Tn*6330* is a composite transposon that improves the transmission of the *mcr-1* gene [35]. The second structure shows the *nikB–mcr1–pap2* composition that has lost IS*Apl1* both upstream and downstream. This structure was found within IncI2 plasmids in the AV4P2D, AV5P5C, AV5P3A and AV8P7A isolates (Figure 3). Interestingly, a BLASTN search of the AV5P3A plasmid carrying *mcr-1* showed a high similarity of this plasmid to the IncI2 plasmid pkpCOL17 (99% of identity and 99.97% of coverage) identified in *K. pneumoniae* isolated from a patient in a Peruvian hospital [15] (Supplementary Figure S2). In a pig isolate (C3P2A), we observed the presence of a downstream copy of IS*Apl1* only. Due to short-read sequencing, we were not able to determine the genetic context of the *mcr-1* gene for six isolates because of incomplete assembly.

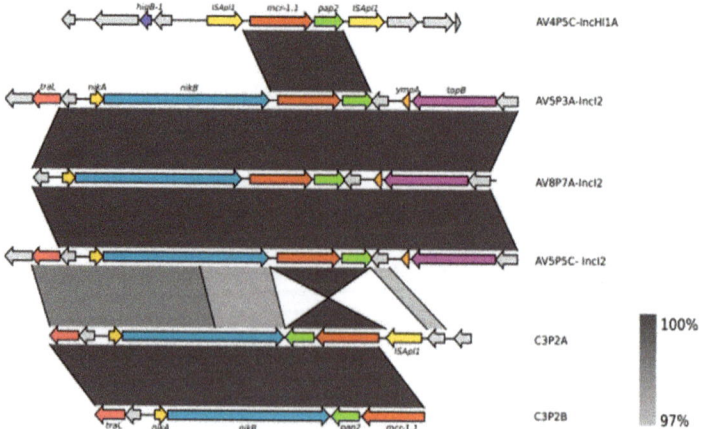

Figure 3. Genetic context of the *mcr-1* gene in *E. coli* genomes isolated from chicken and pig farms in Lima. Six representative sequences show the diversity of the structural context of the *mcr-1* gene from chicken and pig *E. coli* isolates in this study. The *mcr-1* gene is marked in red. IS*Apl1* transposase, *pap2* and *nickB* genes are marked in yellow, green and yellow, respectively. Regions of homology between sequences (>97%) are indicated by the graded shading.

4. Discussion

We studied the occurrence of *E. coli* carrying the *mcr-1* gene in 15 livestock farms in Lima, Peru, from 2019 to 2020. The results of the PCR showed that *E. coli* was positive for *mcr-1* in 9 of the 15 farms evaluated in this study at different rates, i.e., in 21% (42/197) of the isolates from poultry and in 12% (18/144) of the isolates from pigs. To the best of our knowledge, this is the first study to investigate the occurrence of *mcr-1*-positive *E. coli* isolates in farms in Peru. Previous works reported *E. coli* isolates carrying the *mcr-1* gene in samples of clinical and food origin in Peru [12–14,16]. In December 2019, the Ministry of Agriculture and Irrigation of Peru (MINAGRI) published a resolution prohibiting the use of colistin in food-producing animals [36]. The effect of the ban was not evaluated in this study because all samples were collected before the application of the resolution in March 2020. We expect a reduction in *mcr-1* prevalence as was observed in China. After the implementation of the colistin prohibition for veterinary use in China, the prevalence of *E. coli* carrying *mcr-1* decreased from 45% to 19% between 2016 and 2018 in pig farms [37]. In South America, the circulation of *mcr-1*-harboring *Enterobacteriaceae* isolates has a higher prevalence in animals (8.7%) than in food (5.4%) or humans (2.0%), mainly in Brazil, Bolivia and Argentina [38].

All isolates sequenced in this study belong to different sequence types, suggesting an important diversity in *mcr-1*-positive *E. coli*. These isolates were classified as belonging to phylogroup A or B1, with commensal *E. coli* usually found in humans and animal hosts [39,40]. The clones found in our study, ST48, ST602, ST746, ST46, ST345, were previously reported in clinical isolates from humans and other hosts; ST602 is widely distributed internationally [41,42]. This information is concerning, since it suggests that these strains have the ability to move and proliferate in different ecological niches, which may facilitate the genetic exchange of the *mcr-1* gene and other antibiotic resistance genes between a wide range of bacterial species. A highly diverse resistome was revealed, with 39 different genes conferring resistance to 15 different antibiotics including ESBL, chloramphenicol, ciprofloxacin, tetracycline and sulfamethoxazole, indicating an extensive circulation of *E. coli* carrying multiple antibiotic-resistant genes in livestock in Lima; in fact, Peru is considered one of the countries with a high projected increase of antimicrobial consumption by livestock [43]. We detected that *mcr-1* was associated with resistance mechanisms to beta-lactams; five *mcr-1*-positive *E. coli* also encoded $bla_{CTX-M-55}$, while other eight isolates produced the bla_{TEM-1B} gene. The co-occurrence of *mcr-1* and beta-lactam genes was also reported previously in South America, in samples from chicken meat in Brazil and in *E. coli* isolated from pig farms and companion animals in Argentina [44–46].

The composite transposon Tn6330 (IS*Apl1*–*mcr1*–*pap2*–IS*Apl1*) is considered the main vehicle for *mcr-1* mobilization [6,35]. Only one out of fourteen *mcr-1*-positive *E. coli* sequenced in this work contained Tn6330 with both copies of IS*Apl1* within an IncHI1A:IncHI1B plasmid, while in another isolate, we noted the presence of an upstream copy of IS*Apl1*. Cassettes with the Tn6330 structure are generally mobilized by IncHI2 plasmids; however, *E. coli* has been reported harboring *mcr-1* into hybrid plasmids containing the incompatible types IncHI1A and IncHI1B in Asia [47,48]. Up to now, only four plasmids have been described to carry the *mrc-1* gene in Latin America: IncX4, IncP, IncI2 and IncHI2 [49]. On other hand, some *E. coli* genomes from chicken and pigs presented *mcr-1* carried by the IncI2 plasmid lacking the IS*Apl1* copies. The plasmid IncI2 has already been described to spread different *mcr* genes variants in Latin American countries such as Argentina, Brazil and Uruguay [50]. According to global genomic studies, *mcr-1* sequences with two copies of IS*Apl1* are found in lesser frequency than sequences with only a single copy of IS*Apl1*, while the majority of positive *mcr-1* isolates do not present the IS*Apl1* sequence [4,6]. Due to the short-read sequencing method used in this work, we were not able to determine the genetic context of the *mcr-1* gene for six *mcr-1*-positive genomes because of the incomplete assembly of the (plasmid) sequences. Therefore, we cannot exclude the presence of other plasmid types that mobilize the *mcr-1* gene in our isolates.

In conclusion, we determined the occurrence of *mcr-1*-harboring *E. coli* in chicken farms (21.3%) and pig farms (12.5%) in Lima. The genomic analysis showed diverse lineages of *E. coli* carrying the *mcr-1* gene mobilized by the IncI2 and IncHI1A:IncHI1B plasmids, including the presence of IS*Apl1* copies enhancing the dissemination of *mcr-1*. The elevated prevalence of multidrug-resistant strains in farms in Lima could serve as a reservoir of ARGs that can be disseminated by farmers or food, impacting public health. We need to expand the genomic and epidemiological surveillance of colistin resistance in farmers, livestock, the environment, wastewater and hospitals to understand the dynamic of *mcr-1* transmission in Peru.

Supplementary Materials: The following supporting information can be downloaded at: https://www.mdpi.com/article/10.3390/antibiotics11121781/s1, Figure S1: Virulome and plasmid replicons of 14 *mcr-1 E. coli*.; Figure S2: Genetic characteristics of the IncI2 *mcr-1*-carrying plasmid identified in this study. Circular view and alignment comparison of closely related IncI2 plasmids carrying the *mcr-1* gene.; Supplementary Table S1: Sampling information and *mcr-1* positivity by PCR in the farms sampled in this study.; Supplementary Table S2: Accession numbers and sequencing statistics of 14 *E. coli* genomes carrying the *mcr-1* gene.; Supplementary Table S3: Virulence factors and plasmid types predicted by *abricate* using VFDB (Virulence Factor Database) and Plasmidfinder. Values represent the gene coverage.

Author Contributions: L.M.H., L.L.E., D.C. and C.G.D.G. conceived the idea and designed the experiments. L.L.E., G.M.M. and L.M.H. coordinated the sample collection. D.C., C.G.D.G., Y.I.L., T.S.E. and C.L.R.C. performed bacteria isolation and sequencing. D.C., C.G.D.G., C.L.R.C., Y.I.L. and T.S.E. analyzed the data. D.C., C.G.D.G., C.L.R.C., Y.I.L. and T.S.E. wrote the manuscript. D.C., C.G.D.G., C.L.R.C., L.L.E., R.H.R.A., N.L. and L.M.H. performed the manuscript review and editing. L.L.E. and L.M.H. supervised this work. All authors have read and agreed to the published version of the manuscript.

Funding: This study was funded by PROCIENCIA-CONCYTEC, through its executing unit ProCiencia—Proyectos de Investigación Básica 2018-01, Contract number No. 127-2018-FONDECYT. CD and YI were supported by Vicerrectorado de Investigación y Postgrado—Universidad Nacional Mayor de San Marcos (Project Number A21081091).

Institutional Review Board Statement: Not applicable.

Informed Consent Statement: Not applicable.

Data Availability Statement: Genome sequence data analyzed in this study can be found here: https://www.ncbi.nlm.nih.gov/bioproject/PRJNA892251.

Conflicts of Interest: The authors declare no conflict of interest.

References

1. Sulis, G.; Gandra, S. Access to Antibiotics: Not a Problem in Some LMICs. *Lancet Glob. Health* **2021**, *9*, e561–e562. [CrossRef] [PubMed]
2. WHO Critically Important Antimicrobials for Human Medicine: 6th Revision. Available online: https://www.who.int/publications-detail-redirect/9789241515528 (accessed on 20 October 2022).
3. Kempf, I.; Jouy, E.; Chauvin, C. Colistin Use and Colistin Resistance in Bacteria from Animals. *Int. J. Antimicrob. Agents* **2016**, *48*, 598–606. [CrossRef] [PubMed]
4. Matamoros, S.; van Hattem, J.M.; Arcilla, M.S.; Willemse, N.; Melles, D.C.; Penders, J.; Vinh, T.N.; Thi Hoa, N.; Bootsma, M.C.J.; van Genderen, P.J.; et al. Global Phylogenetic Analysis of *Escherichia coli* and Plasmids Carrying the *mcr-1* Gene Indicates Bacterial Diversity but Plasmid Restriction. *Sci. Rep.* **2017**, *7*, 15364. [CrossRef] [PubMed]
5. Liu, Y.-Y.; Wang, Y.; Walsh, T.R.; Yi, L.-X.; Zhang, R.; Spencer, J.; Doi, Y.; Tian, G.; Dong, B.; Huang, X.; et al. Emergence of Plasmid-Mediated Colistin Resistance Mechanism MCR-1 in Animals and Human Beings in China: A Microbiological and Molecular Biological Study. *Lancet Infect. Dis.* **2016**, *16*, 161–168. [CrossRef] [PubMed]
6. Wang, R.; van Dorp, L.; Shaw, L.P.; Bradley, P.; Wang, Q.; Wang, X.; Jin, L.; Zhang, Q.; Liu, Y.; Rieux, A.; et al. The Global Distribution and Spread of the Mobilized Colistin Resistance Gene *mcr-1*. *Nat. Commun.* **2018**, *9*, 1179. [CrossRef]
7. Poirel, L.; Madec, J.-Y.; Lupo, A.; Schink, A.-K.; Kieffer, N.; Nordmann, P.; Schwarz, S. Antimicrobial Resistance in *Escherichia coli*. *Microbiol. Spectr.* **2018**, *6*, 4. [CrossRef]

8. Leekitcharoenphon, P.; Johansson, M.H.K.; Munk, P.; Malorny, B.; Skarżyńska, M.; Wadepohl, K.; Moyano, G.; Hesp, A.; Veldman, K.T.; Bossers, A.; et al. Genomic Evolution of Antimicrobial Resistance in *Escherichia coli*. *Sci. Rep.* **2021**, *11*, 15108. [CrossRef]
9. Brisola, M.C.; Crecencio, R.B.; Bitner, D.S.; Frigo, A.; Rampazzo, L.; Stefani, L.M.; Faria, G.A. *Escherichia coli* Used as a Biomarker of Antimicrobial Resistance in Pig Farms of Southern Brazil. *Sci. Total Environ.* **2019**, *647*, 362–368. [CrossRef]
10. Vu Thi Ngoc, B.; Le Viet, T.; Nguyen Thi Tuyet, M.; Nguyen Thi Hong, T.; Nguyen Thi Ngoc, D.; Le Van, D.; Chu Thi, L.; Tran Huy, H.; Penders, J.; Wertheim, H.; et al. Characterization of Genetic Elements Carrying *mcr-1* Gene in *Escherichia coli* from the Community and Hospital Settings in Vietnam. *Microbiol. Spectr.* **2022**, *10*, e0135621. [CrossRef]
11. Yang, H.; Chen, S.; White, D.G.; Zhao, S.; McDermott, P.; Walker, R.; Meng, J. Characterization of Multiple-Antimicrobial-Resistant *Escherichia coli* Isolates from Diseased Chickens and Swine in China. *J. Clin. Microbiol.* **2004**, *42*, 3483–3489. [CrossRef]
12. Ugarte Silva, R.G.; Olivo López, J.M.; Corso, A.; Pasteran, F.; Albornoz, E.; Sahuanay Blácido, Z.P. Resistencia a Colistín Mediado por el gen *mcr-1* Identificado en Cepas de *Escherichia coli* y *Klebsiella pneumoniae*: Primeros Reportes en el Perú. In *Anales de la Facultad de Medicina*; UNMSM: Lima, Peru, 2018; Volume 79, pp. 213–217. [CrossRef]
13. Deshpande, L.M.; Hubler, C.; Davis, A.P.; Castanheira, M. Updated Prevalence of *mcr*-like Genes among *Escherichia coli* and *Klebsiella pneumoniae* in the SENTRY Program and Characterization of *mcr-1.11* Variant. *Antimicrob. Agents Chemother.* **2019**, *63*, e02450-18. [CrossRef] [PubMed]
14. Yauri-Condor, K.; Zavaleta Apestegui, M.; Sevilla-Andrade, C.R.; Sara, J.P.; Villoslado Espinoza, C.; Taboada, W.V.; Gonzales-Escalante, E. Extended-Spectrum Beta-Lactamase-Producing Enterobacterales Carrying the *mcr-1* Gene in Lima, Peru. *Rev. Peru. Med. Exp. Salud Pública* **2021**, *37*, 711–715. [CrossRef] [PubMed]
15. Gonzales-Escalante, E.; Ruggiero, M.; Cerdeira, L.; Esposito, F.; Fontana, H.; Lincopan, N.; Gutkind, G.; Di Conza, J. Whole-Genome Analysis of a High-Risk Clone of *Klebsiella pneumoniae* ST147 Carrying Both *mcr-1* and bla_{NDM-1} Genes in Peru. *Microb. Drug Resist.* **2022**, *28*, 171–179. [CrossRef] [PubMed]
16. Murray, M.; Salvatierra, G.; Dávila-Barclay, A.; Ayzanoa, B.; Castillo-Vilcahuaman, C.; Huang, M.; Pajuelo, M.J.; Lescano, A.G.; Cabrera, L.; Calderón, M.; et al. Market Chickens as a Source of Antibiotic-Resistant *Escherichia coli* in a Peri-Urban Community in Lima, Peru. *Front. Microbiol.* **2021**, *12*, 635871. [CrossRef] [PubMed]
17. Van Boeckel, T.P.; Pires, J.; Silvester, R.; Zhao, C.; Song, J.; Criscuolo, N.G.; Gilbert, M.; Bonhoeffer, S.; Laxminarayan, R. Global Trends in Antimicrobial Resistance in Animals in Low- and Middle-Income Countries. *Science* **2019**, *365*, eaaw1944. [CrossRef]
18. Rebelo, A.R.; Bortolaia, V.; Kjeldgaard, J.S.; Pedersen, S.K.; Leekitcharoenphon, P.; Hansen, I.M.; Guerra, B.; Malorny, B.; Borowiak, M.; Hammerl, J.A.; et al. Multiplex PCR for Detection of Plasmid-Mediated Colistin Resistance Determinants, *mcr-1*, *mcr-2*, *mcr-3*, *mcr-4* and *mcr-5* for Surveillance Purposes. *Euro Surveill. Bull. Eur. Sur Mal. Transm. Eur. Commun. Dis. Bull.* **2018**, *23*, 17-00672. [CrossRef]
19. Andrews, S. FastQC. A Quality Control Tool for High Throughput Sequence Data. Available online: https://www.bioinformatics.babraham.ac.uk/projects/fastqc/ (accessed on 14 July 2022).
20. Bolger, A.M.; Lohse, M.; Usadel, B. Trimmomatic: A Flexible Trimmer for Illumina Sequence Data. *Bioinformatics* **2014**, *30*, 2114–2120. [CrossRef]
21. Bankevich, A.; Nurk, S.; Antipov, D.; Gurevich, A.A.; Dvorkin, M.; Kulikov, A.S.; Lesin, V.M.; Nikolenko, S.I.; Pham, S.; Prjibelski, A.D.; et al. SPAdes: A New Genome Assembly Algorithm and Its Applications to Single-Cell Sequencing. *J. Comput. Biol.* **2012**, *19*, 455–477. [CrossRef]
22. Seemann, T. Prokka: Rapid Prokaryotic Genome Annotation. *Bioinform. Oxf. Engl.* **2014**, *30*, 2068–2069. [CrossRef]
23. Waters, N.R.; Abram, F.; Brennan, F.; Holmes, A.; Pritchard, L. Easy Phylotyping of *Escherichia coli* via the EzClermont Web App and Command-Line Tool. *Access Microbiol.* **2020**, *2*, acmi000143. [CrossRef]
24. Croucher, N.J.; Page, A.J.; Connor, T.R.; Delaney, A.J.; Keane, J.A.; Bentley, S.D.; Parkhill, J.; Harris, S.R. Rapid Phylogenetic Analysis of Large Samples of Recombinant Bacterial Whole Genome Sequences Using Gubbins. *Nucleic Acids Res.* **2015**, *43*, e15. [CrossRef]
25. Nguyen, L.-T.; Schmidt, H.A.; von Haeseler, A.; Minh, B.Q. IQ-TREE: A Fast and Effective Stochastic Algorithm for Estimating Maximum-Likelihood Phylogenies. *Mol. Biol. Evol.* **2015**, *32*, 268–274. [CrossRef]
26. Yu, G.; Smith, D.K.; Zhu, H.; Guan, Y.; Lam, T.T.-Y. Ggtree: An r Package for Visualization and Annotation of Phylogenetic Trees with Their Covariates and Other Associated Data. *Methods Ecol. Evol.* **2017**, *8*, 28–36. [CrossRef]
27. Sullivan, M.J.; Petty, N.K.; Beatson, S.A. Easyfig: A Genome Comparison Visualizer. *Bioinformatics* **2011**, *27*, 1009–1010. [CrossRef]
28. Antipov, D.; Hartwick, N.; Shen, M.; Raiko, M.; Lapidus, A.; Pevzner, P.A. PlasmidSPAdes: Assembling Plasmids from Whole Genome Sequencing Data. *Bioinformatics* **2016**, *32*, 3380–3387. [CrossRef]
29. Carattoli, A.; Hasman, H. PlasmidFinder and In Silico PMLST: Identification and Typing of Plasmid Replicons in Whole-Genome Sequencing (WGS). In *Horizontal Gene Transfer: Methods and Protocols*; de la Cruz, F., Ed.; Methods in Molecular Biology; Springer US: New York, NY, USA, 2020; pp. 285–294, ISBN 978-1-4939-9877-7.
30. Li, X.; Xie, Y.; Liu, M.; Tai, C.; Sun, J.; Deng, Z.; Ou, H.-Y. OriTfinder: A Web-Based Tool for the Identification of Origin of Transfers in DNA Sequences of Bacterial Mobile Genetic Elements. *Nucleic Acids Res.* **2018**, *46*, W229–W234. [CrossRef]
31. Schmartz, G.P.; Hartung, A.; Hirsch, P.; Kern, F.; Fehlmann, T.; Müller, R.; Keller, A. PLSDB: Advancing a Comprehensive Database of Bacterial Plasmids. *Nucleic Acids Res.* **2022**, *50*, D273–D278. [CrossRef]

32. Alikhan, N.-F.; Petty, N.K.; Ben Zakour, N.L.; Beatson, S.A. BLAST Ring Image Generator (BRIG): Simple Prokaryote Genome Comparisons. *BMC Genom.* **2011**, *12*, 402. [CrossRef]
33. Barbieri, N.L.; Pimenta, R.L.; de Melo, D.A.; Nolan, L.K.; de Souza, M.M.S.; Logue, C.M. mcr-1 Identified in Fecal *Escherichia coli* and Avian Pathogenic *E. coli* (APEC) From Brazil. *Front. Microbiol.* **2021**, *12*, 799. [CrossRef]
34. Sarowska, J.; Futoma-Koloch, B.; Jama-Kmiecik, A.; Frej-Madrzak, M.; Ksiazczyk, M.; Bugla-Ploskonska, G.; Choroszy-Krol, I. Virulence Factors, Prevalence and Potential Transmission of Extraintestinal Pathogenic *Escherichia coli* Isolated from Different Sources: Recent Reports. *Gut Pathog.* **2019**, *11*, 10. [CrossRef]
35. Snesrud, E.; McGann, P.; Chandler, M. The Birth and Demise of the IS*Apl1*-mcr-1-IS*Apl1* Composite Transposon: The Vehicle for Transferable Colistin Resistance. *mBio* **2018**, *9*, e02381-17. [CrossRef] [PubMed]
36. El Peruano. Resolucion Directoral-No 0091-2019-MINAGRI-SENASA-DIAIA. Disponen Prohibir la Importación, Comercialización, Fabricación o Elaboración de Productos Veterinarios que Contengan el Principio Activo Colistina (Polimixina E) o Cualquiera de sus Sales y Dictan Diversas Disposiciones. Available online: http://busquedas.elperuano.pe/normaslegales/disponen-prohibir-la-importacion-comercializacion-fabricac-resolucion-directoral-no-0091-2019-minagri-senasa-diaia-1832393-1/ (accessed on 29 April 2022).
37. Shen, C.; Zhong, L.-L.; Yang, Y.; Doi, Y.; Paterson, D.L.; Stoesser, N.; Ma, F.; Ahmed, M.A.E.-G.E.-S.; Feng, S.; Huang, S.; et al. Dynamics of mcr-1 Prevalence and mcr-1-Positive *Escherichia coli* after the Cessation of Colistin Use as a Feed Additive for Animals in China: A Prospective Cross-Sectional and Whole Genome Sequencing-Based Molecular Epidemiological Study. *Lancet Microbe* **2020**, *1*, e34–e43. [CrossRef] [PubMed]
38. Mendes Oliveira, V.R.; Paiva, M.C.; Lima, W.G. Plasmid-Mediated Colistin Resistance in Latin America and Caribbean: A Systematic Review. *Travel Med. Infect. Dis.* **2019**, *31*, 101459. [CrossRef] [PubMed]
39. Duriez, P.; Clermont, O.; Bonacorsi, S.; Bingen, E.; Chaventré, A.; Elion, J.; Picard, B.; Denamur, E. Commensal *Escherichia coli* Isolates Are Phylogenetically Distributed among Geographically Distinct Human Populations. *Microbiology* **2001**, *147*, 1671–1676. [CrossRef] [PubMed]
40. Madoshi, B.P.; Kudirkiene, E.; Mtambo, M.M.A.; Muhairwa, A.P.; Lupindu, A.M.; Olsen, J.E. Characterisation of Commensal *Escherichia coli* Isolated from Apparently Healthy Cattle and Their Attendants in Tanzania. *PLoS ONE* **2016**, *11*, e0168160. [CrossRef]
41. Fuentes-Castillo, D.; Esposito, F.; Cardoso, B.; Dalazen, G.; Moura, Q.; Fuga, B.; Fontana, H.; Cerdeira, L.; Dropa, M.; Rottmann, J.; et al. Genomic Data Reveal International Lineages of Critical Priority *Escherichia coli* Harbouring Wide Resistome in Andean Condors (Vultur Gryphus Linnaeus, 1758). *Mol. Ecol.* **2020**, *29*, 1919–1935. [CrossRef]
42. Aworh, M.K.; Abiodun-Adewusi, O.; Mba, N.; Helwigh, B.; Hendriksen, R.S. Prevalence and Risk Factors for Faecal Carriage of Multidrug Resistant *Escherichia coli* among Slaughterhouse Workers. *Sci. Rep.* **2021**, *11*, 13362. [CrossRef]
43. Van Boeckel, T.P.; Brower, C.; Gilbert, M.; Grenfell, B.T.; Levin, S.A.; Robinson, T.P.; Teillant, A.; Laxminarayan, R. Global Trends in Antimicrobial Use in Food Animals. *Proc. Natl. Acad. Sci. USA* **2015**, *112*, 5649–5654. [CrossRef]
44. Monte, D.F.; Mem, A.; Fernandes, M.R.; Cerdeira, L.; Esposito, F.; Galvão, J.A.; Franco, B.D.G.M.; Lincopan, N.; Landgraf, M. Chicken Meat as a Reservoir of Colistin-Resistant *Escherichia coli* Strains Carrying mcr-1 Genes in South America. *Antimicrob. Agents Chemother.* **2017**, *61*, e02718-16. [CrossRef]
45. Faccone, D.; Moredo, F.A.; Giacoboni, G.I.; Albornoz, E.; Alarcón, L.; Nievas, V.F.; Corso, A. Multidrug-Resistant *Escherichia coli* Harbouring mcr-1 and bla$_{CTX-M}$ Genes Isolated from Swine in Argentina. *J. Glob. Antimicrob. Resist.* **2019**, *18*, 160–162. [CrossRef]
46. Rumi, M.V.; Mas, J.; Elena, A.; Cerdeira, L.; Muñoz, M.E.; Lincopan, N.; Gentilini, É.R.; Di Conza, J.; Gutkind, G. Co-Occurrence of Clinically Relevant β-Lactamases and MCR-1 Encoding Genes in *Escherichia coli* from Companion Animals in Argentina. *Vet. Microbiol.* **2019**, *230*, 228–234. [CrossRef] [PubMed]
47. Li, R.; Zhang, P.; Yang, X.; Wang, Z.; Fanning, S.; Wang, J.; Du, P.; Bai, L. Identification of a Novel Hybrid Plasmid Coproducing MCR-1 and MCR-3 Variant from an *Escherichia coli* Strain. *J. Antimicrob. Chemother.* **2019**, *74*, 1517–1520. [CrossRef] [PubMed]
48. Li, R.; Du, P.; Zhang, P.; Li, Y.; Yang, X.; Wang, Z.; Wang, J.; Bai, L. Comprehensive Genomic Investigation of Coevolution of Mcr Genes in *Escherichia coli* Strains via Nanopore Sequencing. *Glob. Chall.* **2021**, *5*, 2000014. [CrossRef] [PubMed]
49. Lentz, S.A.M.; Dalmolin, T.V.; Barth, A.L.; Martins, A.F. mcr-1 Gene in Latin America: How Is It Disseminated Among Humans, Animals, and the Environment? *Front. Public Health* **2021**, *9*, 648940. [CrossRef]
50. Papa-Ezdra, R.; Grill Diaz, F.; Vieytes, M.; García-Fulgueiras, V.; Caiata, L.; Ávila, P.; Brasesco, M.; Christophersen, I.; Cordeiro, N.F.; Algorta, G.; et al. First Three *Escherichia coli* Isolates Harbouring mcr-1 in Uruguay. *J. Glob. Antimicrob. Resist.* **2020**, *20*, 187–190. [CrossRef]

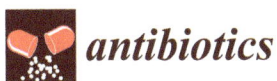

Article

Metabolism Profile of Mequindox in Sea Cucumbers In Vivo Using LC-HRMS

Xin Mao [1], Xiaozhen Zhou [1], Jun He [1], Gongzhen Liu [2], Huihui Liu [3], Han Zhao [1], Pengjie Luo [4], Yongning Wu [4,*] and Yanshen Li [1,*]

1. Department of Marine Product Quality and Safety Inspection Key Laboratory, Yantai University, Yantai 264005, China
2. College of Agriculture and Forestry, Linyi University, Linyi 276000, China
3. Shandong Marine Resource and Environment Research Institute, Yantai 264006, China
4. NHC Key Laboratory of Food Safety Risk Assessment, Chinese Academy of Medical Science Research Unit (2019RU014), China National Center for Food Safety Risk Assessment, Beijing 100017, China
* Correspondence: wuyongning@cfsa.net.cn (Y.W.); liyanshen@ytu.edu.cn (Y.L.)

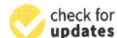

Abstract: In this work, the metabolism behavior of mequindox (MEQ) in sea cucumber in vivo was investigated using LC-HRMS. In total, nine metabolites were detected and identified as well as the precursor in sea cucumber tissues. The metabolic pathways of MEQ in sea cucumber mainly include hydrogenation reduction, deoxidation, carboxylation, deacetylation, and combinations thereof. The most predominant metabolites of MEQ in sea cucumber are 2-iso-BDMEQ and 2-iso-1-DMEQ, with deoxidation and carbonyl reduction as major metabolic pathways. In particular, this work first reported 3-methyl-2-quinoxalinecarboxylic acid (MQCA) as a metabolite of MEQ, and carboxylation is a major metabolic pathway of MEQ in sea cucumber. This work revealed that the metabolism of MEQ in marine animals is different from that in land animals. The metabolism results in this work could facilitate the accurate risk assessment of MEQ in sea cucumber and related marine foods.

Keywords: mequindox; metabolites; metabolic pathway; sea cucumbers; deoxidation; carbonyl reduction

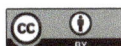

1. Introduction

Quinoxalines, a class of synthetic quinoxaline veterinary drugs with a Quinoxaline 1,4-di-N-oxides structure (QdNOs), were reported with broad-spectrum antimicrobial activity [1]. QdNOs have been applied as food additives in farm animal husbandry. As a major QdNO, Mequindox (3-methyl-2-quinoaxlinacetyl-1,4-dioxide, MEQ) was developed in the 1980s. Due to its high antibacterial activity, MEQ was used as an additive in swine and chicken feed [2]. Recently, QdNOs were reported with potential carcinogenicity and mutagenicity [3,4]. In particular, carbadox (CBX) and olaquindox (OLA), two members of QdNOs, were banned by the European Commission (EC) [5]. Deriving from the same family of QdNOs with a corresponding basic structure, MEQ has attracted increasing attention due to corresponding toxic risk, including induced apoptosis, carcinogenicity, DNA damage, etc. [6,7].

It was reported that MEQ could be easily metabolized after ingestion by animals, and some of the metabolites were detected and their structure identified in previous metabolic investigations in chicken and swine [8,9]. N → O group reduction and carboxylation were the major metabolic pathways in farm animals [10]. In farm animals, the major N → O group reduction metabolites were 1–desoxymequindox (1–DMEQ) and 1,4–bisdesoxymequindox (BDMEQ). Moreover, carboxylation metabolites and hydroxylation metabolites were also detected and identified. However, these metabolic investigations and the metabolites identified were mainly in land farm animal tissues and related products. There are few reports regarding metabolism investigations of QdNOs in aquatic animals. The analytical methods for QdNOs and metabolites detection in aquatic animals and related products were mainly based on metabolic results in land farm animals and the metabolites identified in chicken and swine [11,12]. The potential metabolic enzyme between land farm animals and aquatic animals might lead to different metabolic mechanisms [13,14]. To the best of our knowledge, there have been no related comprehensive metabolic investigations of MEQ in sea cucumber.

As a high-nutrition and high-value marine food, sea cucumbers have been farmed and exploited for commercial use as food and functional food [15,16]. Recently, sea cucumbers have been investigated and processed for different functional foods, and the sea cucumber industry is becoming one of the most important food commodities around the globe for health purposes [17,18]. Bioactive compounds in sea cucumbers were detected and reported with antioxidant, antihypertensive, anti-inflammatory, anticancer, antimicrobial activities [19]. Mequindox has been widely applied and used as a feed additive and antibacterial medicine in the sea cucumber farming industry [20]. Considering the extensive application of sea cucumber in food and health-care food industry, the identification of potentially hazardous compounds in sea cucumber appears to be necessary.

In this metabolism investigation, the major metabolites and metabolic pathways of MEQ in sea cucumber were examined. This work could provide the basis and target compound for further control of sea-cucumber-related food safety.

2. Results and Discussion

2.1. Optimization of Sample Preparation

In order to obtain more comprehensive metabolites, the first and most important step is target compounds and metabolites extraction. In this work, three schemes were optimized according to the previous literature [21–23], with some modification. An experiment group sample and bland control of 2.00 ± 0.02 g were weighed into a 50 mL polypropylene centrifuge tube, respectively. In total, 10 compounds, including MEQ and 9 metabolites, were evaluated in different pretreatment schemes. By comparing the extraction effects of three different schemes, it was obvious that Scheme 1 led to the most optimized results with the highest abundance of all target compounds (Figure 1). Additionally, Scheme 1 was used for MEQ and metabolites pretreatment of sea cucumber.

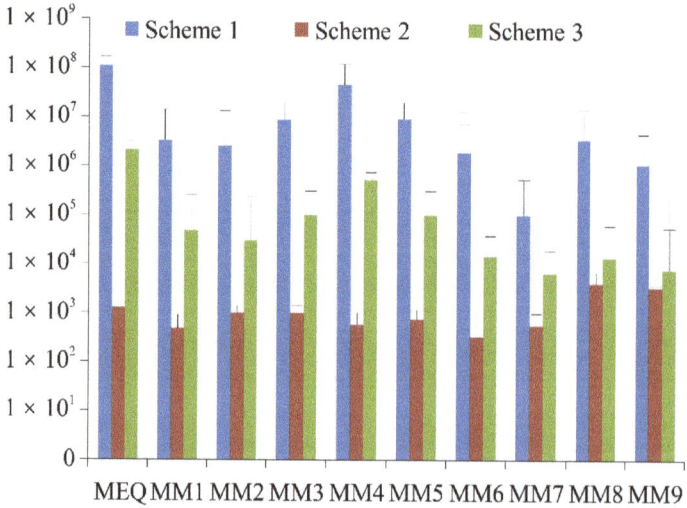

Figure 1. Optimization of extraction efficiency with three different schemes ($n = 6$).

2.2. Identification of Metabolites in Sea Cucumber

After administration, all experimental and control group samples were simply pretreated according to Scheme 2 and determined by HRMS. According to the elemental composition of MEQ and the accuracy mass difference value between the metabolites and MEQ, the elemental composition of metabolites could be speculated. In total, nine metabolites were detected and identified in sea cucumber in vivo. The predicted elemental compositions ($[M + H]^+$), mass errors, retention times (RT), fragmentation ions, and relative percentages of peak area are presented in Table 1. The errors between the measured and predicted masses were within less than 6 ppm, which demonstrated the high mass accuracy of the instrument. The chromatograms of MEQ and metabolites are shown in Figure 2, and the fragmentation ions and potential neutral losses are shown in Figure 3.

Table 1. Retention times (RT), predicted elemental compositions ($[M + H]^+$), mass errors, major fragmentation ions, and relative percentages of protonated MEQ and metabolites.

Compound Name	RT (min)	$[M + H]^+$ (m/z)	Predicted Composition ($[M + H]^+$)	RDB	Error ppm	Major Fragment Ions	Relative Percentage
MEQ, M0	4.56	219.0764	$C_{11}H_{11}O_3N_2$	7.5	0.143	143.0596, 185.0698, 160.0622, 177.0648, 202.0722, 132.0675	33.3%
2-iso-MEQ, M1	4.34	221.0921	$C_{11}H_{13}O_3N_2$	6.5	0.367	169.0760, 187.0866, 203.0815, 160.0632, 177.0659, 143.0604	1.9%
1-DMEQ, M2	5.36	203.0803	$C_{11}H_{11}O_2N_2$	7.5	0.817	203.0803, 186.0777, 161.0701, 144.0674	1.1%
4-DMEQ, M3	5.69	203.0804	$C_{11}H_{11}O_2N_2$	7.5	0.718	186.0778, 144.0674, 158.0829	3.4%
2-iso-1-DMEQ, M4	4.60	205.0960	$C_{11}H_{13}O_2N_2$	6.5	0.370	169.0751, 187.0855, 205.0960, 171.0900, 145.0752	17.4%
BDMEQ, M5	7.32	187.0856	$C_{11}H_{11}ON_2$	7.5	−5.503	159.0909, 145.0752	5.2%
2-iso-BDMEQ, M6	6.52	189.1011	$C_{11}H_{13}ON_2$	6.5	−5.762	171.0907, 143.0598	36.6%
MQCA, M7	5.51	189.0654	$C_{10}H_9O_2N_2$	7.5	−2.507	145.0752, 143.0597, 171.0901	0.4%
deacetyl-MEQ, M8	3.42	177.0651	$C_9H_9O_2N_2$	6.5	2.010	160.0622, 143.0606	0.5%
Deacetyl-1-DMEQ, M9	5.35	161.0706	$C_9H_9ON_2$	6.5	−4.963	144.0644	0.2%

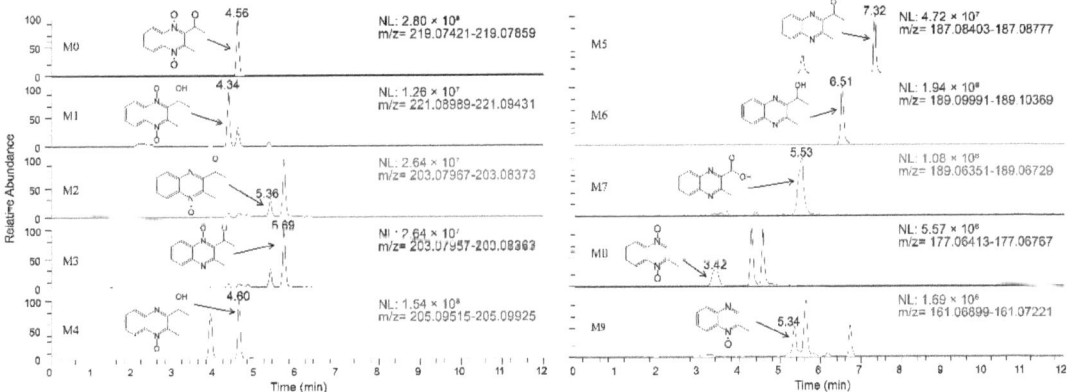

Figure 2. Accurate extracted ion chromatograms (EICs) of mequindox and its major metabolites in sea cucumber in vivo.

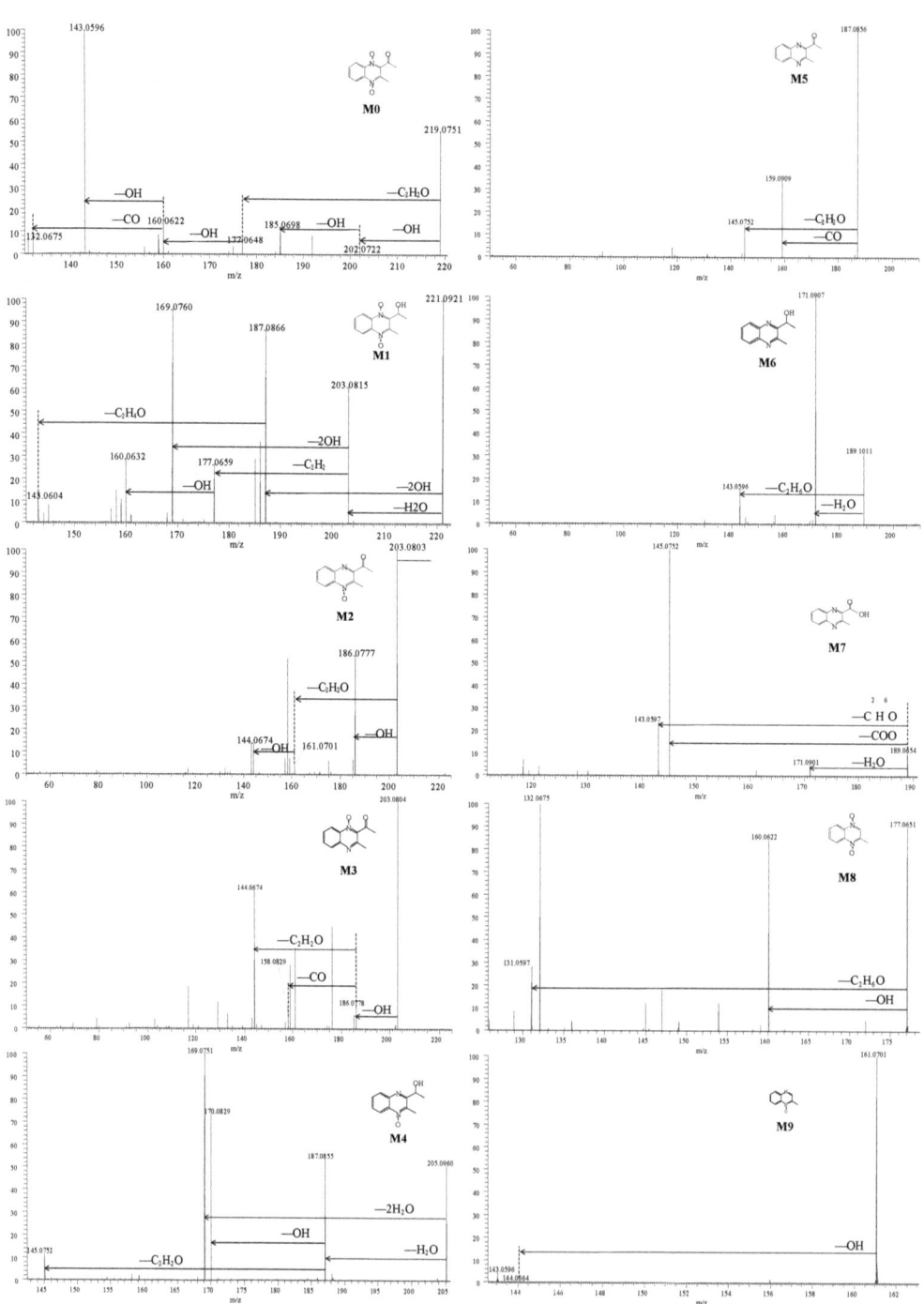

Figure 3. Accurate MS2 spectra and major proposed neutral loss of MEQ and metabolites detected in DDA mode. The MS2 spectra were produced by collision-induced dissociation (CID) of the selected precursor ions with different energies (20, 40, 70).

2.2.1. Performance of MEQ in Mass Spectrum

MEQ is eluted at a retention time of 4.56 min with protonated molecule ($[M + H]^+$) at m/z 219.0764. An MS/MS spectrum of MEQ is acquired under collision-induced dissociation (CID) with fragmentation ions of m/z 143.0596, 185.0698, 160.0622, 177.0648, 202.0722, and 132.0675. The predicted elemental compositions, observed and calculated masses, and mass errors of protonated MEQ and its fragmentation ions are presented in Figure 3.

From the figure, it can be concluded that the loss of the OH radical from MEQ led to formation of a product ion at m/z 202.0722 and 185.0698; further loss of the C_2H_2O side chain resulted in m/z 143.0596. In other words, protonated MEQ led to loss of the C_2H_2O side chain to form the fragment m/z 177.0648; further loss of the OH radical led to formation of m/z 160.0622. Subsequently, the fragment ion at m/z 160.0622 lost the CO radical to form the product radical at m/z 132.0675.

2.2.2. Metabolite MM1

Metabolite MM1 is eluted at a retention time of 4.34 with a protonated molecule at m/z 221.0921. In the accurate MS2 spectra of MM1, the fragment ions are at m/z 169.0760, 187.0866, 203.0815, 160.0632, 177.0659, and 143.0604. The protonated MM1 and product ion m/z 187.0866 are 2 Da higher than MEQ and the metabolites at m/z 185.0709, suggesting a hydrogenation reduction metabolite with two hydrogen additions. The fragment ion at m/z 187.0866 is 34 Da lower than the protonated molecule of MM3 at m/z 221.0920, showing that the m/z 187.0709 is formed by the loss of the 2 OH group, indicating that two N → O groups still exist in MM1 as MEQ. In addition, the fragment ions at m/z 169.0760 and 203.0815 are neutral losses of H2O from the fragment at m/z 187.0866 and protonated MM1 with 18 Da mass shift, which suggests that hydrogenation takes place in the acetyl group of a further side chain. The fragment at m/z 143.0603 is formed by losing the C_2H_4O of the side chain from the fragment at m/z 187.0866 with 44 Da mass shift. The fragment at m/z 177.0659 is formed by losing the side chain of fragment m/z 203.0815 and further loss of the OH group to form fragment m/z 160.0632. From the mass spectra, MM1 is considered as 2-isoethanol-mequindox (2-iso-MEQ).

2.2.3. Metabolites MM2, MM3, and MM4

Metabolites MM2 and MM3 are eluted at a retention time of 5.36 min and 5.69 min with protonated molecules at m/z 203.0803 and 203.0804, which are 16 Da lower than MEQ. For MM2, the MS2 spectra of fragments at 203.0803, 186.0777, 161.0701, and 144.0674 are 1 Da higher than fragments of MEQ, indicating a similar structure between MM2 and MEQ. According to the MEQ mass spectra, the coordination bond oxygen could be eliminated by the OH group with a neutral loss at 17 Da. For MM3, the fragment ion m/z 186.0778 is 17 Da lower than the protonated molecule by losing the OH group. Fragment ions m/z 144.0674 and m/z 158.0829 are further eliminated from the C_2H_2O and CO groups, respectively. From the mass spectra, MM2 and MM3 are identified as the N→O group reduction metabolites of MEQ. The amount of MM3 is higher than MM2 in the chromatogram. From the structure of MEQ, the side chain at position 2 could enhance the steric hindrance of oxygen at position 1. The deoxidation reaction at position 4 is easier than at position 1. Therefore, MM3 is identified as 4-desoxy-MEQ (4-DMEQ), while MM2 is identified as 1-desoxy-MEQ (1-DMEQ).

Metabolite MM4 is eluted at a retention time of 4.60 with protonated molecule at m/z 205.0960. MM4 is 2 Da higher than m/z 203.0816, indicating a hydrogenation reduction metabolite of desoxy-MEQ. The natural loss of 17 and 18 Da might result from the coordination bond oxygen and the hydroxyl group in the structure. Considering that the coordination bond oxygen at position 1 is much more stable than at position 4 as MM3, therefore, MM4 is considered as 2-isoethanol-1-desoxy-MEQ (2-iso-1-DMEQ).

2.2.4. Metabolites MM5, MM6, and MM7

Metabolite MM5 is eluted at a retention time of 7.32 with protonated molecule at m/z 187.0856, which is 32 Da lower than MEQ. In addition, the neutral loss of 28 Da is detected in MS2 spectra, indicating a carbonyl group in the structure. MM5 is considered as a bisdesoxy-MEQ metabolite (BDMEQ).

Metabolites MM6 and MM7 are eluted at a retention time of 6.52 min and 5.51 min with protonated molecule at *m/z* 189.1011 and *m/z* 189.0654. Based on the varied *m/z* value, the elemental composition of MM6 and MM7 might be different. From the Xcalibur platform, the fragment of *m/z* 189.1011 (MM6) is recommended as $C_{11}H_{13}N_2O$, while *m/z* 189.0654 (MM7) is $C_{10}H_9N_2O_2$. In the MS2 spectra of MM6, the neutral losses of 18 Da and 46 Da in MM6 are detected by loss of the H_2O and C_2H_6O side chain. In the MS2 spectra of MM7, the neutral loss of 44 Da is recommended as the loss of the COO group, indicating a carboxyl group in MM7. Therefore, MM6 is considered as 2-isoethanol bisdesoxy-MEQ (2-iso-BDMEQ), and MM7 is considered as 3-methyl-2-quinoxalinecarboxylic acid (MQCA).

2.2.5. Metabolites MM8 and MM9

Metabolite MM8 is eluted at a retention time of 3.42 min with protonated molecule at *m/z* 177.0651. MM8 is 42 Da lower than MEQ, indicating the loss of the acetyl group in the structure. In the MS2 spectra, fragment ions *m/z* 160.0622 and 143.0606 are formed with neutral losses of 17 and 34 Da, which is similar to MEQ losing two N→O groups in turn. Therefore, MM8 is considered as deacetyl-MEQ.

Metabolite MM9 (5.35 min) with protonated molecule at *m/z* 161.0706 is 16 Da lower than MM8. Different from MM8 in the MS2 spectra, only a 17 Da neutral loss is detected without 34 Da. According to the easy deoxidation reaction at position 4, MM9 is considered as deacetyl-1-desoxy-MEQ (Deacetyl-1-DMEQ).

2.3. Metabolic Pathway of MEQ in Sea Cucumber In Vivo

The results show that mequindox can be metabolized in sea cucumber after administration. In total, nine metabolites of MEQ are detected and identified by HRMS in sea cucumber. The metabolic pathways of MEQ in sea cucumber mainly include hydrogenation reduction, deoxidation, carboxylation, deacetylation, and combinations of these metabolic pathways (Figure 4). Table 1 shows the relative percentage of metabolites as well as mequindox in sea cucumber in vivo. The relative percentages of these targets are estimated on the basis of peak areas in HRMS. From the table, M6 and M4 are the predominant metabolites of MEQ in sea cucumber, accounting for 36.6% and 17.4% of all MEQ and metabolites. The percentages are: M5 (5.2%), M3 (3.4%), M1 (1.9%), M2 (1.1%), M8 (0.5%), M7 (0.4%), and M9 (0.2%).

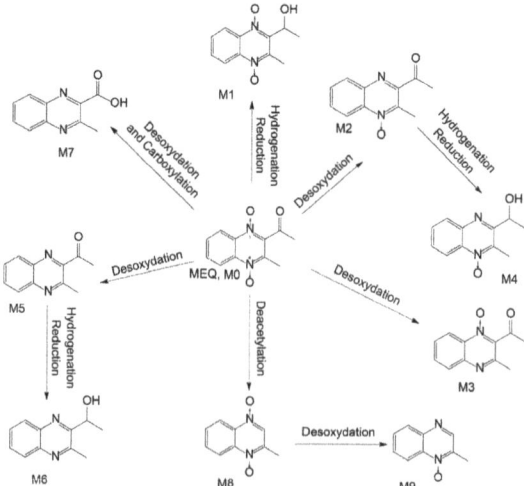

Figure 4. Proposed metabolic pathways of MEQ and metabolites in sea cucumber in vivo (hydrogenation reduction, deoxidation, carboxylation, deacetylation, and combinations thereof).

In the previous literature on MEQ metabolism investigations, the predominant metabolite of MEQ in rat is 1-DMEQ, which takes almost half of total MEQ and metabolites, followed by BDMEQ and 3-hydroxymethyl-1-DMEQ. In chicken, the predominant metabolite is 1-DMEQ, as in rat, followed by BDMEQ, 2-isoethanol-1-DMEQ, and 2'-hydroxyacetyl-1-DMEQ. According to a MEQ metabolism study in pig, the predominant metabolite is 2-isoethanol-1-DMEQ. Additionally, 1-DMEQ, 2-isoethanol-MEQ, and BDMEQ are also reported as major metabolites. From the literature, N→O group reduction is the most predominant metabolic pathway of MEQ metabolism in land animals [21]. Different from land animals, in the metabolism investigation of MEQ in sea cucumber, the most predominant metabolic pathways are deoxidation and carbonyl reduction, with M6 (2-isoethanol-BDMEQ) and M4 (2-isoethanol-1-DMEQ) as major metabolites. In particular, carboxylation is also detected as a major metabolic pathway, with MQCA (M7) as one of the metabolites of MEQ. MQCA was reported as a residue marker of olaquindox in land farm animals in previous literature works [24,25]. This work first reported MQCA as one of the metabolites of MEQ in sea cucumber.

3. Materials and Methods

3.1. Chemicals and Reagents

MEQ (purity > 98%) was purchased from A Chemtek, Inc. (Woburn, MA, USA). Sea cucumber samples were purchased from the local market. Acetonitrile, Methanol, formic acid, and ethyl acetate (HPLC grade) were purchased from Dima Technology Inc. (Muskegon, MI, USA). Metaphosphoric acid (analytical reagent) was purchased from Shanghai Macklin Biochemical Co., Ltd. (Shanghai, China). Hydrochloric acid (analytical reagent) was purchased from Yantai Sanhe Chemical Reagent Co., Ltd. (Yantai, Shandong, China). Oasis HLB cartridges (3 mL/60 mg) were purchased from Agilent Technologies (Palo Alto, CA, USA).

3.2. Apparatus

Ultimate 3000 pumping system coupled with a quadrupole-Orbitrap UHPLC-Q/Exactive Plus was obtained from Thermo Fisher Scientific (Bremen, Germany). A QL-901 vortex mixer was purchased from Haimen Kylin-Bell Lab Instruments Co., Ltd. (Haimen, Jiangsu, China). An HH-6 digital display constant temperature water bath was purchased from Changzhou GuoHua Electric Appliance Co., Ltd. (Changzhou, Jiangsu, China). A KQ5200 ultrasonic cleaner was purchased from Kunshan Ultrasonic Instruments Co., Ltd. (Jiangsu, China). An H2050R centrifuge was obtained from Changsha High-tech Industrial Development Zone Xiangyi Centrifuge Instrument Co., Ltd. (Changsha, Hunan, China). Syringe filters (0.2 μm) were obtained from Waters (Milford, MA, USA). Air-pump nitrogen evaporator was obtained from Hangzhou mio Co., Ltd. (Hangzhou, China).

3.3. Sample Preparation

Live sea cucumbers (150 ± 10 g, 3 years old) were obtained from local aquaculture and raised for 7 days to ensure they were MEQ free. Sea cucumbers were divided into the experimental group and the control group with six replicates each. Sea cucumbers in the experimental group were raised in sea water with 4 mg/L MEQ, while the control group were raised in sea water free of MEQ for 24 h. Afterward, sea cucumbers in the experimental and the control group were collected. Each sea cucumber sample was homogenized with a blender machine for further treatment. For sea cucumber preparation, 2.00 g ± 0.02 g experiment samples and blank control samples were weighed into a 50 mL polypropylene centrifuge tube, respectively. Detailed preparation procedures were optimized with three different schemes based on previous literature works [21–23], and each scheme was run in six repetitions. In Scheme 1, each sample was extracted with 5 mL of methanol by vortexing for 5 min and supersonic extraction for 2 min. Each sample was centrifuged at $10,000 \times g$ for 15 min at 4 °C in a refrigerated centrifuge, and the supernatant was transferred into another 50 mL polypropylene centrifuge tube. The residues were re-extracted with 5 mL of ethyl acetate containing 0.1% formic acid. The supernatant was combined after centrifugation and taken to dry under a stream of nitrogen at 45 °C. Then, the residue was re-dissolved with 1 mL of methanol–water (50:50, v/v) and filtered through a 0.22 μm syringe filter into auto-sampler vials for HRMS analysis. In Scheme 2, 20% metaphosphoric acid was added to each sample and settled in a water bath at 55 °C for 30 min for acidolysis and extraction. After centrifugation at 10,000× g for 15 min at 4 °C in a refrigerated centrifuge, the supernatants were purified with an OASIS HLB column. In Scheme 3, 2 mol/L hydrochloride acid was added, and each sample was put in a water bath at 55 °C for 30 min for acidolysis and extraction. After the water bath and centrifugation at 10,000× g for 15 min at 4 °C in a refrigerated centrifuge, the supernatant was purified with an OASIS HLB column. Each sample was filtered through a 0.22 μm syringe filter into auto-sampler vials for HRMS analysis.

3.4. Instrumental Conditions

The HRMS analysis was operated in a positive mode. Samples were analyzed using liquid chromatography coupled with Q/Exactive high-resolution mass spectrum (HRMS). Samples were separated with a Hypersil GOLD C18 column (100 mm × 2.1 mm, i.e., 1.9 μm) by a gradient elution program with water containing 0.1% formic acid as mobile phase A and acetonitrile containing 0.1% formic acid as mobile phase B. The flow rate of the mobile phase was 0.3 mL/min with injection volume at 5 μL. The gradient elution program was as follows: 0–2 min 95% A, 2–3 min 95–75% A, 3–4 min 70–60% A, 4–5.5 min 60–45% A, 5.5–7.5 min 45–5% A, 7.5–9 min 5–95%, and 9–12 min 95% A.

The mass spectrum parameters for HRMS were operated in a data-dependent acquisition (DDA) mode with negative heated electrospray ionization (HESI+). The parameters for full mass scan in DDA were settled at a resolution of 70,000 FWHM, scan range of m/z 120–900, automatic gain control (AGC) target of 3.0×10^6, and maximum ion implantation time (Maximum IT) of 64 ms. The ddMS2 parameters in the DDA mode were settled at a resolution of 17,500 FWHM, TOP N = 5, maximum IT 64 ms, isolation window 1.2 m/z, and normalized collisional energy (NCE) at 20, 40, and 60 eV.

3.5. Data Processing

In this study, Thermo's in-house software Xcalibur was used to demonstrate the high mass accuracy of the instrument by comparing the measured and predicted masses of targets [26]. Simultaneously, the metabolites could be detected and identified by comparing the precursor, fragment ions, and neutral loss between the experimental and control samples. The mass tolerance window was set to 10.0 ppm. The smoothing setting was enabled. The smoother type Gaussian was selected with 7 smoothing points.

4. Conclusions

In general, the metabolism behavior of MEQ in sea cucumber in vivo was investigated in the current study. The result shows that, in total, nine metabolites were detected and identified, as well as the precursor. Different from the metabolism result in land farm animals, the most predominant metabolites of MEQ in sea cucumbers were 2-iso-BDMEQ and 2-iso-1-DMEQ, with deoxidation and carbonyl reduction as major metabolic pathways in sea cucumber. In particular, this work first reported MQCA as a metabolite of MEQ, and carboxylation is a major metabolic pathway of MEQ in sea cucumbers. This work reveals that the metabolism of MEQ in marine animals is different from that in land animals. The metabolism results in this work could facilitate the accurate risk assessment of MEQ in sea cucumber and related marine foods.

Author Contributions: Conceptualization, J.H., Y.L. and Y.W.; methodology, X.Z. and H.Z.; software, X.M. and X.Z.; validation, X.M. and P.L.; formal analysis, X.M. and X.Z.; investigation, X.Z., J.H. and H.Z.; resources, G.L. and H.L.; data curation, X.M. and X.Z.; writing—original draft preparation, X.M. and X.Z.; writing—review and editing, Y.L.; supervision, Y.L. and Y.W.; funding acquisition, Y.L. and H.L. All authors have read and agreed to the published version of the manuscript.

Funding: This research was funded by the National Natural Science Foundation of China, grant number 22193064, and "Preparation and revision of veterinary drug residue standards in China" project, grant number SCB-21029.

Institutional Review Board Statement: The study was conducted according to the guidelines of the technical specification for ethical review of laboratory animal welfare and approved by the Ethics Committee) of Beijing Municipal Commission of Science and Technology (protocol code DB11/T 1734—2020 and date of approval in 2020).

Informed Consent Statement: Not applicable.

Data Availability Statement: Not applicable.

Conflicts of Interest: The authors declare no conflict of interest.

References

1. Suarez-Torres, J.D.; Orozco, C.A.; Ciangherotti, C.E. The numerical probability of carcinogenicity to humans of some antimicrobials: Nitro-monoaromatics (including 5-nitrofurans and 5-nitroimidazoles), quinoxaline-1,4-dioxides (including carbadox), and chloramphenicol. *Toxicol. Vitr.* **2021**, *75*, 105172. [CrossRef] [PubMed]
2. Zhao, Y.; Cheng., G.; Hao, H.; Pan, Y.; Liu, Z.; Dai, M.; Yuan, Z. In vitro antimicrobial activities of animal-used quinoxaline 1, 4-di-N-oxides against mycobacteria, mycoplasma and fungi. *BMC Vet. Res.* **2016**, *12*, 1–13. [CrossRef] [PubMed]
3. Liu, Q.; Zhang, J.; Luo, X.; Ihsan, A.; Liu, X.; Dai, M.; Cheng, G.; Hao, H.; Wang, X.; Yuan, Z. Further investigations into the genotoxicity of quinoxaline-di-N-oxides and their primary metabolites. *Food Chem. Toxicol.* **2016**, *93*, 145–157. [CrossRef] [PubMed]
4. Liu, Y.; Jiang, W.; Chen, Y.; Liu, Y.; Zeng, P.; Xue, F.; Wang, Q. Cytotoxicity of mequindox and its metabolites in HepG2 cells in vitro and murine hepatocytes in vivo. *Mutat. Res-Gen. Tox. En.* **2016**, *797*, 36–45. [CrossRef] [PubMed]
5. Official Journal of the European Union. Commission Regulation No. 2788/98. *Off. J. Eur. Union Commun.* L347 **1998**, *34*, 3132.
6. Liu, Q.; Lei, Z.; Gu, C.; Guo, J.; Yu, H.; Fatima, Z.; Zhou, K.; Shabbir, M.A.; Maan, M.K.; Wu, Q. Mequindox induces apoptosis, DNA damage, and carcinogenicity in Wistar rats. *Food Chem. Toxicol.* **2019**, *127*, 270–279. [CrossRef]
7. Rivera, G. Quinoxaline 1, 4-di-N-oxide derivatives: Are They Unselective or Selective Inhibitors? *Mini-Rev. Med. Chem.* **2022**, *22*, 15–25. [CrossRef]
8. Shan, Q.; Liu, Y.; He, L.; Ding, H.; Huang, X.; Yang, F.; Li, Y.; Zeng, Z. Metabolism of mequindox and its metabolites identification in chickens using LC-LTQ-Orbitrap mass spectrometry. *J. Chromatogr. B* **2012**, *881*, 96–106. [CrossRef]
9. Liu, Z.; Sun, Z. The metabolism of carbadox, olaquindox, mequindox, quinocetone and cyadox: An overview. *Med. Chem.* **2013**, *9*, 1017–1027. [CrossRef]
10. Mu, P.; Zheng, M.; Xu, M.; Zheng, Y.; Tang, X.; Wang, Y.; Wu, K.; Chen, Q.; Wang, L.; Deng, Y. N-oxide reduction of quinoxaline-1, 4-dioxides catalyzed by porcine aldehyde oxidase SsAOX1. *Drug Metab. Dispos.* **2014**, *42*, 511–519. [CrossRef]
11. Li, Y.; Mao, X.; Jiang, L.; Liu, H.; Nie, X.; Liu, X.; Kong, F.; Luo, P.; Li, Y. Reduction and hydroxylation metabolites of mequindox in holothurian analysis by ultra-performance liquid chromatography-tandem mass spectrometry. *J. Chromatogr. Sci.* **2022**, Online ahead of print. [CrossRef] [PubMed]
12. Liu, H.; Ren, C.; Han, D.; Huang, H.; Zou, R.; Zhang, H.; Xu, Y.; Gong, X.; Zhang, X.; Li, Y. UPLC-MS/MS method for simultaneous determination of three major metabolites of mequindox in holothurian. *J. Anal. Methods Chem.* **2018**, *2018*, 2768047. [CrossRef]
13. Hou, R.; Huang, C.; Rao, K.; Xu, Y.; Wang, Z. Characterized in vitro metabolism kinetics of alkyl organophosphate esters in fish liver and intestinal microsomes. *Environ. Sci. Technol.* **2018**, *52*, 3202–3210. [CrossRef] [PubMed]
14. Koenig, S.; Fernández, P.; Solé, M. Differences in cytochrome P450 enzyme activities between fish and crustacea: Relationship with the bioaccumulation patterns of polychlorobiphenyls (PCBs). *Aquat. Toxicol.* **2012**, *108*, 11–17. [CrossRef] [PubMed]
15. Ru, X.; Zhang, L.; Li, X.; Liu, S.; Yang, H. Development strategies for the sea cucumber industry in China. *J. Oceanol. Limnol.* **2019**, *37*, 300–312. [CrossRef]
16. Yue, H.; Tian, Y.; Feng, X.; Bo, Y.; Leng, Z.; Dong, P.; Xue, C.; Wang, J. Novel peptides from sea cucumber intestinal hydrolysates promote longitudinal bone growth in adolescent mice through accelerating cell cycle progress by regulating glutamine metabolism. *Food Funct.* **2022**, *13*, 7730–7739. [CrossRef]
17. Lu, Z.; Sun, N.; Dong, L.; Gao, Y.; Lin, S. Production of bioactive peptides from sea cucumber and its potential health benefits: A comprehensive review. *J. Agr. Food Chem.* **2022**, *70*, 7607–7625. [CrossRef]
18. Siddiqui, R.; Boghossian, A.; Khan, N.A. Sea cucumber as a therapeutic aquatic resource for human health. *Fish Aquat. Sci.* **2022**, *25*, 251–263. [CrossRef]
19. Hamed, I.; Özogul, F.; Özogul, Y.; Regenstein, J.M. Marine bioactive compounds and their health benefits: A review. *Compr. Rev. Food Sci. F.* **2015**, *14*, 446–465. [CrossRef]
20. Liu, Y.; Gong, X.H.; Xu, Y.J.; An, H.H.; Zhang, H.W.; Zhou, Q.L.; Zhang, X.Z. Effects of mequindox on non-specific immunity, growth performance and stress resistance of juvenile sea cucumber Apostichopus japonicus. *J. Shanghai Ocean Univ.* **2014**, *23*, 848–855.

21. Liu, Z.Y.; Huang, L.L.; Chen, D.M.; Yuan, Z.H. Metabolism of mequindox in liver microsomes of rats, chicken and pigs. *Rapid Commun. Mass. Sp.* **2010**, *24*, 909–918. [CrossRef] [PubMed]
22. Zeng, D.; Shen, X.; He, L.; Ding, H.; Tang, Y.; Sun, Y.; Fang, B.; Zeng, Z. Liquid chromatography tandem mass spectrometry for the simultaneous determination of mequindox and its metabolites in porcine tissues. *J. Sep. Sci.* **2012**, *35*, 1327–1335. [CrossRef]
23. Li, Y.; Sun, M.; Mao, X.; Li, J.; Sumarah, M.W.; You, Y.; Wang, Y. Tracing major metabolites of quinoxaline-1,4-dioxides in abalone with high-performance liquid chromatography tandem positive-mode electrospray ionization mass spectrometry. *J. Sci. Food Agr.* **2019**, *99*, 5550–5557. [CrossRef] [PubMed]
24. Peng, D.; Kavanagh, O.; Gao, H.; Zhang, X.; Deng, S.; Chen, D.; Liu, Z.; Xie, C.; Situ, C.; Yuan, Z. Surface plasmon resonance biosensor for the determination of 3-methyl-quinoxaline-2-carboxylic acid, the marker residue of olaquindox, in swine tissues. *Food Chem.* **2020**, *302*, 124623. [CrossRef]
25. Tan, H.; Pan, Y.; Chen, D.; Tao, Y.; Zhou, K.; Liu, Z.; Yuan, Z.; Huang, L. Discovery of the marker residue of olaquindox in pigs, broilers, and carp. *J. Agr. Food Chem.* **2019**, *67*, 6603–6613. [CrossRef]
26. Li, Y.; Qu, J.; Lin, Y.; Lu, G.; You, Y.; Jiang, G.; Wu, Y. Visible Post-Data analysis protocol for natural mycotoxin production. *J. Agr. Food Chem.* **2020**, *68*, 9603–9611. [CrossRef]

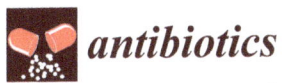

Communication

Effect of Phorate on the Development of Hyperglycaemia in Mouse and Resistance Genes in Intestinal Microbiota

Tingting Cao [1,†], Yajie Guo [2,†], Dan Wang [3], Zhiyang Liu [1], Suli Huang [1], Changfeng Peng [1], Shaolin Wang [4], Yang Wang [4], Qi Lu [1], Fan Xiao [1], Zhaoyi Liang [1], Sijia Zheng [1], Jianzhong Shen [4], Yongning Wu [5], Ziquan Lv [1,*] and Yuebin Ke [1,3,*]

1. Shenzhen Center for Disease Control and Prevention, Shenzhen 518055, China
2. The Eighth Affiliated Hospital, Sun Yat-Sen University, Shenzhen 518033, China
3. School of Public Health, Southern Medical University, Guangzhou 510515, China
4. College of Veterinary Medicine, China Agricultural University, Beijing 100091, China
5. Food Safety Research Unit (2019RU014), Chinese Academy of Medical Science, NHC Key Laboratory of Food Safety Risk Assessment, China National Center for Food Safety Risk Assessment, Beijing 100021, China
* Correspondence: lvziquan1984@126.com (Z.L.); keyke@szu.edu.cn (Y.K.)
† These authors contributed equally to this work.

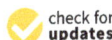

Abstract: Phorate is a systemic, broad-spectrum organophosphorus insecticide. Although it is commonly used worldwide, phorate, like other pesticides, not only causes environmental pollution but also poses serious threats to human and animal health. Herein, we measured the blood glucose concentrations of high-fat-diet-fed mice exposed to various concentrations of phorate (0, 0.005, 0.05, or 0.5 mg/kg); we also assessed the blood glucose concentrations of high-fat-diet-fed mice exposed to phorate; we also assessed the distribution characteristics of the resistance genes in the intestinal microbiota of these mice. We found that 0.005 and 0.5 mg/kg of phorate induced obvious hyperglycaemia in the high-fat-diet-fed mice. Exposure to phorate markedly reduced the abundance of *Akkermansia muciniphila* in the mouse intestine. The resistance genes *vanRG*, *tetW/N/W*, *acrD*, and *evgS* were significantly upregulated in the test group compared with the control group. Efflux pumping was the primary mechanism of drug resistance in the *Firmicutes*, *Proteobacteria*, *Bacteroidetes*, *Verrucomicrobia*, *Synergistetes*, *Spirochaetes*, and *Actinobacteria* found in the mouse intestine. Our findings indicate that changes in the abundance of the intestinal microbiota are closely related to the presence of antibiotic-resistant bacteria in the intestinal tract and the metabolic health of the host.

Keywords: phorate; hyperglycaemia; intestinal microbiota; resistance genes

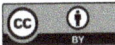

1. Introduction

Organophosphorus (OP) compounds are widely used in China and abroad to protect crops from insects [1]. OP pesticides generally work by irreversibly inhibiting the enzyme acetylcholinesterase [2]. Phorate is a systemic, broad-spectrum OP insecticide and is commonly used in the agricultural sector to control sucking and chewing pests, leaf hoppers, and mites. Phorate is primarily available as a granular formulation that can be applied by banding when planting a crop or by directly placing it in-furrow with a seed [3]. However, the use of OP pesticides leads to varying degrees of environmental pollution, which can originate from various sources. Studies have reported that phorate is found in vegetables (tomatoes, 2.0–98.5 µg/kg; aubergines, 1.0–20.7 µg/kg) and fruits (apples, 1.5–45.1 µg/kg; grapes, 3.4 µg/kg; pears, 1.4–26.4 µg/kg) [4]. The estimated daily intake of phorate ranges from 0.1 to 0.47 µg/kg bw/day in the general population and from 0.18 to 43.73 µg/kg bw/day in farmers [5]. These numbers have raised concerns regarding human exposure to phorate.

Phorate undergoes a P450-mediated desulphurisation reaction to produce oxon metabolites; its primary mechanism of acute toxicity is acetylcholinesterase inhibition mediated mainly by the oxon metabolite phorate–oxon [6]. It remains unknown whether animals can develop resistance after exposure to phorate. Nevertheless, the emergence of resistance is thought to be linked to the use of antibiotics, which pose a threat to human and animal health [7]. In humans and animals, the gut is the key reservoir of microbial communities, comprising both commensal and pathogenic bacteria [8]. A growing number of studies have found that because the gut microbiota is frequently exposed to exogenous antibiotics from drugs or from the food chain, it possesses multiple drug-resistance genes [9]. Moreover, long-term exposure of humans and animals to antibiotics leads to the enrichment of intestinal drug-resistance genes.

A recent review of comprehensive studies on intestinal microbiota and antibiotic resistance conducted in a large human cohort in China found that the antibiotic resistance of the intestinal microbiota is closely associated with faecal metabolites and the host's metabolic health [10]. Antibiotic-resistance gene diversity is associated with a higher risk of type 2 diabetes (T2D). Moreover, a study reported that the pesticide chlorpyrifos impaired mitochondrial function and diet-induced thermogenesis in brown adipose tissue (BAT) and promoted increased obesity, non-alcoholic fatty liver disease (NAFLD), and insulin resistance in high-fat-diet-fed mice [11]. However, to date, no studies have assessed the effects of phorate on glucose metabolism.

To explore the hazards of pesticide residues with respect to host metabolic health and the correlation between the production of resistance genes and glucose metabolism, in this study, we measured the blood glucose concentrations and assessed the distribution characteristics of antibiotic-resistance genes in the intestinal microbiota of HFD-fed mice exposed to phorate.

2. Results

2.1. Phorate Exposure Elevated the Blood Glucose Concentrations in HFD-Fed Mice

To determine the effects of phorate on glucose metabolism, 7–8-week-old male HFD-fed C57Bl/6j mice were exposed to 0, 0.005, 0.05, and 0.5 mg/kg bw/day of phorate by oral gavage each day for 5 weeks. We then measured the blood glucose concentrations of the mice in the natural state (Figure 1a). The blood glucose concentrations of the mice exposed to phorate, especially the 0.005 and 0.5 mg/kg bw/day doses, were significantly higher than those of the control group ($p < 0.05$).

2.2. Effects of Phorate on the Beta Diversity of the Gut Microbiota in HFD-Fed Mice

Principal component analysis was used to study the extent of intergroup similarity or heterogeneity in terms of community structure. A shorter distance between samples indicates a greater similarity in community structure and vice versa. The community similarity was measured based on phylogenetic relatedness using unweighted UniFrac in a principal component analysis plot (Figure 1b). PC1 and PC2, the first two principal components, explain 12.78% and 9.25% of the data variation, respectively, clearly separating each community. Samples of the same group are represented by the same colour. The A group (control group) and the B, C, and D groups (0.005, 0.05, and 0.5 mg/kg group) are clearly separated, indicating that the gut microbiota structure had discernibly changed after exposure to phorate.

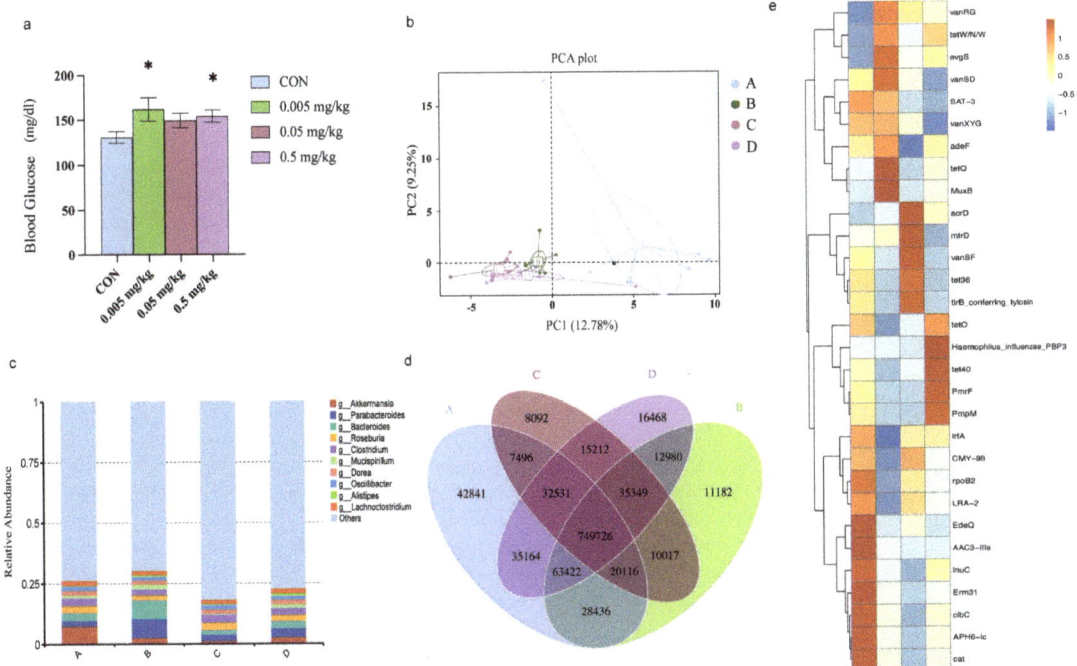

Figure 1. (a) Effect of phorate on the blood glucose concentrations of mice after 35 days of exposure. (b) PCA plots of the different genera. The abscissa is the first principal component, whereas the ordinate is the second principal component. Both percentages represent the contribution of the second principal component to the sample differences. Each point in the figure represents a sample, and samples of the same colour belong to the same group. (c) Relative-abundance bar chart of the genus-annotation results of each sample at different classification levels; the top 10 genera with the largest relative abundances in each group are indicated, whereas the remaining genera are grouped as 'others'. (d) Venn diagrams showing the numbers of unique and common genes in the mouse intestinal tract. (e) Distribution of resistance genes in the phorate-exposed groups. *: $p < 0.05$, as assayed by two-tailed Student's t-test or one-way ANOVA followed by Student-Newman-Keuls test.

2.3. Relative Abundance of the Intestinal Microbiota in Mice Exposed to Phorate

The intergroup analysis identified the enrichment of specific genera, indicated by significant intergroup differences in abundance. Gut microbiota genera having a relative abundance of 0.01% in at least one group were scrutinized. Genera with a relative abundance of >0.01% of the intestinal microbiota genera in each group were selected. Figure 1C shows the abundances of the top 10 bacterial genera. *Akkermansia* was the dominant genus in the control group (7.43%), with the other classifications ignored. However, the abundance of *Akkermansia* was decreased in the phorate-exposed groups (B: 2.54%, C: 2.76%, D: 3.82%). The abundance of Parabacteroides (B: 7.99%, C: 2.76%, D: 2.56%) and that of *Alistipes* (B: 0.87%, C: 0.55%, D: 1.24%) were increased in the phorate-exposed groups compared with the control group (*Parabacteroides*: 2.38%, *Alistipes*: 0.53%).

2.4. Effects of Phorate on Intestinal Microbiota Gene Numbers

A Venn diagram was drawn to investigate the distribution of gene numbers among the designated groups and to analyse the common and unique information of the genes in the different groups. Overall, 749,726 genes were shared among the four groups (Figure 1D). In total, 42,841 genes were unique to the control group. In comparison, 11,182 unique genes were found in the 0.005 mg/kg group, 8092 in the 0.05 mg/kg group, and 16,468 in the 0.5 mg/kg group. Thus, significant differences were found in the microbial compositions of the four groups. Moreover, exposure to phorate reduced the number of intestinal microbiota genes.

2.5. Composition of Intestinal Antibiotic-Resistance Genes after Phorate Exposure

After analysing the drug-resistance genes in the intestinal microbiota in the four groups of mice, the 30 genes with the most obvious expression differences were subjected to further analysis (Figure 1E). The resistance genes *vanRG, tetW/N/W, acrD,* and *evgS* were significantly upregulated in the phorate-exposed groups compared with the control group. However, the resistance genes *lrfA, CMY-98, rpoB2, LRA-2, EdeQ, AAC3-IIa, InuC, Erm31, clbC, APH6-Ic,* and *cat*-resistance genes were significantly downregulated regulated in the phorate-exposed groups.

2.6. Relationship between the Resistance Gene Mechanisms and the Intestinal Microbiota Composition

Figure 2 shows that the most abundant phyla in the mouse intestinal microbiota were *Firmicutes* and *Proteobacteria*. The abundance of *Firmicutes* is mainly attributable to the following three mechanisms of drug resistance: efflux pumping, inactivation, and target alternation. Meanwhile, efflux pumping is the main mechanism of drug resistance in *Proteobacteria*. *Bacteroidetes, Verrucomicrobia, Synergistetes, Spirochaetes,* and *Actinobacteria* were also widely distributed in the intestinal microbiota of the mice. Moreover, target protection, replacement, and other mechanisms exhibited by the above-mentioned strains affect the development of drug resistance by the intestinal microbiota.

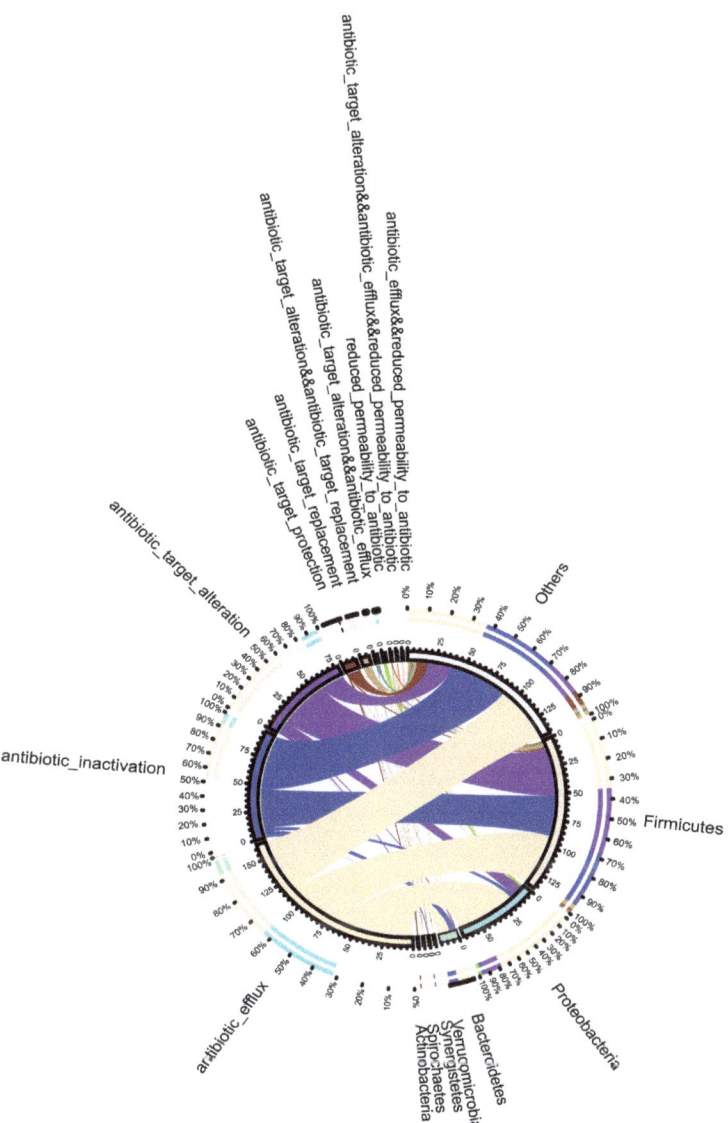

Figure 2. Circular diagram outlining the resistance mechanisms and genera. The circle is divided into two parts, with the genus information at the gate level on the right and the resistance mechanism-related information on the left. The different colours in the inner circle indicate the resistance mechanisms for different genera and resistances, and the scale denotes the number of genes. The left side indicates the sum of the number of resistance genes in the genera that contain the corresponding resistance mechanism, and the right side denotes the sum of the number of resistance genes contained in the genera with different resistance mechanisms. The left side of the outer circle denotes the relative proportion of the resistance genes in each genus to the resistance genes of its resistance mechanism, whereas the right side of the outer circle denotes the relative proportion of the resistance genes in each resistance mechanism to the resistance genes of its genus.

3. Discussion

Phorate is a systemic, broad-spectrum OP insecticide. In this study, for the first time, we found that phorate has a hyperglycaemic effect on HFD-fed mice. Diabetes is reportedly induced by environmental and genetic causes, and increasing evidence has shown that the use of global pesticides has increased the risk of obesity and T2D [12]. A previous study reported that the increased risk of diabetes in humans may be related to the use of phorate [13]. The body weight changes of the four groups of mice were recorded during the whole experiment. However, we did not find a significant difference in body weight between the phorate groups and the control group (data not shown). We felt that there was probably no relationship between weight and blood glucose levels in this study. Among 13,637 farmers' wives who were exposed to phorate, 688 (5%) were found to have diabetes over a 10-year follow-up period. This finding is consistent with our hyperglycaemia results in mice. However, our mouse experiments clearly demonstrated a dose-dependent relationship between phorate and hyperglycaemia. Mice exposed to 0.005 and 0.5 mg/kg phorate had obvious hyperglycaemia. Phorate is a potential risk factor for human health, and the acceptable daily intake recommend by the WHO is 0.0005 mg/kg bw/day [14]. Occupational exposure of farmers to phorate increases their daily intake of pesticides, with a median exposure of 0.69 µg/kg bw/day, the equivalent of which is 0.006279 mg/kg bw/day in mice [5]. Phorate at concentrations of 0.25–2 µg/mL can lead to the splitting and mutation of DNA as well as DNA loss in human lymphocytes [15]. However, the regulatory roles of phorate in glucose metabolism remain unclear.

Upon entry through oral gavage, phorate inevitably affects the intestinal microbiota of mice. The gut microbiome is closely associated with the occurrence and development of chronic diseases [16]. The gut microbiota engages in symbiotic relationships and regulates various metabolic functions, including intestinal barrier homeostasis and glucose homeostasis [17,18]. Preclinical and clinical studies have shown that the abundance of *A. muciniphila* is associated with the development of metabolic disorders, including obesity and T2D [19,20]. *A. muciniphila* secretes a glucagon-like peptide-1-inducing protein to improve glucose homeostasis and regulate metabolic diseases in mice [21]. Similarly, in the present study, we found that the abundance of *A. muciniphila* was significantly reduced after exposure to phorate, and this may have led to the observed increases in blood glucose concentrations. However, the abundances of *Parabacteroides* and *Alistipes* were increased in the phorate-exposed groups compared with those in the control group. *Parabacteroides* can accelerate the development of diabetes in non-obese diabetic mice as well as increase the macrophage, dendritic cell, and destructive CD8+ T cell levels and reduce the Treg cell levels [22]. Feeding on HFDs increases the abundance of *Alistipes* [23]. The enrichment of anti-inflammatory bacteria in *Alistipes* can improve its glucose tolerance and insulin sensitivity [24]. Our results were consistent with those of previous studies and suggested that the changes in the intestinal microbiota induced by phorate were closely associated with glucose metabolism.

Interestingly, we found that phorate may also contribute to the development of resistance genes in the intestinal microbiota as well as the development of hyperglycaemia in mice. According to a recent study [10] that analysed the metagenomic landscape of intestinal antibiotic-resistant microorganisms in a large multiomics human cohort (n = 1210) study, a significant overall change was observed in the intestinal antibiotic-resistance structure of the healthy, prediabetic, and T2D groups. The study reported that the levels of *vanRG*, *tetW/N/W*, *acrD*, and *evgS* were significantly upregulated after exposure to phorate. *vanX* present in vancomycin-resistant genes is reportedly associated with the risk of T2D [10]. *AcrD*, which is paralogous to *AcrB*—which belongs to the RND family of transporters—confers resistance to tetracycline, novobiocin, nalidixic acid, norfloxacin, sodium dodecyl sulfate, and aminoglycosides [25]. We found that hyperglycaemic mice carried the vancomycin-resistance gene *vanRG*, the tetracycline-resistance gene *tetW/N/W*, and the multidrug-resistance genes *acrD* and *evgS*; these genes have not been previously reported in mice. We believe that the increase in the abundances of these resistance genes is attributable to the use of phorate.

For the first time, we found that phorate can lead to the production of drug-resistance genes in the intestinal microbiota. Phorate can also lead to the corresponding drug resistance in bacteria. For instance, tetracycline efflux transporters are a major facilitator of the antibiotic efflux pumps of the aminoglycoside gene superfamily [26]. We found that efflux pumps were the main mechanism of drug resistance in *Firmicutes, Proteobacteria, Bacteroidetes, Verrucomicrobia, Synergistetes, Spirochaetes,* and *Actinobacteria*. Notably, *Firmicutes, Proteobacteria,* and *Bacteroidetes* have been found to be dominant in the microbiota of mice and humans [27]. Therefore, we suspect that phorate causes hyperglycaemia in mice primarily by causing the dominant bacteria in the intestine to produce efflux pumps. Some studies have reported that the gut antibiotic resistome may change earlier than the gut microbiota during T2D progression and/or that changes in the gut antibiotic resistome are more sensitive to the development of T2D [10]. Herein, we propose that phorate can cause hyperglycaemia in mice by influencing the abundance of the intestinal microbiota and by modulating or altering the expression of drug-resistance genes.

4. Materials and Methods

4.1. Chemicals

Phorate was obtained from Tianjin Alta Scientific Co., Ltd. (Tianjin, China) (purity quotient of ≥99%, product no. 298-02-2). Pure corn oil was purchased from Sigma-Aldrich (100%, product no. C116023; Sigma-Aldrich (Shanghai, China) Trading Co, Ltd, Shanghai, China). The mice were fed with a HFD (60 kcal% fat; Cat# D12492; Research Diets Inc., New Brunswick, NJ, USA).

4.2. Animals and Treatments

A total of 28 male C57Bl/6j mice aged 7–8 weeks were obtained from Beijing Vital River Laboratory Animal Technology Co., Ltd. (Beijing, China). The mice were randomly divided into four groups (control, 0.005 mg/kg, 0.05 mg/kg, and 0.5 mg/kg) and fed an HFD. Based on their group, the mice were treated with different doses of phorate or corn oil (control) daily for 5 weeks consecutively. Phorate dissolves well in corn oil and was administered by gavage. All the mice were housed under a 12 h light/dark cycle at 22–25 °C and were provided free access to drinking water and food, except when the food had to be withdrawn for experimental purposes. All of the animal experiments were performed according to the guidelines of Shenzhen TopBiotech Co., Ltd (Shenzhen, China). (TOP-IACUC-2021-0083).

4.3. Blood Glucose Concentrations

Blood glucose concentrations were determined using a FreeStyle Optium Neo meter (Abbott, Shanghai, China) at the fifth week of the treatment period. Blood samples were collected from mice through a small cut made at the tip of the tail.

4.4. Metagenomic Sequencing

Using the QIAamp DNA Stool Kit (Qiagen, Gaithersburg, MD, USA), genomic DNA was extracted from the caecum contents. A Thermo NanoDrop One (Thermo Fisher Scientific Co., Ltd, Waltham, USA) was used to detect the purity and concentration of the extracted DNA (n = 28 C57Bl/6j mice fed an HFD). We used the paired-end sequencing mode of the Illumina HiSeq sequencing platform (Novogene Company Limited Co., Ltd, Tianjin, China) for high-throughput sequencing of multiple samples. The raw data obtained using this platform were pre-processed using Readfq to acquire clean data for subsequent analyses. Bioinformatic analysis of the sequencing data was conducted using the Quantitative Insights into Microbial Ecology software. Low-quality reads, barcodes, and primers as well as chimera sequences were eliminated using the UCHIME software (version 4.2, http://drive5.com/usearch/manual/uchime_algo.html) with the relevant algorithm, and the effective tags were obtained. Clean data were obtained after pre-processing, and the MEGAHIT assembly software (version 1.0.4-beta) was used for assembly analysis. After quality control of each sample, the clean data were compared with the scaftigs after assembly of each sample using the Bowtie2 software (version 2.2.4, http://bowtie-bio.sourceforge.net/bowtie2/index.shtml). For the scaftigs generated upon single-sample assembly, fragments <500 bp were filtered out, and statistical analysis and subsequent gene prediction were conducted. Starting from the scaftigs ($\geq$500 bp) of each sample, MetaGeneMark (version 3.05, http://topaz.gatech.edu/GeneMark/) was used for open reading frame prediction, and hits with <100 nucleotides were filtered out based on the prediction results. For the open reading frame prediction results of each sample assembly, the CD-HIT software (version 4.5.8, http://www.bioinformatics.org/cd-hit/) was used to eliminate redundancies to obtain a non-redundant initial gene catalogue. By default, 95% identity and 90% coverage were maintained for clustering, and the longest sequence was selected as the representative sequence. Based on the abundance information of each gene in each sample in the gene catalogue, basic information statistics, core pan-gene analysis, correlation analysis between samples, and gene-number Wayne diagram analysis were conducted. The 28 gut microbial metagenome sequence data that support the findings are available in the SRA under the NCBI BioProject ID PRJNA892724.

4.5. Annotation of Resistance Genes

Resistance gene identifier (RGI) software (version 6.0.0, https://card.mcmaster.ca/analyze/rgi) in the Comprehensive Antibiotic Resistance Database (v2.0.1) was used to compare unigenes with the CARD data (RGI built-in Blastp); bitcore value comparison was performed to score the results [28]. The relative abundance of each Antibiotic Resistance Ontology was calculated based on the comparison results.

4.6. Statistical Analysis

Based on the data distribution, significance was assessed using the unpaired two-tailed t-test or one-way analysis of variance, as appropriate. Significant differences are indicated in the figures with * $p < 0.05$. All differences are considered statistically significant at $p < 0.05$, unless indicated otherwise. GraphPad Prism version 8.0 (GraphPad Software Co., Ltd, San Diego, CA, USA) was used for graphical illustrations and statistical analyses. The non-parametric factorial Kruskal–Wallis rank sum test was used to detect genera with significant abundance differences between groups, and the Wilcoxon rank sum test was then used to analyse the differences between the two groups. Finally, linear discriminant analysis was performed to achieve dimensionality reduction and assess the impact size of the significantly different genera.

5. Conclusions

We found that phorate can cause hyperglycaemia in mice. An in-depth analysis of the intestinal microbiota in mice revealed that phorate can affect the abundance of the intestinal microbiota and therefore alter the expression of drug-resistance genes. Moreover, changes in the abundance of the intestinal microbiota are closely related to the presence of antibiotic-resistant bacteria in the intestinal tract and the host's metabolic health. Taken together, our results can guide pesticide safety evaluations in future studies.

Author Contributions: Conceptualization, Z.L. (Ziquan Lv) and Y.G.; methodology, Y.K.; software, T.C.; validation, D.W. and Z.L. (Zhiyang Liu; formal analysis, T.C.; investigation, S.H.; resources, F.X.; data curation, C.P.; writing—original draft preparation, T.C.; writing—review and editing, Y.G., Y.K. and Z.L. (Ziquan Lv); visualization, S.W.; supervision, Y.W. (Yang Wang), Q.L., Z.L. (Zhaoyi Liang), S.Z. and J.S.; project administration, Y.W. (Yongning Wu), Z.L. (Ziquan Lv) and Y.K.; funding acquisition, Y.K. All authors have read and agreed to the published version of the manuscript.

Funding: This research was funded by the National Key R&D Program of China (2019YFC1605104), National Natural Science Foundation of China (22193064), Shenzhen Science and Technology Program (JCYJ20210324124201004), Sanming Project of Medicine in Shenzhen (SZSM202011008), Shenzhen Key Medical Discipline Construction Fund (SZXK066), and Shenzhen Science and Technology Planning Project (JCYJ20170413101841798).

Institutional Review Board Statement: The animal study protocol was approved by Shenzhen TopBiotech Co., Ltd. (TOP-IACUC-2022-0021, 28 February 2022).

Informed Consent Statement: Not applicable.

Data Availability Statement: Not applicable.

Conflicts of Interest: The authors declare no conflict of interest.

References

1. Du, L.; Li, S.; Qi, L.; Hou, Y.; Zeng, Y.; Xu, W.; Wang, H.; Zhao, X.; Sun, C. Metabonomic analysis of the joint toxic action of long-term low-level exposure to a mixture of four organophosphate pesticides in rat plasma. *Mol. Biosyst.* **2014**, *10*, 1153–1161. [CrossRef] [PubMed]
2. De Bleecker, J.L. Organophosphate and carbamate poisoning. *Handb. Clin. Neurol.* **2008**, *91*, 401–432. [PubMed]
3. Saquib, Q.; Attia, S.M.; Siddiqui, M.A.; Aboul-Soud, M.A.; Al-Khedhairy, A.A.; Giesy, J.P.; Musarrat, J. Phorate-induced oxidative stress, DNA damage and transcriptional activation of p53 and caspase genes in male Wistar rats. *Toxicol. Appl. Pharmacol.* **2012**, *259*, 54–65. [CrossRef] [PubMed]
4. Li, H.; Chang, Q.; Bai, R.; Lv, X.; Cao, T.; Shen, S.; Liang, S.; Pang, G. Simultaneous determination and risk assessment of highly toxic pesticides in the market-sold vegetables and fruits in China: A 4-year investigational study. *Ecotoxicol. Environ. Saf.* **2021**, *221*, 112428. [CrossRef] [PubMed]
5. Katsikantami, I.; Colosio, C.; Alegakis, A.; Tzatzarakis, M.N.; Vakonaki, E.; Rizos, A.K.; Sarigiannis, D.A.; Tsatsakis, A.M. Estimation of daily intake and risk assessment of organophosphorus pesticides based on biomonitoring data—The internal exposure approach. *Food. Chem. Toxicol.* **2019**, *123*, 57–71. [CrossRef] [PubMed]
6. Moyer, R.A.; McGarry, K.G., Jr.; Babin, M.C.; Platoff, G.E., Jr.; Jett, D.A.; Yeung, D.T. Kinetic analysis of oxime-assisted reactivation of human, Guinea pig, and rat acetylcholinesterase inhibited by the organophosphorus pesticide metabolite phorate oxon (PHO). *Pestic. Biochem. Physiol.* **2018**, *145*, 93–99. [CrossRef] [PubMed]
7. Bueno, T.S.; Loiko, M.R.; Vidaletti, M.R.; de Oliveira, J.A.; Fetzner, T.; Cerva, C.; de Moraes, L.B.; De Carli, S.; Siqueira, F.M.; Rodrigues, R.O.; et al. Multidrug-resistant *Escherichia coli* from free-living pigeons (*Columba livia*): Insights into antibiotic environmental contamination and detection of resistance genes. *Zoonoses Public Health* **2022**, *69*, 682–693. [CrossRef]
8. Salyers, A.A.; Gupta, A.; Wang, Y. Human intestinal bacteria as reservoirs for antibiotic resistance genes. *Trends Microbiol.* **2004**, *12*, 412–416. [CrossRef]
9. Isles, N.S.; Mu, A.; Kwong, J.C.; Howden, B.P.; Stinear, T.P. Gut microbiome signatures and host colonization with multidrug-resistant bacteria. *Trends Microbiol.* **2022**, *30*, 853–865. [CrossRef]
10. Shuai, M.; Zhang, G.; Zeng, F.F.; Fu, Y.; Liang, X.; Yuan, L.; Xu, F.; Gou, W.; Miao, Z.; Jiang, Z.; et al. Human Gut Antibiotic Resistome and Progression of Diabetes. *Adv. Sci.* **2022**, *9*, e2104965. [CrossRef]
11. Wang, B.; Tsakiridis, E.E.; Zhang, S.; Llanos, A.; Desjardins, E.M.; Yabut, J.M.; Green, A.E.; Day, E.A.; Smith, B.K.; Lally, J.S.V.; et al. The pesticide chlorpyrifos promotes obesity by inhibiting diet-induced thermogenesis in brown adipose tissue. *Nat. Commun.* **2021**, *12*, 5163. [CrossRef] [PubMed]
12. Thayer, K.A.; Heindel, J.J.; Bucher, J.R.; Gallo, M.A. Role of environmental chemicals in diabetes and obesity: A National Toxicology Program workshop review. *Environ. Health Perspect.* **2012**, *120*, 779–789. [CrossRef] [PubMed]
13. Starling, A.P.; Umbach, D.M.; Kamel, F.; Long, S.; Sandler, D.P.; Hoppin, J.A. Pesticide use and incident diabetes among wives of farmers in the Agricultural Health Study. *Occup. Environ. Med.* **2014**, *71*, 629–635. [CrossRef] [PubMed]
14. Mansour, S.A.; Belal, M.H.; Abou-Arab, A.A.K.; Gad, M.F. Monitoring of pesticides and heavy metals in cucumber fruits produced from different farming systems. *Chemosphere* **2009**, *75*, 601–609. [CrossRef] [PubMed]
15. Timoroglu, I.; Yuzbasioglu, D.; Unal, F.; Yilmaz, S.; Aksoy, H.; Celik, M. Assessment of the genotoxic effects of organophosphorus insecticides phorate and trichlorfon in human lymphocytes. *Environ. Toxicol.* **2014**, *29*, 577–587. [CrossRef] [PubMed]
16. Aron-Wisnewsky, J.; Clement, K. The gut microbiome, diet, and links to cardiometabolic and chronic disorders. *Nat. Rev. Nephrol.* **2016**, *12*, 169–181. [CrossRef] [PubMed]
17. Geach, T. Gut microbiota: Mucin-munching bacteria modulate glucose metabolism. *Nat. Rev. Endocrinol.* **2017**, *13*, 66. [CrossRef] [PubMed]
18. Sonnenburg, J.L.; Backhed, F. Diet-microbiota interactions as moderators of human metabolism. *Nature* **2016**, *535*, 56–64. [CrossRef]
19. Dao, M.C.; Belda, E.; Prifti, E.; Everard, A.; Kayser, B.D.; Bouillot, J.L.; Chevallier, J.M.; Pons, N.; Le Chatelier, E.; Ehrlich, S.D.; et al. *Akkermansia muciniphila* abundance is lower in severe obesity, but its increased level after bariatric surgery is not associated with metabolic health improvement. *Am. J. Physiol. Endocrinol. Metab.* **2019**, *317*, E446–E459. [CrossRef]

20. Zhang, L.; Qin, Q.; Liu, M.; Zhang, X.; He, F.; Wang, G. *Akkermansia muciniphila* can reduce the damage of gluco/lipotoxicity, oxidative stress and inflammation, and normalize intestine microbiota in streptozotocin-induced diabetic rats. *Pathog. Dis.* **2018**, *76*, fty028. [CrossRef]
21. Yoon, H.S.; Cho, C.H.; Yun, M.S.; Jang, S.J.; You, H.J.; Kim, J.H.; Han, D.; Cha, K.H.; Moon, S.H.; Lee, K.; et al. *Akkermansia muciniphila* secretes a glucagon-like peptide-1-inducing protein that improves glucose homeostasis and ameliorates metabolic disease in mice. *Nat. Microbiol.* **2021**, *6*, 563–573. [CrossRef] [PubMed]
22. Girdhar, K.; Huang, Q.; Chow, I.T.; Vatanen, T.; Brady, C.; Raisingani, A.; Autissier, P.; Atkinson, M.A.; Kwok, W.W.; Kahn, C.R.; et al. A gut microbial peptide and molecular mimicry in the pathogenesis of type 1 diabetes. *Proc. Natl. Acad. Sci. USA* **2022**, *119*, e2120028119. [CrossRef] [PubMed]
23. Wan, Y.; Wang, F.; Yuan, J.; Li, J.; Jiang, D.; Zhang, J.; Li, H.; Wang, R.; Tang, J.; Huang, T.; et al. Effects of dietary fat on gut microbiota and faecal metabolites, and their relationship with cardiometabolic risk factors: A 6-month randomised controlled-feeding trial. *Gut* **2019**, *68*, 1417–1429. [CrossRef] [PubMed]
24. Zhang, L.; Zhang, T.; Sun, J.; Huang, Y.; Liu, T.; Ye, Z.; Hu, J.; Zhang, G.; Chen, H.; Ye, Z.; et al. Calorie restriction ameliorates hyperglycemia, modulates the disordered gut microbiota, and mitigates metabolic endotoxemia and inflammation in type 2 diabetic rats. *J. Endocrinol. Investig.* **2022**. [CrossRef] [PubMed]
25. Yu, L.; Li, W.; Liu, Z.; Yu, J.; Wang, W.; Shang, F.; Xue, T. Role of McbR in the regulation of antibiotic susceptibility in avian pathogenic *Escherichia coli*. *Poult Sci.* **2020**, *99*, 6390–6401. [CrossRef] [PubMed]
26. Kazimierczak, K.A.; Scott, K.P.; Kelly, D.; Aminov, R.I. Tetracycline resistome of the organic pig gut. *Appl. Environ. Microbiol.* **2009**, *75*, 1717–1722. [CrossRef] [PubMed]
27. Ruuskanen, M.O.; Erawijantari, P.P.; Havulinna, A.S.; Liu, Y.; Meric, G.; Tuomilehto, J.; Inouye, M.; Jousilahti, P.; Salomaa, V.; Jain, M.; et al. Gut Microbiome Composition Is Predictive of Incident Type 2 Diabetes in a Population Cohort of 5572 Finnish Adults. *Diabetes Care* **2022**, *45*, 811–818. [CrossRef]
28. McArthur, A.G.; Waglechner, N.; Nizam, F.; Yan, A.; Azad, M.A.; Baylay, A.J.; Bhullar, K.; Canova, M.J.; De Pascale, G.; Ejim, L.; et al. The comprehensive antibiotic resistance database. *Antimicrob. Agents Chemother.* **2013**, *57*, 3348–3357. [CrossRef]

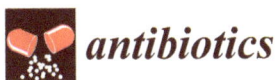

Article

Occurrence and Risk Assessment of Fluoroquinolone Residues in Chicken and Pork in China

Zhixin Fei [1,2,†], Shufeng Song [1,†], Xin Yang [1], Dingguo Jiang [1], Jie Gao [1,*] and Dajin Yang [1,*]

1 NHC Key Laboratory of Food Safety Risk Assessment, China National Center for Food Safety Risk Assessment, Beijing 100022, China
2 Yunnan Center for Disease Control and Prevention, Kunming 650022, China
* Correspondence: gaojie@cfsa.net.cn (J.G.); yangdajin@cfsa.net.cn (D.Y.)
† These authors contributed equally to this work.

Abstract: Antibiotics, especially fluoroquinolones, have been exhaustively used in animal husbandry. However, very limited information on the occurrence and exposure assessment of fluoroquinolone residues in chicken and pork in China is available to date. Thus, a total of 1754 chicken samples and 1712 pork samples were collected from 25 provinces in China and tested by ultra-high performance liquid chromatography-tandem mass spectrometry (UPLC–MS/MS) for residual determination of six common fluoroquinolones. The results revealed that the detection frequencies of fluoroquinolone residues were 3.99% and 1.69% in chicken and pork samples. The overall violation frequencies were 0.68% and 0.41% for chicken and pork. Enrofloxacin and its metabolite ciprofloxacin were found to be the most predominant fluoroquinolones. The occurrence of these antibiotics in different sampling regions and market types was analyzed. The %ADI values of enrofloxacin and ciprofloxacin were far less than 100, indicating the health risk associated with the exposure to these aforementioned fluoroquinolone residues via chicken and pork for Chinese children, adolescents, and adults was acceptable. The results provided useful references for Chinese consumers, and helped to appropriately use these antibiotics in poultry and livestock industry.

Keywords: occurrence; risk assessment; fluoroquinolone; chicken; pork; China

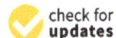

Citation: Fei, Z.; Song, S.; Yang, X.; Jiang, D.; Gao, J.; Yang, D. Occurrence and Risk Assessment of Fluoroquinolone Residues in Chicken and Pork in China. *Antibiotics* **2022**, *11*, 1292. https://doi.org/10.3390/antibiotics11101292

Academic Editor: Carlos M. Franco

Received: 5 August 2022
Accepted: 5 September 2022
Published: 22 September 2022

Publisher's Note: MDPI stays neutral with regard to jurisdictional claims in published maps and institutional affiliations.

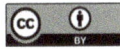

Copyright: © 2022 by the authors. Licensee MDPI, Basel, Switzerland. This article is an open access article distributed under the terms and conditions of the Creative Commons Attribution (CC BY) license (https:// creativecommons.org/licenses/by/ 4.0/).

1. Introduction

Chicken and pork are two of the most commonly consumed meats in China. Over the past 30 years, the per capita consumption of meat in China has increased by 50% [1]. The growth in demand has meant that the poultry and livestock industries have shifted from traditional family farming to intensive farming [2]. Nevertheless, as any intensive animal production system, the risk of the emergence and spread of infectious diseases are high [3]. Antibiotics have become an increasingly indispensable solution to protect food-producing animals from disease endangerments, either prophylactically or therapeutically, and avoid economic losses. Unfortunately, the use of huge amounts of antibiotics can result in the presence of their residues, and adverse effects on consumers and the environment. Antibiotic residues in the tissues of animals have raised several safety questions regarding allergenic potential, toxic effects (neurotoxicity, hepatotoxicity, nephrotoxicity, genotoxic effects and arthrotoxicity) and, more alarming, the development of antimicrobial resistance [4–9]. In addition, more than 70% of the antibiotics applied are then excreted into the environment via urine and feces [10]. The residual antibiotics in the environment may lead to potentially negative impacts on nontarget organisms, contamination of food and drinking water, and increase antibiotic resistance [11]. Because of long-term antibiotic use during animal breeding, antibiotic resistance has markedly increased in recent decades, which currently has become one of the most serious threats to human health [12–14].

Fluoroquinolones are a group of antibiotics exhaustively used in human and veterinary medicine, and act by inhibiting bacterial DNA gyrase and/or topoisomerase IV. After administration, fluoroquinolones exhibit rapid absorption with wide tissue dissemination and are excreted through urine and bile [15]. Usually, higher concentrations of drug residues are found in the liver and kidney, considering that the hepatobiliary system and the kidneys are the main routes by which drugs and their metabolites leave the body [16]. Owing to fluoroquinolones' lipophilic characteristics, they possess a long half-life, and their metabolization is slow [17]. Fluoroquinolone residues can pose health hazards to consumers, and cause joint injury and allergic reactions, inducing unscheduled DNA synthesis, DNA strand breakage, and chromosome damage [15,18]. Furthermore, fluoroquinolone-resistance bacterial strains have been widely reported [6,19]. Many studies demonstrated that the resistant strains of *Campylobacter* spp., *Salmonella* spp., and *Escherichia coli* toward fluoroquinolones have been positively correlated with their use in animal production [20–22]. There is a high risk of transmitting these resistant strains to humans via the food chain, which makes infections difficult to treat [5].

Enrofloxacin is one of the most commonly used fluoroquinolone drugs in food-producing animals, and one of its major metabolites, ciprofloxacin is often found in animal tissue [4,23]. Although enrofloxacin has not been approved for use in poultry in the United States, it is extensively used in Latin America, Asia, and the European Union [4,6]. To standardize the use of enrofloxacin and ensure its residual concentration in animal-derived foods at an acceptable level, China has established a maximum residue level (MRL), which is calculated as the sum of enrofloxacin and ciprofloxacin. In poultry and pig, the defined MRLs are 100, 200, and 300 µg/kg for muscle, liver, and kidney tissues, respectively [24]. It is noteworthy that the withdrawal periods of 8 days for chicken and 10 days for pigs were enough to decrease the levels of enrofloxacin and ciprofloxacin below the permitted MRLs [25]. However, a longer time is needed from the last administration until residues are no longer detected. Moreover, for fluoroquinolone drugs without MRLs, a zero-tolerance principle applies. For example, norfloxacin, ofloxacin, pefloxacin, and lomefloxacin are used in human medicine, but are not allowed as veterinary medicine in food-producing animals in China [26].

In light of the above, monitoring and assessing dietary exposure risk to fluoroquinolone residues are essential to ensure the safety of the animal-based foods available to consumers. Several studies have reported fluoroquinolone residue levels in chicken or/and pork from other countries [4,27–34]. However, so far, limited information on the occurrence and exposure assessment of fluoroquinolone residues in chicken and pork in China is available.

The primary goal of the present work was to investigate the occurrence and exposure risk of fluoroquinolone residues in chicken and pork in China. A national survey was conducted and 1754 chicken and 1712 pork samples were collected from 25 provinces across China. The presence and levels of six common fluoroquinolones were acquired using ultra-high performance liquid chromatography-tandem mass spectrometry (UPLC–MS/MS). Additionally, the residual levels acquired were further combined with food consumption data so as to estimate the exposure of fluoroquinolone residues to the consumers in China, and the potential health risks were conducted. To the best of our knowledge, this is the first comprehensive study on the occurrence and risk assessment of fluoroquinolones in chicken and pork in China.

2. Results and Discussion

2.1. Occurrence of Fluoroquinolone Residues in Chicken and Pork

The occurrence and residue levels of six fluoroquinolones in chicken and pork are summarized in Table 1. Overall, the detection frequencies of these antibiotics were 3.99% and 1.69% in chicken and pork samples, respectively. The overall violation frequencies of exceeding MRLs and misusing banned antibiotics in samples were 0.68% and 0.41% for chicken and pork. It can be easily seen that the occurrence and levels of fluoroquinolone residues in chicken were higher than those in pork in China.

Table 1. Occurrence and residue levels of the selected antibiotics and their MRLs.

Antibiotic	Chicken (n = 1754)					Pork (n = 1712)				
	DF (n, %)	Mean (µg/kg)	Min (µg/kg)	Max (µg/kg)	VF (m, %)	DF (n, %)	Mean (µg/kg)	Min (µg/kg)	Max (µg/kg)	VF (m, %)
Enrofloxacin	59, 3.36	2.07	3.05	1280	-	25, 1.46	0.74	4.81	529	-
Ciprofloxacin	20, 1.14	0.20	3.88	45.3	-	13, 0.76	0.14	3.88	89.9	-
Ciprofloxacin + Enrofloxacin	67, 3.82	2.26	3.05	1280	9, 0.51	26, 1.52	0.88	4.81	618.9	4, 0.23
Ofloxacin	1, 0.06	0.05	92.6	92.6	1, 0.06	5, 0.29	0.65	3.48	848	5, 0.29
Norfloxacin	0, 0.00	<LOD	<LOD	<LOD	0, 0.00	0, 0.00	<LOD	<LOD	<LOD	0, 0.00
Pefloxacin	0, 0.00	<LOD	<LOD	<LOD	0, 0.00	0, 0.00	<LOD	<LOD	<LOD	0, 0.00
Lomefloxacin	2, 0.11	0.01	10.5	10.8	2, 0.11	0, 0.00	<LOD	<LOD	<LOD	0, 0.00
Fluoroquinolones	70, 3.99	-	-	-	12, 0.68	29, 1.69	-	-	-	7, 0.41

Abbreviations: DF, detection frequency; VF, violation frequency; Mean, mean concentration; Min, minimum concentration; Max, maximum concentration; ND, non-detectable, NA, not available; not calculated; LOD, limits of detection.

It was found that the detection frequency of enrofloxacin was the highest among all the individual fluoroquinolones, followed by ciprofloxacin, in both pork and chicken (Table 1). In chicken, enrofloxacin occurred with a detection frequency of 3.36%, a mean concentration of 2.07 µg/kg, and a maximum concentration of 1280 µg/kg. In contrast, ciprofloxacin occurred with a lower detection frequency of 1.14%, a mean concentration of 0.20 µg/kg, and a maximum concentration of 45.3 µg/kg. A sum of enrofloxacin and ciprofloxacin residue was detected in 3.82% of chicken samples. In pork, enrofloxacin was detected in 25 samples (1.46%) with a mean concentration of 0.74 µg/kg and a maximum concentration of 529 µg/kg, and ciprofloxacin was found in 13 samples (0.76%), with a mean concentration of 0.14 µg/kg and a maximum concentration of 89.9 µg/kg. Enrofloxacin and/or ciprofloxacin were detected in 1.52% of pork samples. Moreover, 9 chicken samples (0.51%) and 4 pork samples (0.23%) exceeded the MRL of 100 µg/kg for the sum of enrofloxacin and ciprofloxacin (Table 1), which might result from inadequate withdrawal periods before slaughter, and/or inappropriate dosage [35].

Because ciprofloxacin is a primary metabolite of enrofloxacin, the amount of ciprofloxacin increases according to the dose and duration of enrofloxacin administration. In this study, enrofloxacin and ciprofloxacin were simultaneously detected in 12 chicken and 12 pork samples, and concentrations of the two fluoroquinolones were compared in Figure 1. Almost all of the concentrations detected of enrofloxacin were high than ciprofloxacin except for one sample that the detection values of enrofloxacin and ciprofloxacin were 17.1 and 19.7 µg/kg, respectively. This result was in accordance with those of studies on pharmacokinetic in poultry and pigs, in which the concentrations of ciprofloxacin were lower than those of the parent drug enrofloxacin in the muscle after treated with enrofloxacin [36–39].

Meanwhile, we also detected prohibited fluoroquinolones in samples (Table 1). Ofloxacin was detected in one chicken sample with a concentration of 92.6 µg/kg, and in five pork samples with a maximum concentration of 848 µg/kg, respectively. Lomefloxacin was present in two chicken samples with a maximum concentration of 10.8 µg/kg. It is noteworthy that those prohibited fluoroquinolones were also detected in livestock and poultry products from some provinces of China in recent years, such as Shanghai [23], Fujian [40], and Xinjiang [41]. These results demonstrated that the illegal use of antibiotics still existed.

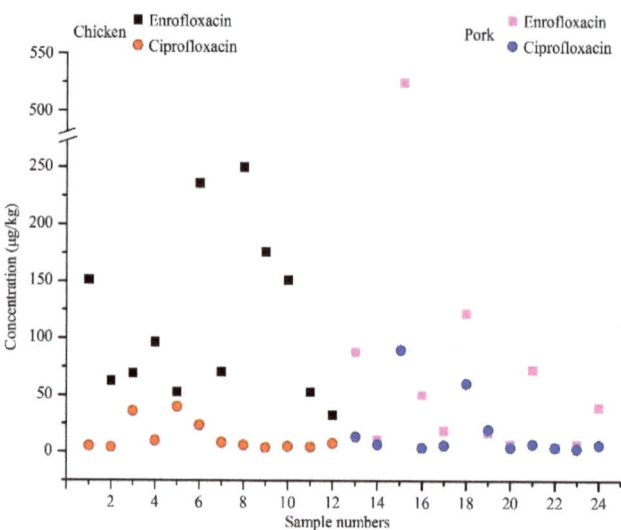

Figure 1. Concentrations of enrofloxacin and ciprofloxacin in the chicken and pork samples with the two fluoroquinolones detected simultaneously.

2.2. Occurrence of Fluoroquinolone Residues in Different Regions

The regional distribution of fluoroquinolone residues in chicken and pork can be observed in Figure 1. The red (Figure 2A) and green (Figure 2B) coloring illustrate the detection frequencies of fluoroquinolone residues in chicken and pork, respectively, with darker colors representing higher detection frequency. In addition, the blanks indicate missing data. In chicken, Yunnan (35.00%) presented the highest detection frequency of fluoroquinolone, followed by Liaoning (10.00%), Fujian (8.33%), and Zhejiang (7.23%). The occurrence of fluoroquinolones in pork was lower than that in chicken with the exception of Anhui, Beijing, Guangdong, Henan, and Shaanxi. The provinces with higher detection frequencies in pork were mainly Henan (11.11%), Tianjing (4.29%), Shaanxi (4.23%), and Guangdong (4.05%). One should note that no antibiotics were detected in pork and chicken in Hubei, Jilin, Jiangsu, and Jiangxi. This study indicated that the occurrence of fluoroquinolone residues in chicken and pork varied considerably among different regions. Chicken in Yunnan and pork in Henan should be given more attention. It is necessary to strengthen the monitoring by expanding sample size in key provinces.

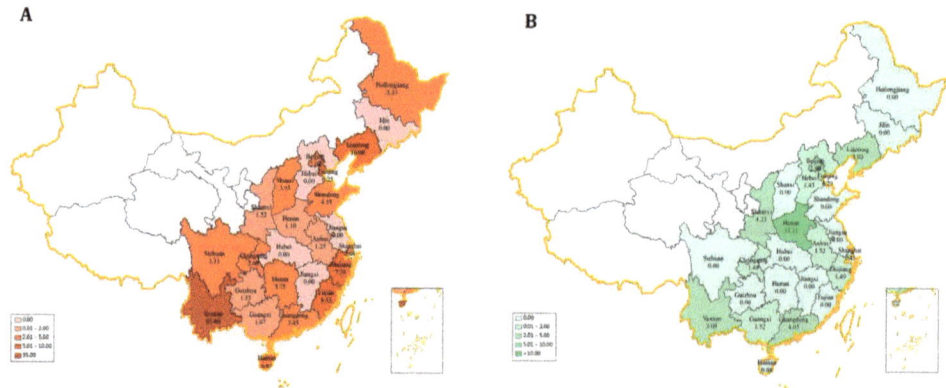

Figure 2. Occurrence of fluoroquinolone residues in different provinces (%). (**A**) chicken; (**B**) pork.

2.3. Occurrence of Fluoroquinolone Residues in Different Sampling Site Types

Table 2 shows the difference in fluoroquinolone residue occurrence between sampling site types. Regarding the samples from country fairs, fluoroquinolones were detected in 4.47% and 1.88% of the chicken and pork, respectively, and violation frequencies were 0.98% and 0.22%. Concerning samples from stores, fluoroquinolones were found in 3.46% and 1.48% of chicken and pork, respectively, and violation frequencies were 0.36% and 0.62%. Although there were higher detection frequencies in samples from country fairs, the results of statistical analysis showed that there was no significant difference in fluoroquinolone contaminations of chicken and pork between country fairs and stores ($p > 0.05$).

Table 2. Occurrence of fluoroquinolone residues in country fairs and stores.

Sampling Site Types	Chicken		Pork	
	DF [a]	VF [b]	DF [c]	VF [d]
Country fairs	4.47% (41/917)	0.98% (9/917)	1.88% (17/903)	0.22% (2/903)
Stores	3.46% (29/837)	0.36% (3/837)	1.48% (12/809)	0.62% (5/809)

Abbreviations: DF, detection frequency; VF, violation frequency; [a] Within a column, there was no significant difference ($\chi^2 = 1.157$, $p = 0.282$, $p > 0.05$). [b] Within a column, there was no significant difference ($\chi^2 = 2.500$, $p = 0.114$, $p > 0.05$). [c] Within a column, there was no significant difference ($\chi^2 = 0.409$, $p = 0.523$, $p > 0.05$). [d] Within a column, there was no significant difference ($\chi^2 = 0.818$, $p = 0.366$, $p > 0.05$).

2.4. Comparison with Other Studies

The findings of this study were further compared to some of the data presented in other studies regarding the measurement of quinolones or fluoroquinolones in chicken meat. In a previous study, a total of 127 chicken meat samples were studied to detect quinolones from Ankara, Turkey, where 45.7% of samples were positive for quinolones and the mean level of quinolones was found to be 30.81 µg/kg [42]. In other studies, data on the occurrence of enrofloxacin or/and ciprofloxacin in chicken were found for Portugal [4,27], Indonesia [28], Korea [29], Lebanon [30], Sri Lanka [31], South Africa [32], and Vietnam [33], with a detected frequency in the range of 4.2–51.9% and 5.17–67.3%, respectively, which was higher than that observed in our study (3.36% and 1.14%). This result indicated that these antibiotics are widely used in the world. Moreover, there is a huge difference in the enrofloxacin and ciprofloxacin residues among different countries. For example, enrofloxacin was detected in Sri Lanka at a higher frequency of 51.9% compared to ciprofloxacin (7.0%) [31]. Similarly, seven (12.1%) of the chicken meat samples were positive for enrofloxacin, but only three (5.2%) of the chicken meat samples were positive for ciprofloxacin in Korea [29]. On the contrary, the detection frequencies of enrofloxacin residues were found to be lower than that of ciprofloxacin in chicken samples in Indonesia (41.8% and 67.3%), Lebanon (12.5% and 32.5%), and Portugal (51.0% and 60.4%) [4,28,30].

To our knowledge, there are only two reports on the residues of enrofloxacin and ciprofloxacin in pork. Ciprofloxacin residues were detected at mean concentrations of 315.30 µg/kg in 28 out of 80 pork samples collected from open markets in Ibadan, Nigeria [34]. Another study showed that enrofloxacin and ciprofloxacin were not detected in 19 pork samples in Shanghai, China [23].

Norfloxacin was found in 11.1% of the chicken samples from school canteens in Portugal, whereas it was not found in samples from supermarkets from 2013–2015 [4]. However, also in Portugal, 16% of the supermarket samples showed contamination with norfloxacin in 2010 [27]. The highest detection frequency for norfloxacin was observed in Nigeria, with 55 and 30% in chicken and pork, respectively [34]. Another study showed that the detection frequency for norfloxacin in chicken in Lebanon was 5%; furthermore, ofloxacin and lomefloxacin were detected at a frequency of 18.75% and 7.5% [30]. These studies reported a higher occurrence of the prohibited fluoroquinolones than that in our study.

Although there were lower occurrences and levels of fluoroquinolone residue frequencies in chicken and pork meat in this study, the high frequencies of fluoroquinolone contaminations were found in other meat in China, such as beef, mutton, and fish. Zhang et al.

analyzed 22 cattle muscle and 24 sheep muscle samples obtained from southern Xinjiang of China and found fluoroquinolone residue rates up to 63.64% and 62.50% [41]. Wang et al. reported detection frequencies of fluoroquinolones as 58.5% in fish from a total of 53 samples in Shanghai, China [23]. In addition, high detection frequencies for some prohibited fluoroquinolones were also observed in those studies, such as norfloxacin (18.18% in cattle muscle and 29.17% in sheep muscle) and ofloxacin (15.1% in fish). These results suggest that a national survey of fluoroquinolone residues in other animal-derived foods should be conducted in the future.

2.5. Risk Assessment

In general, risk assessment is the systematic characterization of potential adverse effects caused by exposure to hazardous agents. Dietary exposure assessment study is an important step for risk assessment procedure [43]. In our work, dietary exposure assessment of fluoroquinolones was performed using the residue levels of the fluoroquinolones in meat and food consumption of target specific groups of the population, including children, adolescents and adults. As norfloxacin and pefloxacin were not detected in chicken or pork, this study only estimated the dietary exposure to the other four fluoroquinolones.

The results are summarized In Table 3. Regarding chicken and pork, the average EDIs of the four individual fluoroquinolones ranged from 0.003 to 0.965 ng/kg bw/day and from 0.155 to 1.328 ng/kg bw/day in all population groups, respectively. Although the residue levels of enrofloxacin and ciprofloxacin were higher in chicken than those in pork, and the exposure values of the two antibiotics in chicken were lower, owing to higher consumption of pork. The average EDIs for the sum of consumption of chicken and pork ranged from 0.003 to 2.633 ng/kg bw/day, while the EDIs in the worst-case scenario ranged from 2.8 to 1707.0 ng/kg bw/day, which was an extremely conservative estimation. In addition, we could clearly observe that the EDI values of each antibiotic in different age groups of the population followed the order of children > adolescents > adults, and all EDIs for children were ~70% higher than those for adults. This indicated that young consumers were more susceptible to various residues than adults [4,44]. Therefore, systematic exposure of antibiotics even in low concentrations, especially in early life, may have a negative impact in human health [43].

Table 3. Estimated daily exposure and risk assessment of fluoroquinolones in chicken and pork.

Sample	Antibiotic	Average Scenario Approach						Worst-Case Scenario Approach					
		Children		Adolescents		Adult		Children		Adolescents		Adult	
		EDI (ng/kg bw/day)	% ADI ($\times 10^{-2}$)	EDI (ng/kg bw/day)	% ADI ($\times 10^{-2}$)	EDI (ng/kg bw/day)	% ADI ($\times 10^{-2}$)	EDI (ng/kg bw/day)	% ADI	EDI (ng/kg bw/day)	% ADI	EDI (ng/kg bw/day)	% ADI
Chicken	Ciprofloxacin	0.965	-	0.664	-	0.538	-	596.8	-	410.8	-	332.8	-
	Enrofloxacin	0.093	-	0.064	-	0.052	-	21.1	-	14.5	-	11.8	-
	Ciprofloxacin + Enrofloxacin	1.054	1.70	0.725	1.17	0.588	0.95	596.8	9.62	410.8	6.62	332.8	5.37
	Lomefloxacin	0.005	-	0.003	-	0.003	-	5.0	-	3.5	-	2.8	-
	Ofloxacin	0.023	-	0.016	-	0.013	-	43.2	-	29.7	-	24.1	-
Pork	Ciprofloxacin	1.328	-	0.880	-	0.819	-	949.0	-	629.1	-	585.4	-
	Enrofloxacin	0.251	-	0.166	-	0.155	-	161.3	-	106.9	-	99.5	-
	Ciprofloxacin + Enrofloxacin	1.579	2.55	1.046	1.69	0.974	1.57	1110.2	17.91	736	11.87	684.9	11.05
	Lomefloxacin	ND	-	ND	-	ND	-	ND	-	ND	-	ND	-
	Ofloxacin	1.166	-	0.773	-	0.719	-	1521.2	-	1008.5	-	938.4	-
Chicken + Pork	Ciprofloxacin	2.293	-	1.544	-	1.357	-	1545.8	-	1039.9	-	918.2	-
	Enrofloxacin	0.344	-	0.230	-	0.207	-	182.4	-	121.4	-	111.3	-
	Ciprofloxacin + Enrofloxacin	2.633	4.25	1.771	2.86	1.562	2.52	1707.0	27.53	1146.8	18.50	1017.7	16.41
	Lomefloxacin	0.005	-	0.003	-	0.003	-	5.0	-	3.5	-	2.8	-
	Ofloxacin	1.189	-	0.789	-	0.732	-	1564.4	-	1038.2	-	962.5	-

Due to the lack of health guidance value, it was not possible to undertake risk characterization of ofloxacin and lomefloxacin. The acceptable daily intake (ADI) of enrofloxacin (6.2 μg/kg bw/day) set by China [24] was used for risk characterization of enrofloxacin and its metabolite ciprofloxacin. Considering the consumption of chicken and pork, the

%ADI values in the average scenario were 4.25×10^{-2}, 2.86×10^{-2}, and 2.52×10^{-2} for children, adolescents, and adults, respectively, which indicated a low health risk. Using the worst-case scenario approach, the consumption of chicken and pork accounted for 16.41–27.53% of the ADI, suggesting that the exposure risk is still acceptable for different age groups of the Chinese population.

Nevertheless, in the present study, other food items that might contain fluoroquinolones, such as beef, fish, lamb, and eggs, were not considered. Further evaluation of dietary exposure to fluoroquinolones should be conducted. Furthermore, those drug residues in food may lead to the development of bacterial resistance to human antibiotics, even if the contaminant concentration is low [3]. Consequently, continuous monitoring and risk assessment for fluoroquinolones in animal food is still greatly needed.

3. Materials and Methods

3.1. Sample Collection and Preparation

A total of 1754 raw chicken samples and 1712 raw pork samples were randomly collected from stores and country fairs located in 25 provinces (Anhui, Beijing, Fujian, Guangdong, Guangxi, Guizhou, Hainan, Hebei, Henan, Heilongjiang, Hubei, Hunan, Jilin, Jiangsu, Jiangxi, Liaoning, Shandong, Shanxi, Shaanxi, Shanghai, Sichuan, Tianjin, Yunnan, Zhejiang, and Chongqing) across China in 2019. These samples were later subjected to grinding in a laboratory blender and stored at $-18\ °C$ until the extraction procedure.

3.2. Chemicals and Reagents

The standards of six fluoroquinolones, enrofloxacin, ciprofloxacin, ofloxacin, norfloxacin, pefloxacin, and lomefloxacin were of high purity grade (>95%) and purchased from Sigma-Aldrich (St. Louis, MO, USA) and Dr. Ehrenstorfer (Augsburg, Germany). Methanol and acetonitrile were of HPLC grade and purchased from Thermo Fisher (Thermo Fisher Scientific, Waltham, MA, USA) and J. T. Baker (Phillipsburg, NJ, USA). Formic acid was of HPLC grade and citrate, sodium hydrogen phosphate, and disodium ethylenediaminetetraacetate dihydrate (Na_2EDTA) were all analytical grade. Ultra-pure water was prepared using a Milli-Q system (Bedford, MA, USA).

3.3. Extraction Procedures

All samples from different regions were analyzed using a confirmatory UPLC–MS/MS method as described by Shao et al. in local laboratories with some minor modifications [45]. Briefly, 2.0 g of the samples were separately weighed into a 50 mL polypropylene centrifuge tube with a screw cap. Subsequently, 20 mL of EDTA-McIlvaine buffer (0.1 mol/L) was added to the tube, followed by vortex mixing for 1 min. The sample was ultrasonically extracted for 10 min at room temperature, and centrifuged at 10,000 rpm for 5 min. Afterward, the supernatant was subjected to solid-phase extraction on an OASIS HLB cartridge (200 mg, 6 mL; Waters, Milford, MA, USA). The cartridge was sequentially preconditioned with 6 mL of methanol and 6 mL of ultrapure water. Then, the extract was applied to the cartridge at a flow rate of 2–3 mL/min and washed with 2 mL of a mixture of methanol/water 5/95 (v/v). The analytes were eluted with 6 mL of methanol into a new centrifuge tube. The eluate was evaporated to dryness under a flow of nitrogen, and 1 mL of 0.1% formic acid was added. The reconstituted solution was filtered through 0.22 µm filters for analysis.

3.4. Instrumental Analysis

Analysis was performed by UPLC–MS/MS system using an ACQUITY UPLC BEH C18 column (100 mm × 2.1 mm, 1.7 µm, Waters, Dublin, Ireland) at a flow rate of 0.2 mL/min; the column temperature was kept at 40 °C. The mobile phases consisted of 40% (v/v) methanol/acetonitrile (A) and 0.2% (v/v) formic acid solution (B). A gradient elution program was used: It started with 10% A; increased linearly to 30% A from 0 to 6.0 min; increased linearly to 50% A from 6.0 to 9.0 min; and increased linearly to 100% A from 9.0 to 9.5 min; kept at 100% A for 1.0 min, returned to the initial conditions at 11 min. The run time was 15 min for each injection.

MS/MS acquisition was performed using electrospray ionization (ESI) in positive ion mode, and multiple reaction monitoring (MRM) mode was used to quantitatively determine. The source temperature and desolvation temperature were 110 and 350 °C, respectively. The capillary voltage was 2.0 kV. Mass parameters of six fluoroquinolones are shown in Table 4.

Table 4. UPLC–MS/MS parameters for six fluoroquinolones.

Antibiotic	Formula	Parention (m/z)	Daughter Ion (m/z)	Cone Voltage (V)	Collision Energy (eV)
Ciprofloxacin	$C_{17}H_{18}N_3FO_3$	332.2	314.3 */288.3	36/36	19/17
Enrofloxacin	$C_{19}H_{22}FN_3O_3$	360.3	316.4 */342.3	38/38	19/23
Lomefloxacin	$C_{17}H_{19}F_2N_3O_3$	352.3	265.2 */308.3	36/36	23/17
Norfloxacin	$C_{16}H_{18}FN_3O_3$	320.3	302.3 */276.3	50/50	19/17
Ofloxacin	$C_{18}H_{20}FN_3O_4$	362.2	318.3 */261.2	38/38	18/27
Pefloxacin	$C_{17}H_{20}FN_3O_3$	334.3	290.3 */233.2	38/38	17/25

* Quantitative ion.

3.5. Quality Control and Quality Assurance

For each batch of 10~15 samples, one blank control and one matrix-spiked sample were analyzed. The mean recovery rates for all target analytes in the sample spiked were in the range of 75–125% with a relative standard deviation (RSD) of <20%. Linearity was confirmed on the basis of correlation coefficients $R^2 > 0.990$ for all analytes. The limits of detection and quantitation (LOQ) were regarded as the concentrations that produced a signal-to-noise (S/N) ratio of 3 and 10, respectively, which were estimated from the matrix-spiked sample with the lowest fortification level for the individual analyte. The LODs and LOQs of the six fluoroquinolones were 3 and 10 µg/kg, respectively.

3.6. Statistical Analysis

All statistical analysis was performed using R statistical software (Version 4.1.1, R Core Team). The chi-square test and *t*-test were applied to test for differences. Results with a *p*-value of <0.05 were considered significant.

3.7. Risk Assessment

To obtain comprehensive information about consumer exposure, the estimated daily intake (EDI) of antibiotics for children, adolescents, and adults was calculated according to the following Equation (1) [3].

$$\text{EDI} = \frac{C \times IR}{BW \times 1000} \qquad (1)$$

where C (µg/kg) is the content of the target fluoroquinolones in the chicken/pork samples. The mean and maximum concentrations of antibiotics were applied to set the average and the worst-case scenario [46], respectively. IR represents the daily consumption of meat for the population. According to the monitoring report on the nutrition and health status of Chinese residents from 2010 to 2013, the mean daily consumption of poultry/pork was 15.6/66.4, 17.3/64.1, and 13.8/53.1 g/day for an adult, 14–17 years for adolescents, and 7–10 years for children [47], respectively, which was used in this study. Finally, the term BW refers to the average body weight, which was 60 kg for adults, 53.9 kg for adolescents, and 29.6 kg for children [48,49].

The resulting dietary exposure estimate was then compared with the recommended ADI value obtained from toxicological assessments, as shown below the Equation (2):

$$\%ADI = \frac{EDI}{ADI} \times 100 \qquad (2)$$

when %ADI < 100, the risk is acceptable or low risk; otherwise, %ADI > 100 indicates an unacceptable risk [43,48].

4. Conclusions

In this study, the occurrence and exposure risk of fluoroquinolone residues in chicken and pork in China was investigated. On the whole, the levels of fluoroquinolone residues in chicken were higher than those in pork, with detection frequencies of 3.99% and 1.69%, respectively. It is clear that the detection frequencies and mean concentrations were found to be highest for enrofloxacin, followed by ciprofloxacin, both in chicken and pork. Moreover, we detected prohibited fluoroquinolones (ofloxacin and lomefloxacin) in samples. The violation frequencies of fluoroquinolones in chicken and pork were found to be 0.68% and 0.41%, respectively. Due to higher consumption of pork, the EDI of enrofloxacin and ciprofloxacin from pork was higher than that from chicken. All EDI values of enrofloxacin and ciprofloxacin (0.588 to 1707.0 ng/kg bw/day) were lower than the ADI. Although the results of the dietary risk assessment indicated an acceptable risk for enrofloxacin and ciprofloxacin from chicken and pork in the different age groups of China population, continuous residue monitoring and risk evaluation of fluoroquinolones in animal food should be increased.

Author Contributions: Conceptualization, J.G. and D.Y.; methodology, X.Y. and D.J.; visualization and software, Z.F.; formal analysis, J.G., Z.F. and S.S.; investigation, S.S. and J.G.; resources, D.Y.; data curation, X.Y. and D.J.; writing—original draft, Z.F.; writing—review and editing, J.G., Z.F. and D.Y.; supervision, S.S. and D.Y.; funding acquisition, J.G. All authors have read and agreed to the published version of the manuscript.

Funding: This study was supported by the National Key Research and Development Program of China (2019YFC1605703) and the National Natural Science Foundation of China (22193064).

Institutional Review Board Statement: Not applicable.

Informed Consent Statement: Not applicable.

Data Availability Statement: All of the data supporting this article are included in the main text.

Acknowledgments: The authors would like to thank all of the participants of this study and their great contributions.

Conflicts of Interest: The authors declare no conflict of interest.

References

1. Chang, Y.; Zhao, H.; Sun, L.; Cui, J.; Liu, J.; Tang, Q.; Du, F.; Liu, X.; Yao, D. Resource Utilization of Biogas Waste as Fertilizer in China Needs More Inspections Due to the Risk of Heavy Metals. *Agriculture* **2022**, *12*, 72. [CrossRef]
2. Shimokawa, S. Sustainable meat consumption in China. *J. Integr. Agric.* **2015**, *14*, 1023–1032. [CrossRef]
3. Griboff, J.; Carrizo, J.C.; Bonansea, R.I.; Valdés, M.E.; Wunderlin, D.A.; Amé, M.V. Multiantibiotic residues in commercial fish from Argentina. The presence of mixtures of antibiotics in edible fish, a challenge to health risk assessment. *Food Chem.* **2020**, *332*, 127380. [CrossRef]
4. Pereira, A.M.; Silva, L.J.; Rodrigues, J.; Lino, C.; Pena, A. Risk assessment of fluoroquinolones from poultry muscle consumption: Comparing healthy adult and pre-school populations. *Food Chem. Toxicol.* **2018**, *118*, 340–347. [CrossRef]
5. Bacanlı, M.; Başaran, N. Importance of antibiotic residues in animal food. *Food Chem. Toxicol.* **2019**, *125*, 462–466. [CrossRef]
6. Muaz, K.; Riaz, M.; Akhtar, S.; Park, S.; Ismail, A. Antibiotic residues in chicken meat: Global prevalence, threats, and decontamination strategies: A review. *J. Food Prot.* **2018**, *81*, 619–627. [CrossRef]
7. Bhogoju, S.; Nahashon, S. Recent Advances in Probiotic Application in Animal Health and Nutrition: A Review. *Agriculture* **2022**, *12*, 304. [CrossRef]
8. Arsène, M.; Davares, A.; Viktorovna, P.I.; Andreevna, S.L.; Sarra, S.; Khelifi, I.; Sergueïevna, D.M. The public health issue of antibiotic residues in food and feed: Causes, consequences, and potential solutions. *Vet. World* **2022**, *15*, 662–671. [CrossRef]
9. Falagas, M.E.; Rizos, M.; Bliziotis, I.A.; Rellos, K.; Kasiakou, S.K.; Michalopoulos, A. Toxicity after prolonged (more than four weeks) administration of intravenous colistin. *BMC. Infect. Dis.* **2005**, *5*, 1. [CrossRef]
10. Zhang, L.; Shen, L.; Qin, S.; Cui, J.; Liu, Y. Quinolones antibiotics in the Baiyangdian Lake, China: Occurrence, distribution, predicted no-effect concentrations (PNECs) and ecological risks by three methods. *Environ. Pollut.* **2020**, *256*, 113458. [CrossRef]

11. Zhang, Q.; Ying, G.; Pan, C.; Liu, Y.; Zhao, J. Comprehensive evaluation of antibiotics emission and fate in the river basins of china: Source analysis, multimedia modeling, and linkage to bacterial resistance. *Environ. Sci. Technol.* **2015**, *49*, 6772–6782. [CrossRef] [PubMed]
12. Qiao, M.; Ying, G.G.; Singer, A.C.; Zhu, Y.G. Review of antibiotic resistance in China and its environment. *Environ. Int.* **2018**, *110*, 160–172. [CrossRef] [PubMed]
13. Bortolotte, A.R.; Daniel, D.; Reyes, F.G.R. Occurrence of antimicrobial residues in tilapia (*Oreochromis niloticus*) fillets produced in Brazil and available at the retail market. *Food Res. Int.* **2021**, *140*, 109865. [CrossRef] [PubMed]
14. Zhang, L.; Fu, Y.; Xiong, Z.; Ma, Y.; Wei, Y.; Qu, X.; Zhang, H.; Zhang, J.; Liao, M.; Fu, Y. Highly prevalent multidrug-resistant Salmonella from chicken and pork meat at retail markets in Guangdong, China. *Front. Microbiol.* **2018**, *9*, 2104. [CrossRef]
15. Gouvêa, R.; Dos Santos, F.F.; De Aquino, M.H.C. Fluoroquinolones in industrial poultry production, bacterial resistance and food residues: A review. *Braz. J. Poult. Sci.* **2015**, *17*, 1–10. [CrossRef]
16. Montfoort, J.V.; Hagenbuch, B.; Groothuis, G.; Koepsell, H.; Meier, P.; Meijer, D. Drug uptake systems in liver and kidney. *Curr. Drug Metab.* **2003**, *4*, 185–211. [CrossRef]
17. Teglia, C.M.; Guiñez, M.; Culzoni, M.J.; Cerutti, S. Determination of residual enrofloxacin in eggs due to long term administration to laying hens. Analysis of the consumer exposure assessment to egg derivatives. *Food Chem.* **2021**, *351*, 129279. [CrossRef]
18. Khadra, A.; Pinelli, E.; Lacroix, M.Z.; Bousquet-Mélou, A.; Hamdi, H.; Merlina, G.; Guiresse, M.; Hafidi, M. Assessment of the genotoxicity of quinolone and fluoroquinolones contaminated soil with the Vicia faba micronucleus test. *Ecotoxicol. Environ. Saf.* **2012**, *76*, 187–192. [CrossRef]
19. Barton, M.D. Antibiotic use in animal feed and its impact on human healt. *Nutr. Res. Rev.* **2000**, *13*, 279–299. [CrossRef]
20. Griggs, D.J.; Johnson, M.M.; Frost, J.A.; Humphrey, T.; Jørgensen, F.; Piddock, L.J. Incidence and mechanism of ciprofloxacin resistance in *Campylobacter* spp. isolated from commercial poultry flocks in the United Kingdom before, during, and after fluoroquinolone treatment. *Antimicrob. Agents Chemother.* **2005**, *49*, 699–707. [CrossRef]
21. European Food Safety Authority. The European Union Summary Report on antimicrobial resistance in Antimicrobial resistance in zoonotic and indicator bacteria from humans, animals and food in 2011. *EFSA J.* **2013**, *11*, 3196. [CrossRef]
22. Joint Inter-agency Antimicrobial Consumption and Resistance Analysis. ECDC/EFSA/EMA second joint report on the integrated analysis of the consumption of antimicrobial agents and occurrence of antimicrobial resistance in bacteria from humans and food-producing animals. *EFSA J.* **2017**, *15*, 7. [CrossRef]
23. Wang, H.; Ren, L.; Yu, X.; Hu, J.; Chen, Y.; He, G.; Jiang, Q. Antibiotic residues in meat, milk and aquatic products in Shanghai and human exposure assessment. *Food Control* **2017**, *80*, 217–225. [CrossRef]
24. GB 31650-2019; Maximum Residue Limits for Veterinary Drugs in Foods. Ministry of Agriculture and Rural Affairs of the People's Republic of China: Beijing, China, 2019.
25. Chinese Veterinary Pharmacopoeia Committee. *Veterinary Pharmacopoeia of the People's Republic of China: Version 2020*; China Agricultural Press: Beijing, China, 2021; ISBN 9787109275881.
26. Ministry of Agriculture and Rural Affairs of the People's Republic of China. 2292 Bulletin of the Ministry of Agriculture of the People's Republic of China. Available online: http://www.moa.gov.cn/nybgb/2015/jiuqi/201712/t20171219_6103873.htm (accessed on 6 May 2022).
27. Pena, A.; Silva, L.J.G.; Pereira, A.; Meisel, L.; Lino, C.M. Determination of fluoroquinolone residues in poultry muscle in Portugal. *Anal. Bioanal. Chem.* **2010**, *397*, 2615–2621. [CrossRef]
28. Widiastuti, R.; Martindah, E.; Anastasia, Y. Detection and Dietary Exposure Assessment of Fluoroquinolones Residues in Chicken Meat from the Districts of Malang and Blitar, Indonesia. *Trop. Anim. Sci. J.* **2022**, *45*, 98–103. [CrossRef]
29. Lee, H.J.; Cho, S.H.; Shin, D.; Kang, H.S. Prevalence of antibiotic residues and antibiotic resistance in isolates of chicken meat in Korea. *Korean J. Food Sci. Anim. Resour.* **2018**, *38*, 1055. [CrossRef]
30. Jammoul, A.; El Darra, N. Evaluation of Antibiotics Residues in Chicken Meat Samples in Lebanon. *Antibiotics* **2019**, *8*, 69. [CrossRef]
31. Karunarathna, N.B.; Perera, I.A.; Nayomi, N.T.; Munasinghe, D.M.S.; Silva, S.S.P.; Strashnov, I.; Fernando, B.R. Occurrence of enrofloxacin and ciprofloxacin residues in broiler meat sold in Sri Lanka. *J. Natn. Sci. Found. Sri Lanka* **2021**, *49*, 479–492. [CrossRef]
32. Ramatla, T.; Ngoma, L.; Adetunji, M.; Mwanza, M. Evaluation of Antibiotic Residues in Raw Meat Using Different Analytical Methods. *Antibiotics* **2017**, *6*, 34. [CrossRef]
33. Yamaguchi, T.; Okihashi, M.; Harada, K.; Konishi, Y.; Uchida, K.; Do, M.H.N.; Bui, H.D.; Nguyen, T.D.; Nguyen, P.D.; Chau, V.V.; et al. Antibiotic residue monitoring results for pork, chicken, and beef samples in Vietnam in 2012–2013. *J. Agric. Food Chem.* **2015**, *63*, 5141–5145. [CrossRef]
34. Omotoso, A.B.; Omojola, A.B. Fluoroquinolone residues in raw meat from open markets in Ibadan, Southwest, Nigeria. *Int. J. Health Anim. Sci. Food Saf.* **2015**, *2*, 32–40. [CrossRef]
35. Mehl, A.; Schmidt, L.J.; Schmidt, L.; Morlock, G.E. High-throughput planar solid-phase extraction coupled to orbitrap high-resolution mass spectrometry via the autoTLC-MS interface for screening of 66 multi-class antibiotic residues in food of animal origin. *Food Chem.* **2021**, *351*, 129211. [CrossRef] [PubMed]
36. Lei, Z.; Liu, Q.; Yang, B.; Xiong, J.; Li, K.; Ahmed, S.; Hong, L.; Chen, P.; He, Q.; Cao, J. Clinical efficacy and residue depletion of 10% enrofloxacin enteric-coated granules in pigs. *Front. Pharmacol.* **2017**, *8*, 294. [CrossRef] [PubMed]

37. Dimitrova, D.J.; Lashev, L.D.; Yanev, S.G.; Pandova, B. Pharmacokinetics of enrofloxacin in turkeys. *Res. Vet. Sci.* **2007**, *82*, 392–397. [CrossRef] [PubMed]
38. San Martín, B.; Cornejo, J.; Lapierre, L.; Iragüen, D.; Pérez, F.; Hidalgo, H.; Andre, F. Withdrawal time of four pharmaceutical formulations of enrofloxacin in poultry according to different maximum residues limits. *J. Vet. Pharmacol. Therap.* **2010**, *33*, 246–251. [CrossRef]
39. Schneider, M.J. Multiresidue analysis of fluoroquinolone antibiotics in chicken tissue using automated microdialysis-liquid chromatography. *J. Chromatogr. Sci.* **2001**, *39*, 351–356. [CrossRef]
40. Yang, Y.; Qiu, W.; Li, Y.; Liu, L. Antibiotic residues in poultry food in Fujian Province of China. *Food Addit. Contam. Part B* **2020**, *13*, 177–184. [CrossRef]
41. Zhang, Y.; Lu, J.; Yan, Y.; Liu, J.; Wang, M. Antibiotic residues in cattle and sheep meat and human exposure assessment in southern Xinjiang, China. *Food Sci. Nutr.* **2021**, *9*, 6152–6161. [CrossRef]
42. Er, B.; Onurdağ, F.K.; Demirhan, B.; Özgacar, S.Ö.; Öktem, A.B.; Abbasoğlu, U. Screening of quinolone antibiotic residues in chicken meat and beef sold in the markets of Ankara, Turkey. *Poult. Sci.* **2013**, *92*, 2212–2215. [CrossRef]
43. Kyriakides, D.; Lazaris, A.C.; Arsenoglou, K.; Emmanouil, M.; Kyriakides, O.; Kavantzas, N.; Panderi, I. Dietary Exposure Assessment of Veterinary Antibiotics in Pork Meat on Children and Adolescents in Cyprus. *Foods* **2020**, *9*, 1479. [CrossRef] [PubMed]
44. Sallam, K.I.; Saad, F.S.S.; Abdelkhalek, A. Health risk assessment of antimicrobial residues in sheep carcasses marketed in Kuwait. *Food Chem.* **2022**, *383*, 132401. [CrossRef] [PubMed]
45. Shao, B.; Jia, X.; Wu, Y.; Hu, J.; Tu, X.; Zhang, J. Multi-class confirmatory method for analyzing trace levels of tetracyline and quinolone antibiotics in pig tissues by ultra-performance liquid chromatography coupled with tandem mass spectrometry. *Rapid Commun. Mass Spectrom.* **2007**, *21*, 3487–3496. [CrossRef]
46. World Health Organization. Evaluation of Certain Veterinary Drug Residues in Food. Available online: http://apps.who.int/iris/bitstream/10665/42127/1/WHO_TRS_879.pdf (accessed on 6 May 2022).
47. Zhao, L.; He, Y. *The Monitoring Report on Nutrition and Health Status of Chinese Residents (2010–2013) No. 1 Dietary and Nutrient Intake*; People's Medical Publishing House: Beijing, China, 2018; p. 129, ISBN 9787117274333.
48. Liu, S.; Dong, G.; Zhao, H.; Chen, M.; Quan, W.; Qu, B. Occurrence and risk assessment of fluoroquinolones and tetracyclines in cultured fish from a coastal region of northern China. *Environ. Sci. Pollut. Res.* **2018**, *25*, 8035–8043. [CrossRef] [PubMed]
49. Fang, H.; Zhao, L.; Guo, Q.; Ju, L.; Xu, X.; Li, S.; Pu, W.; Cheng, X.; Yu, W.; Yu, D. Trends of Height, Weight and BMI in Chinese Children and Adolescents Aged 6~17. *Food Nutr. China* **2021**, *27*, 16–20.

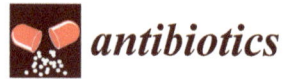

Article

Identification of a Novel IncHI1B Plasmid in MDR *Klebsiella pneumoniae* 200 from Swine in China

Huixian Liang [1], Xinhui Li [2] and He Yan [1,3,*]

1. School of Food Science and Engineering, South China University of Technology, Guangzhou 510641, China
2. Department of Microbiology, University of Wisconsin-La Crosse, La Crosse, WI 54601, USA
3. Guangdong Province Key Laboratory for Green Processing of Natural Products and Product Safety, Guangzhou 510641, China
* Correspondence: yanhe@scut.edu.cn; Tel.: +86-20-87113848

Abstract: Multidrug-resistant (MDR) *Klebsiella pneumoniae* poses a seriously threat to public health. The aim of this study was to better understand the genetic structure of its plasmids and chromosomes. The whole-genome sequence of *K. pneumoniae* 200 isolated from the liver of a swine with diarrhea in China was determined using PacBio RS II and Illumina MiSeq sequencing. The complete sequences of the chromosomal DNA and the plasmids were analyzed for the presence of resistance genes. The phylogenetic trees revealed that *K. pneumoniae* 200 displayed the closest relationship to a human-associated *K. pneumoniae* strain from Thailand. *K. pneumoniae* 200 contained two plasmids, pYhe2001 and pYhe2002, belonging to the incompatibility groups IncH-HI1B and IncF-FIA. The plasmid pYhe2001 was a novel plasmid containing four types of heavy metal resistance genes and a novel Tn6897 transposon flanked by two copies of IS26 at both ends. Mixed plasmids could be transferred from *K. pneumoniae* 200 to *Escherichia coli* DH5α through transformation together. This study reported the first time a novel plasmid pYhe2001 from swine origin *K. pneumoniae* 200, suggesting that the plasmids may act as reservoirs for various antimicrobial resistance genes and transport multiple resistance genes in *K. pneumoniae* of both animal and human origin.

Keywords: *Klebsiella pneumoniae*; plasmid; antibiotic resistance genes; whole genome sequencing

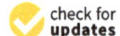

Citation: Liang, H.; Li, X.; Yan, H. Identification of a Novel IncHI1B Plasmid in MDR *Klebsiella pneumoniae* 200 from Swine in China. *Antibiotics* **2022**, *11*, 1225. https://doi.org/10.3390/antibiotics11091225

Academic Editors: Yongning Wu and Zhenling Zeng

Received: 9 August 2022
Accepted: 5 September 2022
Published: 9 September 2022

Publisher's Note: MDPI stays neutral with regard to jurisdictional claims in published maps and institutional affiliations.

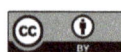

Copyright: © 2022 by the authors. Licensee MDPI, Basel, Switzerland. This article is an open access article distributed under the terms and conditions of the Creative Commons Attribution (CC BY) license (https://creativecommons.org/licenses/by/4.0/).

1. Introduction

Klebsiella pneumoniae, a gram-negative bacterium, is an opportunistic pathogen that can not only colonize the gastrointestinal tracts of healthy humans and animals [1] but also causes invasive diseases in swine [2]. With an increasing number of antibiotics used in livestock farms, *K. pneumoniae* has shown the ability to resist multiple antibiotics, even some last-resort ones (e.g., carbapenem and colistin) [3,4], commonly through acquiring preexisting resistance and virulence genes via plasmids and transposable elements [5].

Spread of resistance and virulence genes in *K. pneumoniae* can result from the conjugation or mobilization functions of plasmids. For example, hypervirulent *K. pneumoniae* from the sputum of an older male patient was found to harbor a $bla_{CTX-M-24}$ carrying an IncFII-type plasmid and a pK2044-like virulent plasmid isolated from blood of a patient with liver abscess and meningitis, due to plasmid conjugation [6]. Furthermore, other transposable elements, such as transposons, play an important role in the spread of resistance genes [5]. For example, the bla_{KPC} gene has been identified within a Tn3-family transposon, Tn4401, in clinical *K. pneumoniae* [7]. Moreover, antibiotic resistance genes could transfer between plasmids and chromosomes through transposable elements. For example, a multidrug-resistant *K. pneumoniae* CN1 from a patient was found to carry both $bla_{CTX-M-15}$ and bla_{KPC-2} genes in the chromosome with the $bla_{CTX-M-15}$ gene linked to an insertion sequence, IS*Ecp1*, and the bla_{KPC-2} gene in Tn4401a [8], while IS*Ecp1*-$bla_{CTX-M-15}$ and Tn4401a could be also found in plasmid pNY9_3 from *K. pneumoniae* NY9 and plasmid pCR14_3 from *K. pneumoniae* CR14, respectively.

Whole-genome sequencing (WGS) is rapidly becoming a powerful tool for identifying pathogenic features in *K. pneumoniae*, particularly for understanding the relative evolution of strains and the potential course of spread of mobile elements [9]. Through WGS, a previous study found that the megaplasmid in the *K. pneumoniae* isolate was a result of cointegration of an IncA/C2-type plasmid harboring $bla_{OXA-427}$ with an IncF1b-type plasmid [10].

So far, most studies have focused on clinical isolates by detecting emerging resistance genes, such as carbapenemase genes or mobile colistin resistance genes in *K. pneumoniae*. However, researchers have rarely aimed to identify genomic elements of isolates from animals in plasmids or in the chromosome of nonhypervirulence *K. pneumoniae*. In this study, we identified an MDR *K. pneumoniae* 200 isolate from swine liver with a novel IncHI1B plasmid and an IncFIA plasmid with the $bla_{CTX-M-27}$ gene, and investigated the mobile elements of *K. pneumoniae* to expand the understanding of MDR *K. pneumoniae*.

2. Results and Discussion

2.1. Characterization of K. pneumoniae 200

K. pneumoniae 200 exhibited resistance to β-lactams, aminoglycosides, florfenicol, streptomycin, quinolones, and sulfonamides (Table S1). The complete genome of *K. pneumoniae* 200 contained a circular 5,257,665 bp chromosome with a total of 5106 ORFs and G + C content of 58.78% and two plasmids: pYhe2001 (213,254 bp) with a total of 290 ORFs and GC content of 50.10% and pYhe2002 (75,320 bp) with a total of 107 ORFs and GC content of 51.65%. Multilocus sequence typing analysis showed that *K. pneumoniae* 200 belonged to sequence type 37 (ST37) [11,12].

2.2. Characterization of Chromosome of K. pneumoniae 200

There were 71 resistance genes and 65 virulence genes in the chromosome. Resistance genes identified in the chromosome included genes for β-lactamases, efflux pumps, quinolone, fosfomycin, multidrug resistance genes (mdtK, tolC, and acrAB), the multiple antibiotic resistance operon (marRA), and resistance to heavy metals (copper, silver, and arsenic). In *K. pneumoniae*, the best-characterized efflux pump systems include acrAB and mdtK complexes [13]. Furthermore, the multidrug efflux pump system (acrAB-tolC) in *K. pneumoniae* isolates was related to resistance to quinolones, tetracyclines, tigecycline, and β-lactams leading to MDR [14]. Overall, the combination of the acrAB-tolC and mdtK genes was strongly associated with the MDR function of K. pneumoniae. The more detailed features of the *K. pneumoniae* 200 genome are listed in Table S2.

Genome analyses revealed that T6SS components of *K. pneumoniae* 200 were highly similar (99% nucleotide sequence identity) to that of *K. pneumoniae* ZYST1 [15] (accession number CP031613): A main cluster and an auxiliary cluster were similar to those found in K. pneumoniae HS11286 and *K. pneumoniae* ZYST1 (Figure S1). Compared with strains HS11286 and ZYST1, the main T6SS cluster in *K. pneumoniae* 200 was conserved except for a portion of the effector and immunity genes and the paaR region. Furthermore, IS4 was found to be inserted upstream of the vipA gene in the main T6SS cluster. The auxiliary T6SS cluster also showed a conserved region and variable effector and immunity genes compared to strains HS11286 and ZYST1. BLASTN analyses revealed that there were protein homologs of the regulatory proteins TfoX and QstR as well as the competence proteins ComEA and ComEC in K. pneumoniae 200, suggesting the potential ability of uptaking genes and recombination consequences via the combination of natural competence and target cell killing mediated by T6SS [15]. The phylogenetic trees of all ST37 *K. pneumoniae* strains in GenBank revealed that the isolates from the same countries clustered on the same branches and were closely related (Figure 1). *K. pneumoniae* 200 branched from *K. pneumoniae* F10 (AN) from China and displayed the closest relationship to human-associated *K. pneumoniae* 4300STDY6470454 (UFHS01) from Thailand, suggesting that they may share a common origin.

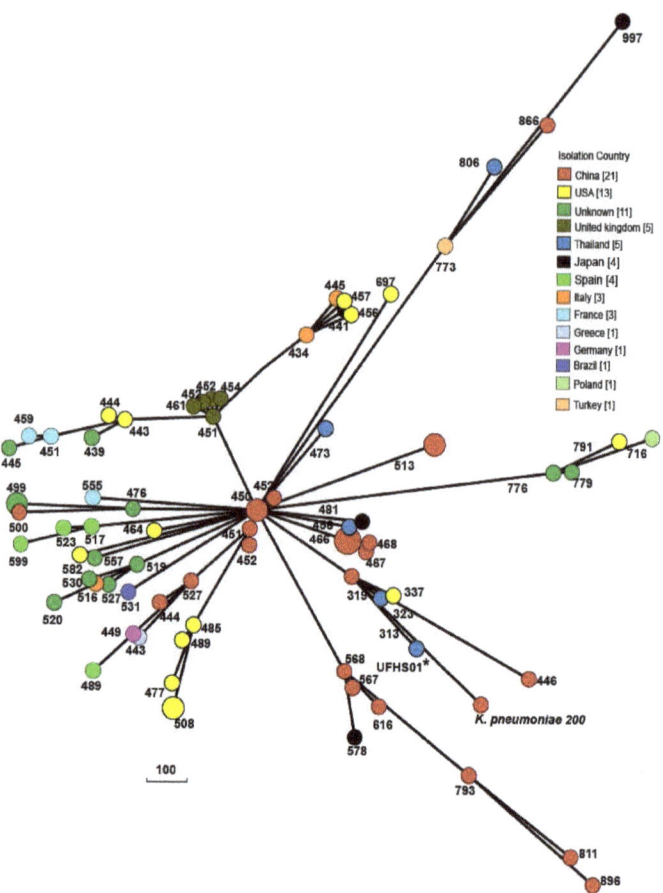

Figure 1. Phylogenetic trees of all ST37 K. pneumoniae strains of released public sequences based on cgMLST. The evolutionary distance showed that *K. pneumoniae* 200 was related to human-associated *K. pneumoniae* 4300STDY6470454 (UFHS01) from Thailand. The numbers indicate the number of allele differences between *K. pneumoniae* 200 and other isolates.

2.3. Characterization of Plasmids Carried by K. pneumoniae 200

K. pneumoniae 200 contained two plasmids, pYhe2001 and pYhe2002. The plasmid pYhe2002 belonged to the IncF type and contained IncFIA replicon: FIA. The IncF-type plasmids were narrow-host range plasmids that are frequently identified among *Enterobacteriaceae* strains, especially *K. pneumoniae* [16]. BLASTN comparison revealed that the backbone of pYhe2002 was highly similar (99% nucleotide sequence identity with a query coverage of 98%) to that of the plasmid p19110124-2 (accession number NZ_CP064179.1), which originated from a *K. pneumoniae* strain isolated from an anal swab of swine in China. Comparison of the plasmid sequence with the plasmid records in PLSDB [15,17,18] using mash dist with maximal *p* value and distance thresholds set to 0.1, showed a result with 681 hits (Table S3). The plasmids included in the hits were mostly from *K. pneumoniae* and the remaining plasmids were from other *Enterobacteriaceae* species (e.g., *Escherichia coli*, *Salmonella enterica*, and *Citrobacter freundii*). These plasmids were in isolates from humans (e.g., clinical patients), food (e.g., pork and milk), the environment (e.g., rivers and air), and animals (e.g., ducks, rabbits, chickens, and swine). The plasmid pYhe2002 contained antibiotic resistance genes *tetA*, *floR*, $bla_{CTX-M-27}$, *sul1*, *qnrB2*, $\Delta qacE$, *aadA16*, *dfrA27*, *arr-6*, and *aac(6′)-Ib-cr* (Figure S2). The IncF transmissible novel plasmid with $bla_{CTX-M-27}$ was identified as *E. coli* isolated from swine in China [19]. In a previous study, of the 24 IncF-type plasmids analyzed, 22 $bla_{CTX-M-27}$-carrying plasmids were identified in *E. coli* [20], suggesting that the backbone of the IncF plasmid may be a major transport for dissemination of the $bla_{CTX-M-27}$ gene. The expression of CTX-M β-lactamase genes were found commonly in *K. pneumoniae* strains all over the world. Many kinds of CTX-M allele were found, such as $bla_{CTX-M-55}$ [21], $bla_{CTX-M-63}$ [22], and $bla_{CTX-M-15}$ [23,24]. The predominant ESBL allele $bla_{CTX-M-15}$ was commonly detected in IncF plasmids from *K. pneumoniae* [23,24]. From the results of PLSDB, among the 681 hits, gene $bla_{CTX-M-27}$ could be found in plasmids carried by *K. pneumoniae* from different sources but not liver source (Table S3). This is the first report that an IncFIA plasmid with the $bla_{CTX-M-27}$ gene from swine liver *K. pneumoniae* isolate. The plasmid pYhe2002 carried a *sul1*-type class 1 integron that has a 5′CS and four cassettes, *aadA16-dfrA27-arr-6-aac(6′)-Ib-cr*, and 3′CS. The *sul1*-type class 1 integron was flanked by a gene for IS6 family transposase in the upstream and a gene encoding DUF4440 domain-containing protein, a gene encoding peptide ABC transport, and an IS91 family transposase gene in the downstream.

The plasmid pYhe2001 belonged to the IncH type and contains IncH replicon: HI1B. For comparison of the plasmid with plasmid records in PLSDB using mash dist with maximal *p* value and distance thresholds set to 0.1, the search resulted in 915 hits (Table S4). The plasmids included in the hits were mostly from *K. pneumoniae*, and the remaining plasmids were from other Enterobacteriaceae species (e.g., *Escherichia coli*, *Salmonella enterica*, and *Citrobacter freundii*). These plasmids were collected from humans (e.g., clinical patients), food (e.g., pork and milk), the environment (e.g., rivers and air), and animals (e.g., chickens and swine). Previous studies showed that the plasmids from *K. pneumoniae* shared more than 85% query coverage with plasmid records [15,25]. Combining BLASTN comparison with PLSDB, the backbone of these plasmids is currently lower than 80% query coverage of pYhe2001, suggesting that pYhe2001 is a novel plasmid. Figure 2 shows the four plasmids with the highest similarity compared with pYhe2001.

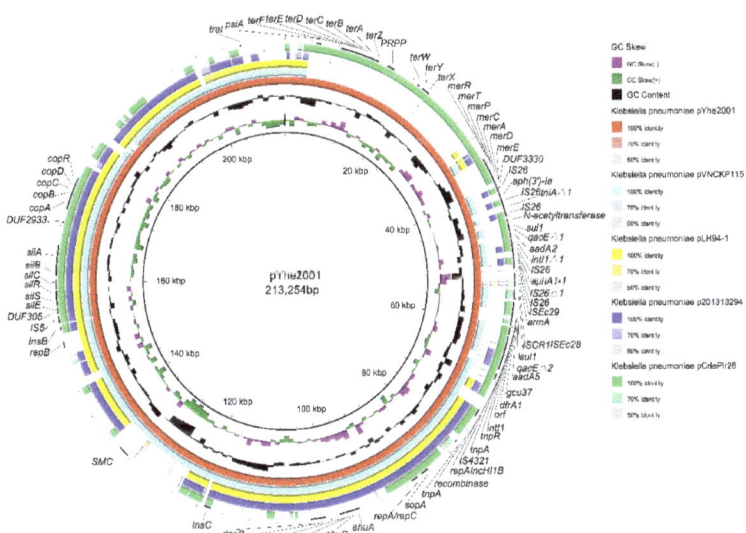

Figure 2. Comparisons of pYhe2001 complete genome sequences with NCBI-published complete plasmid sequences of another four *K. pneumoniae* strains using BRIG. The innermost circles represent the GC skew (purple/green) and GC content (black). Rings 1–5 represent *K. pneumoniae* pYhe2001, *K. pneumoniae* pVNCKp115, *K. pneumoniae* pLH94-1, *K. pneumoniae* p201313294, *K. pneumoniae* pCriePir26, respectively.

The plasmid pYhe2001 showed query coverage of 78% in the plasmid pVNCKp115 (accession number LC549807.1), a plasmid from a *K. pneumoniae* isolate in Vietnam. Compared with pVNCKp115, four types of heavy metal resistance genes and a novel transposon, Tn6897, were specific to the plasmid pYhe2001. The plasmid pYhe2001 consisted of partition (parB/parA), transfer (traI) functions, a 26.5 kb MDR region as well as tellurium resistance-associated, mercury resistance-associated, silver resistance-associated [26,27], and copper resistance-associated genes. The MDR region comprised two modules: module one was a novel transposon and module two comprised a Tn1696-like transposon. The MDR region showed an organization very similar (99% nucleotide sequence identity with a query coverage of 90%) to the plasmid pOZ181 (accession number CP016764), a plasmid from a C. freundii B38 isolate from a hospital in 1998 in China (Figure S3).

The tellurium resistance-associated region located from 8380 bp to 23,064 bp consists of terF-terE-terD-terC-terB-terA-terZ as well as terW-terY-terX. Seven intervening ORFs were identified between terZ and terW. The ter cluster was highly (100%) similar to the ter cluster in p362713-HI3 from K. pneumoniae 362713, the plasmid unnamed1 from K. pneumoniae FDAARGOS_439, p1 from K. oxytoca pKOX3, and p1 from K. pneumoniae 20467, among others. The mercury resistance cluster located from 35,301 bp to 39,277 bp consists of merR-merT-merP-merC-merA-merD-merE. The mer cluster is identical (100%) to those of p1 from *K. pneumoniae* BA2275, pSW37-267106 from S. Worthington OLF-FSR1, the plasmid from *E. coli* S15FP06257, and pMS-37 from *Enterobacter hormaechei* EGYMCRVIM, among others. The silver resistance cluster located from 155,928 bp to 165,278 bp, consisted of silE-silS-silR-silC-silB-silA, which was identical (100%) to those of pLH94-1 from *K. pneumoniae*, the plasmid unnamed1 from *K. pneumoniae* KSB1_7F-sc-2280268, pVNCKp115 from *K. pneumoniae* VNCKp115, and pCAV2018-177 from *K. pneumoniae* CAV2018, among others. The copper resistance-associated region located from 169,677 bp to 175,162 bp consisted of copE-copA-copB-copC-copD-copR. The cop operon was highly (100%) similar to the cop operon in plasmids unnamed1 from *K. pneumoniae* KSB1_7F-sc-2280268, pVNCKp115 from *K. pneumoniae* VNCKp115, pLH94-1 from K. pneumoniae, and the chromosome from *K. pneumoniae* NCTC9180, among others. It has been reported that tellurium, mercury, and copper heavy metal resistance genes have been identified in the IncH plasmid pH11 from a clinical *K. pneumoniae* isolate [28]. A large virulence IncH plasmid, pLVPK, harboring copper, silver, and tellurite resistance genes was previously detected in a bacteremic isolate of K. pneumoniae CG43 [29]. To the best of our knowledge, this is the first report that the IncH plasmid from K. pneumoniae contained these four kinds of heavy metal resistance genes, suggesting that the IncH plasmid from *K. pneumoniae* may be a major reservoir for heavy metal resistance genes. Since heavy metal resistance is not the main focus of this study, we did not investigate the phenotype of the resistance to heavy metals of *K. pneumoniae* 200.

We identified a novel transposon in module one of the MDR regions in pYhe2001, designated Tn6897 in the Tn Number Registry (https://transposon.lstmed.ac.uk/ (accessed on 22 June 2020). Tn6897, flanked by direct copies of intact IS26, contained four direction-similar IS26 and one direction-reverse IS26. IS6 family elements, IS26, have played a pivotal role in the dissemination of resistance determinants in gram-negative bacteria [5,30]. This transposon harbored two transposons, mutated Tn4352 and Tn6020b-1 (Figure 3).

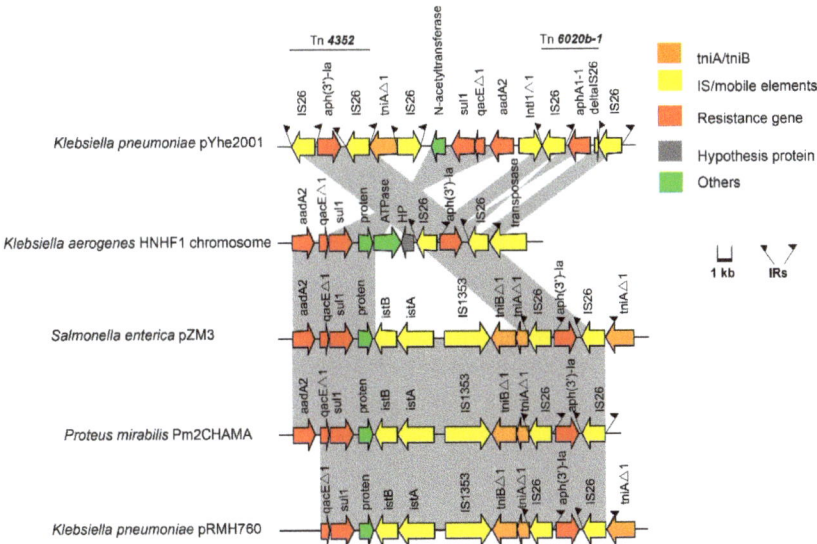

Figure 3. Organization of the Tn6897 transposon in the plasmid pYhe2001 and comparison with a similar structure. ORFs are shown as arrows, indicating the transcription direction, and the colors of the arrows represent different fragments. Intact ISs are represented by arrows, showing the direction of transcription of the transposase genes. Flags represent the IRs of ISs and transposons. Homologous gene clusters in different isolates are shaded in gray (>97%).

Mutated Tn4352 was bound by an 8-bp repeat region (CATCGGCG) on the right; however, the left target site (GATTGGG) was truncated, and the base was mutated. Mutated Tn4352 comprised two intact IS26 sequences that flanked the kanamycin resistance gene aph(3')-Ia in Tn6897. Because of Tn4352, tniAΔ1 was interrupted in the downstream, leading to an 8 bp repeat region (CATCGGCG) on the left. The two IS26 flanked tniAΔ1 in different directions. Tn6897 comprised a part of a class 1 integron that included the truncated 5'-CS (including truncated intI1 gene), the gene cassette aadA2, and the qacEΔ1 and sul1 genes in the 3'-CS. It has been reported that truncated class 1 integrons still have the ability to resist to a greater number of antimicrobials in *E. coli* [31]; therefore, the truncated class 1 integron in Tn6897 may confer resistance to antibiotics. The truncated class 1 integron was between the gene for puromycin N-acetyltransferase protein and an IS26. Further upstream included an intact reverse Tn6020b-1 transposon, which included an intact IS26, an IS26Δ1, and aminoglycoside resistance gene aphA1-1. Through BLASTN searches, a portion of Tn6897 (97% nucleotide sequence similarity) was identified in three different strains, including *K. pneumoniae*, *S. enterica*, and *Proteus mirabilis*. Although high nucleotide sequence similarity occurred in chromosomes or plasmids of different strains, no similar structure was found. Tn6897 had two completely similar repeats of IS26 flanked by 14-bp repeats at both ends (Figure 3), indicating mobility potential. Since Tn6897 contained transposons and truncated class 1 integrons, it has the potential to transfer antibiotic resistance genes in different strains.

We found that the tniA gene was interrupted by Tn4352, leading to an 8-bp repeat region (CATCGGCG) downstream. Furthermore, tniAΔ1 was inserted by IS26, leading to a left inverted repeat (IRL) of IS26. In addition, an intact sul1-type class 1 integron was inserted by an IS26 leading to a right inverted repeat (IRR) of IS26. Reverse Tn6020b-1 had a truncated IS26. Furthermore, we failed to observe direct repeats (DRs) flanking IS26 as well as specific target site duplication patterns, suggesting that the Tn6897 conformation may have occurred by IS26-mediated homologous recombination rather than transposition [32]. These observations revealed that Tn6897 could be formed with the help of IS26 and other transposons. Here, we put forward a hypothesis (Figure 4). To explain the evolution of Tn6896, a hypothetical sequence of 4065 bp, comprising a gene encoding N-acetyltransferase and an intact sul1-type class 1 integron, was sent to BLASTn analysis. The analysis identified matches (100% coverage) to those in plasmids from S. Dublin CVM 22429, S. Anatum str. USDA-ARS-USMARC-1736, and S. Dublin 853. Figure 4 depicts a reverse IS26 inserted in the 5′CS of tniA. Additionally, a Tn4352 inserted into the 3′CS of tniA generating an 8-bp repeat region (CATCGGCG). On the other hand, a Tn6023-like including two IS26 in reverse directions and gene aphA1-1 was inserted downstream of the hypothetical sequence, with a reverse IS26 inserted into intI1 of the hypothetical sequence, and another IS26 was inserted in the upstream of the N-acetyltransferase gene. The sequences described above have one copy of IS26 at both ends. Then, two sequences were recombined by recombination between the copies of IS26 in the same orientation. Finally, the sequence above is inserted by IS26 into the downstream IS26, leading to the generation of Tn6897.

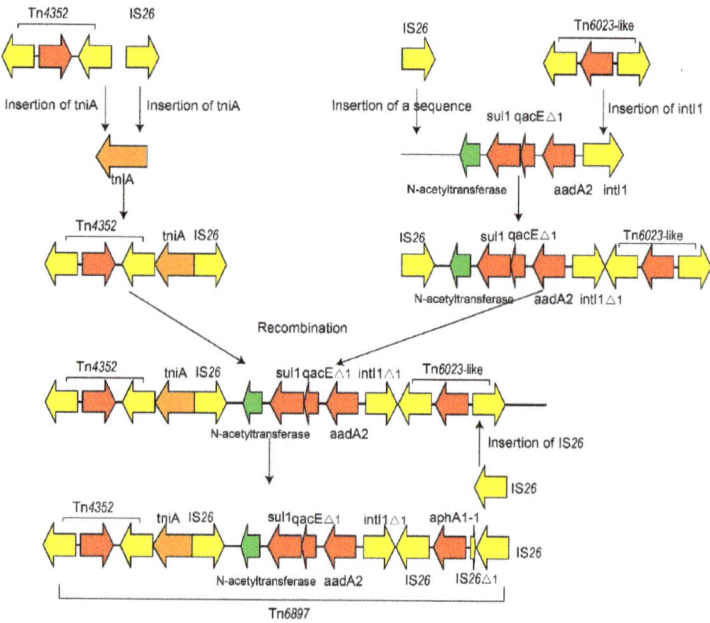

Figure 4. Genealogy of Tn6897 in plasmid pYhe2001. Due to the lack of DRs flanking IS26 as well as specific target site duplication patterns, the novel Tn6897 could be hypothesized to produce by IS26 recombination and other transposons.

Module two was reversed compared with the plasmid pOZ181 from a *C. freundii* B38, which consists of a Tn1696-like transposon (Figure S3). The right IR was interrupted by IS4321, and there was no left IR because of interruption of ISCR1 in the Tn1696-like transposon. Furthermore, a sul1-type class 1 integron that had a 5′CS and four cassettes, aadA5-gcu37-dfrA1-orf, was flanked upstream by a Tn1696-like tnpR-tnpA and downstream by 3′ CS and an ISCR1 transposase. In addition, other resistance genes included the 16S rRNA methylase gene armA downstream of ISCR1. Truncated ISEc29 was located downstream of armA; however, intact ISEc28 was located upstream of armA. Module two showed 99% similarity to the plasmid pBSI034-MCR9 from E. cloacae BSI034, the plasmid pOZ181 from *C. freundii* B38, the plasmid pSIM-1-BJ01 from K. pneumoniae 13624, and the plasmid pWLK-238550 from Raoultella ornithinolytica WLK218, which means that Tn1696-like transposons can be found among different bacteria.

2.4. Transformation Experiment

Transformation of plasmids into E. coli DH5α was achieved at a frequency of 10^{-11} cells per recipient cell. Genes aadA5 and aac(6')-Ib-cr were detected in transformant. The MICs of K. pneumoniae 200, transformant and DH5α, are shown in Table 1. The MIC of gentamicin for K. pneumoniae 200 was 256 mg/L, while the MIC of gentamicin for E. coli DH5α was 0.125 mg/L. In particular, the MIC of gentamicin for the transformant was higher than that of E. coli DH5α, which corresponds to a 256-fold increase in gentamicin MIC because of the presence of plasmids.

Table 1. MICs * of K. pneumonia and transformant.

MIC (mg/L)	K. pneumonia 200	Transformant	DH5α
Amikacin	>256	128	1
Ampicillin	>256	>256	2
Ciprofloxacin	>256	32	0.008
Chloramphenicol	>256	32	2
Gentamicin	256	32	0.125
Kanamycin	>256	128	0.75
Oxacillin	>256	64	0.25
Streptomycin	64	16	1

* minimum inhibitory concentration.

3. Materials and Methods

3.1. Bacterial Strain

The MDR K. pneumoniae 200 examined in this study was originally isolated from the liver of a swine suffering from diarrhea at a commercial swine farm in Guangzhou City, Guangdong Province, China, in 2017. E. coli DH5α was used as the recipient strain in transformation experiments.

3.2. Antimicrobial Susceptibility Testing

Antibiotic susceptibility was determined using the disk diffusion method [11] following the guidelines of the Clinical Laboratory Standards Institute [33]. The disks (OXOID, Hampshire, UK) used in the test were cefotaxime (30 µg), ceftazidime (30 µg), cefoxitin (30 µg), oxacillin (50 µg), meropenem (10 µg), imipenem (10 µg), amikacin (30 µg), gentamicin (10 µg), kanamycin (30 µg), streptomycin (10 µg), ciprofloxacin (5 µg), chloramphenicol (30 µg), erythromycin (15 µg), tetracycline(30 µg), and trimethoprim-sulfamethoxazole (1.25/23.75 µg). E. coli ATCC 25922 was used for quality control.

3.3. Genome Sequencing, Genome Assembly and Bioinformatics

To comprehensively understand the genetic basis of the resistance of K. pneumoniae 200, the complete genome sequence was generated by WGS using PacBio RSII (Pacific Biosciences, Menlo Park, CA, USA) and Illumina MiSeq (Illumina, San Diego, CA, USA) platforms as previously described [34]. WGS data were assembled using SOAPdenovo v1.05 software. Circularization was achieved by manual comparison and removal of a region of overlap, and the final genome was confirmed by remapping the sequence data. The assemblies yielded a circular chromosome and two circular plasmids. Gene prediction was performed using GeneMarkS, and whole-genome BLAST searches (E-value $\leq 1 \times 10^{-5}$, minimal alignment length percentage $\geq 80\%$) were performed against 5 databases: Kyoto Encyclopedia of Genes and Genomes (KEGG), Clusters of Orthologous Groups (COG), NCBI nonredundant protein database (NR), Swiss-Prot, and Gene Ontology (GO). Plasmid incompatibility groups were identified using the online database PlasmidFinder (https://cge.cbs.dtu.dk/services/PlasmidFinder/ (accessed on

2 February 2020). Antimicrobial resistance genes were identified using the ResFinder 3.1 tool (https://cge.cbs.dtu.dk/services/ResFinder/ (accessed on 2 February 2020) with an identity threshold of 96%. Integrons were analyzed using the integron identification tool INTEGRALL (http://integrall.bio.ua.pt/ (accessed on 2 February 2020). *K. pneumoniae* virulence genes were identified with the aid of the *K. pneumoniae* section of the Institut Pasteur MLST and whole genome MLST databases (http://bigsdb.Pasteur.fr (accessed on 2 February 2020). For sequence comparisons, the BLAST algorithm (www.ncbi.nlm.nih.gov/BLAST (accessed on 2 February 2020) was used. Multilocus sequence typing (MLST) analysis of *K. pneumoniae* 200 and cgMLST phylogenetic relationship analyses of all public genomesequences of ST37 were performed using the BacWGSTdb server with a threshold of 1000. The DNA sequences of chromosomes and plasmids of *K. pneumoniae* 200 were deposited in NCBI GenBank with the accession numbers CP055293, CP062278, and CP063211, respectively.

3.4. Transformation Experiments

Transformation of plasmid DNA isolated from *K. pneumoniae* 200 into *E. coli* DH5α was performed as described previously [35]. *K. pneumoniae* 200 and DH5α strains were first grown in 25 mL of LB liquid medium overnight at 37 °C with shaking. Plasmid DNA was extracted from *K. pneumoniae* 200 with a Plasmid Mini Purification Kit (Amersham Biosciences, Uppsala, Sweden). Then, a 1-mL culture of *E. coli* DH5α was diluted in 100 mL of LB liquid medium and incubated at 37 °C until the cells reached the early exponential growth phase. Cells were then centrifuged twice within cooled 0.1 M $CaCl_2$ for 10 min at $2700\times g$ and finally resuspended in 500 μL of LB liquid medium. All centrifugation steps were performed at room temperature (RT) at approximately 25 °C. Four aliquots of 100 μL of cells were prepared, and plasmidic DNA were added and gently mixed, respectively. The remaining 100-μL cell aliquot was used as a negative control (no DNA was added). Samples were incubated at 37 °C for 1 h. After that, three aliquots were plated on LB plates supplemented with gentamicin (32 μg/mL), while the fourth aliquot was serially diluted and plated on LB plates without antibiotic to enumerate recipient cells. Negative control was also plated on LB plates supplemented with gentamicin (32 μg/mL). All the plates were incubated at 37 °C overnight. Transformation efficiency was calculated based on the ratio of transformants to the total number of viable cells. Experiments were performed with three biological replicates. To identify the *aadA5* gene in transformants, primers 5'-CGCTCAACGCAAGATTCTCT-3' (forward), and 5'-ATGGGTGAATTTTTCCCTGCAC-3' (reverse) for *aadA5* (792 bp) were used in PCR. Furthermore, the presence of the *aac(6')-Ib-cr* gene in transformants was confirmed by PCR amplification followed by DNA sequence analysis. Primers for *aac(6')-Ib-cr* (612 bp) were 5'-AAGGGTTAGGCATCACTGCG-3' (forward) and 5'-AGACATCATGAGCAACGCAA-3' (reverse). The primers were designed using NCBI Primer-BLAST. PCR conditions were: initial denaturation at 95 °C for 5 min, 30 cycles of amplification (30 s at 95 °C, 30 s at 55 °C, and 90 s at 72 °C), followed by an extension at 72 °C for 10 min. PCR products were purified and sequenced by Majorbio Company (Shanghai, China). MICs of *E. coli* DH5α and five transformants were determined by Etest (Liofilchem S.R.L.) according to the manufacturer's instructions. *E. coli* ATCC 25922 served as a quality control strain.

4. Conclusions

To the best of our knowledge, we described a novel plasmid pYhe2001 in a *K. pneumoniae* isolate of swine origin for the first time. A novel Tn*6897* that was identified in the plasmid pYhe2001 likely underwent a recombination event and showed a high potential for resistance development. Heavy metal resistance genes were identified in the plasmid pYhe2001, which expanded the spectrum of IncH plasmids. This is the first time that the IncF plasmid carrying $bla_{CTX-M-27}$ was discovered in the liver of a swine, which warrants investigation of the prevalence of $bla_{CTX-M-57}$ harboring *K. pneumoniae*. The results of this study provide additional evidence of the variation in MDR *K. pneumoniae* that threatens the health of humans and animals.

Supplementary Materials: The following supporting information can be downloaded at: https://www.mdpi.com/article/10.3390/antibiotics11091225/s1, Figure S1: linear illustration of the T6SS gene clusters of 200 and comparative analysis of this region with that of *K. pneumoniae* HS11286 and *K. pneumoniae* ZYST1; Figure S2: Circular representation of plasmid pYhe2002; Figure S3: Linear illustration of the MDR region of plasmid pYhe2001 and comparative analysis of this region in pOZ181 from *Citrobactere freundii* B38; Table S1: Antimicrobial resistance profile of *K. pneumoniae* 200; Table S2: Characteristics of *K. pneumonia* strain 200; Table S3: Compared plasmid pYhe2002 with the plasmid records contained in PLSDB; Table S4: Compared plasmid pYhe2001 with the plasmid records contained in PLSDB.

Author Contributions: H.L. designed the research, executed the experiments, analyzed the data, and wrote the draft of the manuscript. X.L. designed, authored, and reviewed drafts of the manuscript and approved the final draft. H.Y. designed the research, supervised the study, provided guidance on the purpose of the project, published studies used to build the conclusion, reviewed the results, and revised the manuscript. All authors have read and agreed to the published version of the manuscript.

Funding: This work was supported by the National Key Basic Research Program [grant number 2016YFD0500606], Construction of the First Class Universities (Subject) and Special Development Guidance Special Fund [grant number K5174960], and Fundamental Research Funds for the Central Universities, SCUT [grant number D2170320].

Data Availability Statement: The chromosomal DNA and plasmids of *K. pneumoniae* 200 were deposited in NCBI GenBank with the accession numbers CP055293, CP062278, and CP063211, respectively.

Acknowledgments: We thank members of our laboratories for fruitful discussions.

Conflicts of Interest: The authors declare no conflict of interest.

References

1. Davis, G.S.; Price, L.B. Recent research examining links among *Klebsiella pneumoniae* from food, food animals, and human extraintestinal infections. *Curr. Environ. Health Rep.* **2016**, *3*, 128–135. [CrossRef] [PubMed]
2. Thomas, E.; Grandemange, E.; Pommier, P.; Wessel-Robert, S.; Davot, J.L. Field evaluation of efficacy and tolerance of a 2% marbofloxacin injectable solution for the treatment of respiratory disease in fattening swines. *Vet. Q.* **2000**, *22*, 131–135. [CrossRef] [PubMed]
3. Fournier, C.; Aires-de-Sousa, M.; Nordmann, P.; Poirel, L. Occurrence of CTX-M-15- and MCR-1-producing Enterobacterales in swines in Portugal: Evidence of direct links with antibiotic selective pressure. *Int. J. Antimicrob. Agents* **2020**, *55*, 105802. [CrossRef] [PubMed]
4. Dong, N.; Liu, L.; Zhang, R.; Chen, K.; Xie, M.; Chan, E.; Chen, S. An IncR plasmid harbored by a hypervirulent carbapenem-resistant *Klebsiella pneumoniae* strain possesses five tandem repeats of the bla(KPC-2): NTEKPC-Id fragment. *Antimicrob. Agents Chemother.* **2019**, *63*, e01775-18. [CrossRef] [PubMed]
5. Partridge, S.R.; Kwong, S.M.; Firth, N.; Jensen, S.O. Mobile genetic elements associated with antimicrobial resistance. *Clin. Microbiol. Rev.* **2018**, *31*, e00088-17. [CrossRef] [PubMed]
6. Yang, Y.; Li, X.; Zhang, Y.; Liu, J.; Hu, X.; Nie, T.; Yang, X.; Wang, X.; Li, C.; You, X. Characterization of a hypervirulent multidrug-resistant ST23 *Klebsiella pneumoniae* carrying a *bla*CTX-M-24 IncFII plasmid and a pK2044-like plasmid. *J. Glob. Antimicrob. Resist.* **2020**, *22*, 674–679. [CrossRef]
7. Naas, T.; Cuzon, G.; Villegas, M.V.; Lartigue, M.F.; Quinn, J.P.; Nordmann, P. Genetic structures at the origin of acquisition of the beta-lactamase *bla*KPC gene. *Antimicrob. Agents Chemother.* **2008**, *52*, 1257–1263. [CrossRef]
8. Huang, W.; Wang, G.; Sebra, R.; Zhuge, J.; Yin, C.; Aguero-Rosenfeld, M.E.; Schuetz, A.N.; Dimitrova, N.; Fallon, J.T. Emergence and evolution of multidrug-resistant *Klebsiella pneumoniae* with both *bla*KPC and *bla*CTX-M integrated in the chromosome. *Antimicrob. Agents Chemother.* **2017**, *61*, e00076-17. [CrossRef]
9. Wyres, K.L.; Lam, M.M.C.; Holt, K.E. Population genomics of *Klebsiella pneumoniae*. *Nat. Rev. Microbiol.* **2020**, *18*, 344–359. [CrossRef] [PubMed]
10. Desmet, S.; Nepal, S.; van Dijl, J.M.; Van Ranst, M.; Chlebowicz, M.A.; Rossen, J.W.; Van Houdt, J.; Maes, P.; Lagrou, K.; Bathoorn, E. Antibiotic resistance plasmids cointegrated into a megaplasmid harboring the *bla*OXA-427 carbapenemase gene. *Antimicrob. Agents Chemother.* **2018**, *62*, e01448-17. [CrossRef]
11. Guo, Q.; Spychala, C.N.; McElheny, C.L.; Doi, Y. Comparative analysis of an IncR plasmid carrying *armA*, *bla*DHA-1 and *qnrB4* from *Klebsiella pneumoniae* ST37 isolates. *J. Antimicrob. Chemother.* **2016**, *71*, 882–886. [CrossRef] [PubMed]
12. Lu, J.; Dong, N.; Liu, C.; Zeng, Y.; Sun, Q.; Zhou, H.; Hu, Y.; Chen, S.; Shen, Z.; Zhang, R. Prevalence and molecular epidemiology of *mcr-1*-positive *Klebsiella pneumoniae* in healthy adults from China. *J. Antimicrob. Chemother.* **2020**, *75*, 2485–2494. [CrossRef] [PubMed]

13. Wasfi, R.; Elkhatib, W.F.; Ashour, H.M. Molecular typing and virulence analysis of multidrug resistant *Klebsiella pneumoniae* clinical isolates recovered from Egyptian hospitals. *Sci. Rep.* **2016**, *6*, 38929. [CrossRef] [PubMed]
14. Yuhan, Y.; Ziyun, Y.; Yongbo, Z.; Fuqiang, L.; Qinghua, Z. Overexpression of AdeABC and AcrAB-TolC efflux systems confers tigecycline resistance in clinical isolates of *Acinetobacter baumannii* and *Klebsiella pneumoniae*. *Rev. Soc. Bras. Med. Trop.* **2016**, *49*, 165–171. [CrossRef]
15. Chen, F.; Zhang, W.; Schwarz, S.; Zhu, Y.; Li, R.; Hua, X.; Liu, S. Genetic characterization of an MDR/virulence genomic element carrying two T6SS gene clusters in a clinical *Klebsiella pneumoniae* isolate of swine origin. *J. Antimicrob. Chemother.* **2019**, *74*, 1539–1544. [CrossRef]
16. Kopotsa, K.; Osei Sekyere, J.; Mbelle, N.M. Plasmid evolution in carbapenemase-producing Enterobacteriaceae: A review. *Ann. N. Y. Acad. Sci.* **2019**, *1457*, 61–91. [CrossRef] [PubMed]
17. Schmartz, G.P.; Hartung, A.; Hirsch, P.; Kern, F.; Fehlmann, T.; Müller, R.; Keller, A. PLSDB: Advancing a comprehensive database of bacterial plasmids. *Nucleic Acids Res.* **2022**, *50*, D273–D278. [CrossRef]
18. Khezri, A.; Avershina, E.; Ahmad, R. Plasmid Identification and Plasmid-Mediated Antimicrobial Gene Detection in Norwegian Isolates. *Microorganisms* **2020**, *9*, 52. [CrossRef]
19. Zhang, Y.; Sun, Y.-H.; Wang, J.-Y.; Chang, M.-X.; Zhao, Q.-Y.; Jiang, H.-X. A Novel Structure Harboring $bla_{CTX-M-27}$ on IncF Plasmids in *Escherichia coli* Isolated from Swine in China. *Antibiotics* **2021**, *10*, 387. [CrossRef]
20. Kawamura, K.; Hayashi, K.; Matsuo, N.; Kitaoka, K.; Kimura, K.; Wachino, J.-I.; Kondo, T.; Iinuma, Y.; Murakami, N.; Fujimoto, S.; et al. Prevalence of CTX-M-Type Extended-Spectrum β-Lactamase-Producing *Escherichia coli* B2-O25-ST131 *H30R* Among Residents in Nonacute Care Facilities in Japan. *Microb. Drug Resist.* **2018**, *24*, 1513–1520. [CrossRef] [PubMed]
21. Cao, X.; Zhong, Q.; Guo, Y.; Hang, Y.; Chen, Y.; Fang, X.; Xiao, Y.; Zhu, H.; Luo, H.; Yu, F.; et al. Emergence of the coexistence of *mcr-1*, *bla*NDM-5, and *bla*CTX-M-55 in *Klebsiella pneumoniae* ST485 clinical isolates in China. *Infect. Drug Resist.* **2021**, *14*, 3449–3458. [CrossRef]
22. Stosic, M.S.; Leangapichart, T.; Lunha, K.; Jiwakanon, J.; Angkititrakul, S.; Järhult, J.D.; Magnusson, U.; Sunde, M. Novel mcr-3.40 variant co-located with mcr-2.3 and blaCTX-M-63 on an IncHI1B/IncFIB plasmid found in Klebsiella pneumoniae from a healthy carrier in Thailand. *J. Antimicrob. Chemother.* **2021**, *76*, 2218–2220. [CrossRef] [PubMed]
23. Gancz, A.; Kondratyeva, K.; Cohen-Eli, D.; Navon-Venezia, S. Genomics and virulence of *Klebsiella pneumoniae* Kpnu95 ST1412 harboring a novel Incf plasmid encoding blactx-M-15 and *qnrs1* causing community urinary tract infection. *Microorganisms* **2021**, *9*, 1022. [CrossRef]
24. Mshana, E.S.; Hain, T.; Domann, E.; Lyamuya, E.F.; Chakraborty, T.; Imirzalioglu, C. Predominance of Klebsiella pneumoniaeST14 carrying CTX-M-15 causing neonatal sepsis in Tanzania. *BMC Infect. Dis.* **2013**, *13*, 466. [CrossRef]
25. Yao, H.; Cheng, J.; Li, A.; Yu, R.; Zhao, W.; Qin, S.; Du, X. Molecular characterization of an IncFII(k) plasmid coharboring *bla*IMP-26 and *tet(A)* variant in a clinical *Klebsiella pneumoniae* isolate. *Front. Microbiol.* **2020**, *11*, 1610. [CrossRef] [PubMed]
26. Hanczvikkel, A.; Fuzi, M.; Ungvari, E.; Toth, A. Transmissible silver resistance readily evolves in high-risk clone isolates of *Klebsiella pneumoniae*. *Acta Microbiol. Immunol. Hung.* **2018**, *65*, 387–403. [CrossRef] [PubMed]
27. Finley, P.J.; Norton, R.; Austin, C.; Mitchell, A.; Zank, S.; Durham, P. Unprecedented silver resistance in clinically isolated Enterobacteriaceae: Major implications for burn and wound management. *Antimicrob. Agents Chemother.* **2015**, *59*, 4734–4741. [CrossRef] [PubMed]
28. Zhai, Y.; He, Z.; Kang, Y.; Yu, H.; Wang, J.; Du, P.; Zhang, Z.; Hu, S.; Gao, Z. Complete nucleotide sequence of pH11, an IncHI2 plasmid conferring multiantibiotic resistance and multiheavy metal resistance genes in a clinical *Klebsiella pneumoniae* isolate. *Plasmid* **2016**, *86*, 26–31. [CrossRef] [PubMed]
29. Chen, Y.-T.; Chang, H.-Y.; Lai, Y.-C.; Pan, C.-C.; Tsai, S.-F.; Peng, H.-L. Sequencing and analysis of the large virulence plasmid pLVPK of Klebsiella pneumoniae CG43. *Gene* **2004**, *337*, 189–198. [CrossRef] [PubMed]
30. He, S.; Hickman, A.B.; Varani, A.M.; Siguier, P.; Chandler, M.; Dekker, J.P.; Dyda, F. Insertion Sequence IS 26 Reorganizes Plasmids in Clinically Isolated Multidrug-Resistant Bacteria by Replicative Transposition. *mBio* **2015**, *6*, e00762. [CrossRef] [PubMed]
31. Kubomura, A.; Sekizuka, T.; Onozuka, D.; Murakami, K.; Kimura, H.; Sakaguchi, M.; Oishi, K.; Hirai, S.; Kuroda, M.; Okabe, N. Truncated class 1 integron gene cassette arrays contribute to antimicrobial resistance of diarrheagenic *Escherichia coli*. *BioMed Res. Int.* **2020**, *2020*, 4908189. [CrossRef]
32. Wang, J.; Zeng, Z.-L.; Huang, X.-Y.; Ma, Z.-B.; Guo, Z.-W.; Lv, L.-C.; Xia, Y.-B.; Zeng, L.; Song, Q.-H.; Liu, J.-H. Evolution and Comparative Genomics of F33:A−:B− Plasmids Carrying $bla_{CTX-M-55}$ or $bla_{CTX-M-65}$ in *Escherichia coli* and *Klebsiella pneumoniae* Isolated from Animals, Food Products, and Humans in China. *mSphere* **2018**, *3*, e00137-18. [CrossRef] [PubMed]
33. dos Santos, E.J.E.; Azevedo, R.P.; Lopes, A.T.S.; Rocha, J.M.; Albuquerque, G.R.; Wenceslau, A.A.; Miranda, F.R.; Rodrigues, D.D.P.; Maciel, B.M. *Salmonella* spp. in Wild Free-Living Birds from Atlantic Forest Fragments in Southern Bahia, Brazil. *BioMed Res. Int.* **2020**, *2020*, 7594136. [CrossRef] [PubMed]
34. Zheng, B.; Yu, X.; Xu, H.; Guo, L.; Zhang, J.; Huang, C.; Shen, P.; Jiang, X.; Xiao, Y.; Li, L. Complete genome sequencing and genomic characterization of two Escherichia coli strains co-producing MCR-1 and NDM-1 from bloodstream infection. *Sci. Rep.* **2017**, *7*, 17885. [CrossRef] [PubMed]
35. Sun, D.; Zhang, Y.; Mei, Y.; Jiang, H.; Xie, Z.; Liu, H.; Chen, X.; Shen, P. *Escherichia coli* is naturally transformable in a novel transformation system. *FEMS Microbiol. Lett.* **2006**, *265*, 249–255. [CrossRef] [PubMed]

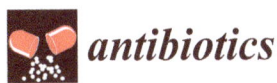

Article

Impact of Raised without Antibiotics Measures on Antimicrobial Resistance and Prevalence of Pathogens in Sow Barns

Alvin C. Alvarado [1,2,†], Samuel M. Chekabab [2,3,†], Bernardo Z. Predicala [1,2] and Darren R. Korber [3,*]

1. Chemical and Biological Engineering, University of Saskatchewan, 57 Campus Dr., Saskatoon, SK S7N 5A9, Canada
2. Prairie Swine Centre Inc., Box 21057, 2105–8th St. East, Saskatoon, SK S7H 5N9, Canada
3. Food and Bioproduct Sciences, University of Saskatchewan, 51 Campus Drive, Saskatoon, SK S7N 5A8, Canada
* Correspondence: darren.korber@usask.ca
† These authors contributed equally to this work.

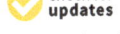

Citation: Alvarado, A.C.; Chekabab, S.M.; Predicala, B.Z.; Korber, D.R. Impact of Raised without Antibiotics Measures on Antimicrobial Resistance and Prevalence of Pathogens in Sow Barns. *Antibiotics* **2022**, *11*, 1221. https://doi.org/10.3390/antibiotics11091221

Academic Editor: Carlo Corino

Received: 26 July 2022
Accepted: 29 August 2022
Published: 8 September 2022

Publisher's Note: MDPI stays neutral with regard to jurisdictional claims in published maps and institutional affiliations.

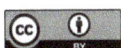

Copyright: © 2022 by the authors. Licensee MDPI, Basel, Switzerland. This article is an open access article distributed under the terms and conditions of the Creative Commons Attribution (CC BY) license (https://creativecommons.org/licenses/by/4.0/).

Abstract: The growing concern over the emergence of antimicrobial resistance (AMR) in animal production as a result of extensive and inappropriate antibiotic use has prompted many swine farmers to raise their animals without antibiotics (RWA). In this study, the impact of implementing an RWA production approach in sow barns on actual on-farm antibiotic use, the emergence of AMR, and the abundance of pathogens was investigated. Over a 13-month period, fecal and nasopharynx samples were collected at 3-month intervals from sows raised in RWA barns and sows in conventional barns using antibiotics in accordance with the new regulations (non-RWA). Whole genome sequencing (WGS) was used to determine the prevalence of AMR and the presence of pathogens in those samples. Records of all drug use from the 13-month longitudinal study indicated a significant reduction in antimicrobial usage in sows from RWA barns compared to conventional non-RWA barns. Antifolates were commonly administered to non-RWA sows, whereas β-lactams were widely used to treat sows in RWA barns. Metagenomic analyses demonstrated an increased abundance of pathogenic *Actinobacteria*, *Firmicutes*, and *Proteobacteria* in the nasopharynx microbiome of RWA sows relative to non-RWA sows. However, WGS analyses revealed that the nasal microbiome of sows raised under RWA production exhibited a significant increase in the frequency of resistance genes coding for β-lactams, MDR, and tetracycline.

Keywords: raised without antibiotics; WGS metagenomics; antimicrobial resistance genes; gut microbiome; nasopharynx microbiome

1. Introduction

Antibiotic overuse and misuse in human and veterinary medicine as well as in agriculture has intensified the emergence and spread of antimicrobial-resistant diseases, making it one of the most serious risks to public health according to World Health Organization [1]. Globally, animal agriculture accounts for more than half of all antibiotic use, which was estimated to be about 131,000 tons in 2013 and is expected to exceed 200,000 tons by 2030 [2]. In Canada, 78% of antimicrobials sold in 2019 (~1.0 million kg) were intended for use in food-producing animals, with the majority (both in kilograms and adjusted for the number of animals and their weights (biomass)) were distributed for use in pig production [3]. This trend has been consistent worldwide [4–9]. Tetracyclines, macrolides, and penicillins (β-lactams) are among the top classes of antimicrobial sold to the Canadian swine sector [3].

Due to risks associated with antimicrobial resistance (AMR) as a result of increased antibiotic use, Canada has implemented more stringent regulations on the use of antibiotics in livestock production. Since December 2018, all medically important antimicrobials for veterinary use must be sold by prescription only, and the use of antibiotics in animal feed is prohibited. Additionally, a number of pig producers have shifted to raising pigs without using any antibiotics (RWA), motivated by the premium price paid by processors for pigs raised completely without antibiotics. However, it has been reported that as swine producers transitioned to antibiotic-free production, the microbial load in the production environment gradually increased, eventually leading to the animals succumbing to the increased microbial challenge, after which severe disease outbreaks began to occur. Thus, the impact of RWA production on the emergence of AMR and prevalence of pathogens in the barn was explored further in this study.

According to Statistics Canada, the Canadian hog industry had a total inventory of around 14.11 million hogs in January 2022, including 5.17 million piglets, 7.68 million grower–finishers, and 1.24 million sows and gilts [10]. Sows, or adult female pigs who have given birth (farrowed) at least once, play a critical role in swine production. Sows are among the oldest animals in a swine barn. They are first bred at the age of 24–30 weeks and have a gestation period of about 115 days. When sows are about to farrow, they are moved to a farrowing room where they stay for 3–4 weeks until they wean their litter, and then they are bred again. Broad-spectrum antibiotics are usually fed or given by injection at farrowing and for a few days afterwards, because sows are susceptible to a number of infections during this period [11]. Given that sows stay longer in the barn, they are more likely to have been exposed to most antibiotics as well as pathogens [12], making the sow stage significant to investigate the impacts of RWA.

Furthermore, the Canadian Integrated Program for Antimicrobial Resistance Surveillance (CIPARS), which monitors antimicrobial usage in the Canadian swine industry, is mostly focused on grower-finisher pigs, with no data on sows available [13]. The impact of antibiotic treatments on the prevalence of pathogens and antimicrobial-resistant genes (ARGs) in the gut microbiome of piglets and grower-finisher pigs has previously been examined [14–17]; however, little is known about the potential differential effects of these treatments on the abundance of pathogens and ARGs in the gut and nasal microbiome of sows [12]. Additionally, while the gut microbiome of pigs has been extensively studied, the impact of antimicrobial treatment on the nasal microbiome has yet to be investigated [18,19]. There is mounting evidence that the nasal microbiota regulates local immunity and contributes to swine respiratory health [19]. Hence, the main objectives of this study were to characterize the gut and nasopharynx microbiome of sows raised under two different production conditions (RWA vs. non-RWA), monitor their antimicrobial usage, and investigate the impact of RWA measures on the prevalence of AMR and the occurrence of pathogens found in the gut and nasopharynx of sows.

2. Results

2.1. Antifolates Are Largely Administered to Non-RWA Sows While β-Lactams Are Still Widely Used for Treatment of Sows in RWA Barns

Records of all drug use for animal treatments as well the actual use of antibiotics in the participating barns were collected regularly from November 2019 to November 2020. These records included the type of drug, dosage, the number and age of treated animals, the cause of treatment, location in the barn, and the date of drug administration. The information and amounts of drugs given were cross-referenced against the Provincial Veterinary Services and swine drug treatment databases (https://www.drugs.com/vet/swine-a.html, accessed on 9 July 2021). The antibiotics mostly given to sows during the monitoring period belonged to three classes: antifolates (Trimidox), β-lactams (Penicillin G, Ampicillin, Ceftiofur), and tetracyclines (Biomycin).

Table 1 shows a list of antibiotics that were administered in RWA and non-RWA barns along with their corresponding quantity in milligrams (mg) and DDDvetCA, which is the Canadian defined daily dose (average labeled dose) in milligrams per kilogram pig weight per day (mg drug/kg animal/day), in accordance with the Canadian Integrated Program for Antimicrobial Resistance Surveillance 2016 report [20]. The data on antibiotic type and dosages were normalized using the number of sows treated during the surveillance period in order to report the values as DDDvetCA. On average, a total of 553 g of antibiotics were administered to 78 non-RWA sows, corresponding to 1285 mg/day/kg cumulative DDDvetCA. However, RWA sows (n = 22) received a total of 130 g of antibiotics, corresponding to 204 mg/day/kg cumulative DDDvetCA. The estimated total antimicrobial usage for sows in RWA barns was reduced by nearly 4.3-fold compared to usage in non-RWA barns. The number of treated sows in RWA barns was 3.5-fold lower and received 6.3-fold less cumulative DDDvetCA value than the sows in non-RWA barns. Sows in non-RWA barns were treated with antifolates (77% of total antibiotics administered), β-lactams (1.4%), and tetracycline (22%), which respectively corresponded to 72%, 1.3%, and 27% of the cumulative DDDvetCA value. In contrast, RWA sows were treated with β-lactams (82%) and tetracycline (18%), which respectively corresponded to 85% and 15% of the cumulative DDDvetCA value (Table 1). Due to potential interpretation bias caused by the lack of consistent criteria for the different treatment categories/reasons across participating barns (e.g., one barn may call the reason for treatment 'infection', while others may list the same symptoms as 'limping' or 'respiratory'), these data were not included in the analysis. Nevertheless, the six most prevalent reasons for treatment recorded during the 13-month monitoring period included infection, injury, limping, respiratory impairment, and symptoms associated with gestation such as difficulty farrowing, vaginal discharge, and mastitis.

Table 1. Quantification of antibiotics administered to sows in the participating barns.

Numbers of Animals	Type of Antibiotics	Antibiotics Used			
		Absolute Quantity		Relative Amount	
		mg	Percent	DDDvetCA [1]	Percent
Non-RWA					
Sow (n = 78)	Antifolate	425,496	77%	925	72%
	B-lactam	8000	1%	13	1%
	Tetracycline	119,500	22%	347	27%
	Total antibiotics (mg)	552,996		1285	
RWA					
Sow (n = 22)	β-lactam	107,085	82%	173	85%
	Tetracycline	23,250	18%	31	15%
	Total antibiotics (mg)	130,335		204	

[1] DDDvetCA is the Canadian defined daily dose (average labeled dose) in milligrams per kilogram pig weight per day (mg drug/kg animal/day).

2.2. RWA Sows Exhibit More Pathogenic Actinobacteria, Firmicutes, and Proteobacteria in Nasopharynx Samples

Metagenomic taxonomy profiling was performed on samples from sow feces and nasal swab samples collected from RWA and non-RWA barns. Bacterial sequences accounted for nearly 99% of all sequenced reads matching the k-mer markers. Analysis through the CosmosID bioinformatics platform resulted in the identification of 395 bacterial species belonging to 150 genera, 24 classes, and 13 phyla (data not shown). The sows' fecal microbiomes were dominated by *Firmicutes* (65–68%), followed by *Actinobacteria* (9–13%), and *Bacteriodetes* (6–7%). The nasal swab samples, however, exhibited a fairly comparable relative abundance at the phylum level, including *Firmicutes* (39–54%) and *Proteobacteria* (19–31%).

The total species/strains present in the microbiome were further analyzed to determine the prevalence of pathogens (the pathome) which is represented by the subset of human and/or animal risk group (RG) 2 and RG3 organisms. From our analysis, 89 and 96 pathogenic strains were found in feces and nasal swabs samples, respectively (See Supplemental Table S1). The total prevalence of pathogens (sequence frequency) in the sow feces was comparable between the non-RWA and RWA barns with an overall reduction in the RWA samples (Figure 1). However, at the phylum level, sow feces in RWA barns exhibited a significant decrease in the frequency of pathogens over time, including microorganisms belonging to *Firmicutes* (Figure 2A, Table S1). Alternatively, the total prevalence of pathogens in the nasal swab samples collected from sows was remarkably higher in RWA barns compared to non-RWA (Figure 1). At the phylum level (Figure 2B), the pathogenic *Actinobacteria*, *Firmicutes*, and *Proteobacteria* were significantly more frequent in the nasal swab samples collected from RWA sows (Table S1).

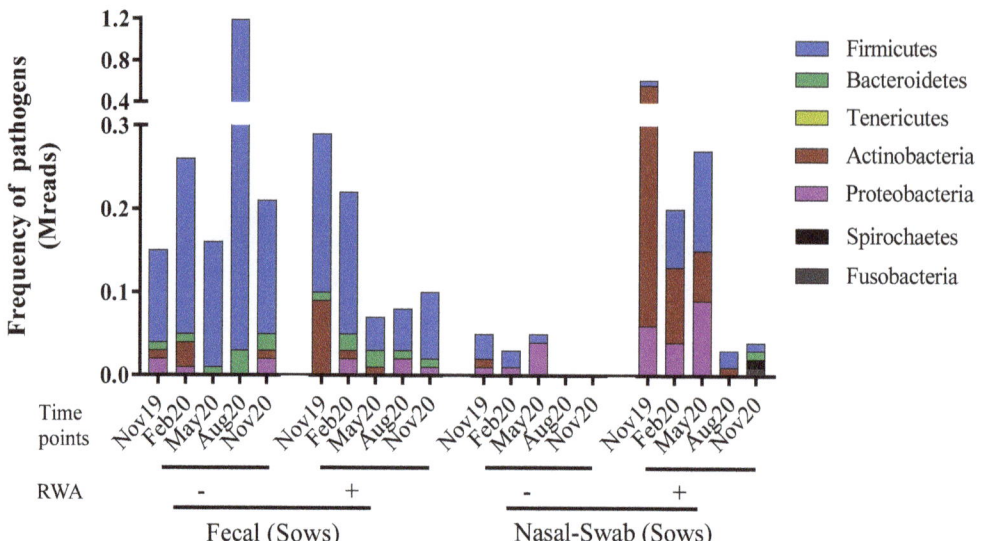

Figure 1. Metagenomic taxonomy profiling at the phylum level from sow feces and nasal swab samples collected from non-RWA − (minus sign) and RWA + (plus sign) barns. The stacked bars represent the average frequency of the major bacteriomes from each type of barn.

2.3. RWA Practices Increased AMR in the Sow Nasopharynx but Not in the Sow Gut

To determine the effect of the RWA production approach on the prevalence of ARGs over time in both the gut and nasopharynx microbiomes of sows, the resistome profiles from the WGS data were compared and yielded the frequency of ARGs present in the samples based on absolute number of reads. As shown in Figure 3, the ARGs were found to belong to six main classes: aminoglycoside (11–32%), β-lactam (2–26%), macrolide (16–32%), phenicol (0.04–0.88%), multi-drug resistance (MDR; 3–13%), and tetracycline (22–46%). Over 13 months of surveillance monitoring, the ARG frequency in sow feces in RWA barns was not significantly different ($p = 0.072$) from non-RWA barns (Figures 3 and 4A). However, the ARG frequency in samples collected from sow nasopharynx was significantly higher ($p = 0.016$) in RWA barns compared to non-RWA barns (Figure 3). Relative to sows raised under non-RWA conditions, the frequency of ARGs in the nasal swab samples from sows in RWA barns significantly increased for β-lactam ($p = 0.004$), MDR ($p = 0.03$), and tetracycline ($p < 0.002$) drug classes (Figure 4B).

Figure 5 shows the frequencies of the ten most abundant ARGs in sow feces and nasal swab samples from RWA and non-RWA barns. Through comparative gene frequency (heat map) analysis of ARG clusters, tetracycline resistance genes *tetW* and *tetQ* were the most frequently found in fecal samples, and the β-lactam resistance gene *blaROB1* was the most frequently found in nasal swab samples, followed by Aminoglycoside (*ant9 la*) and then by MDR (*lsaE*) (Figure 5A). Furthermore, PCoA ordination of ARGs significantly clustered the effect of RWA on the resistome from sow nasal swab samples ($p = 0.016$), but not from sow feces ($p = 0.072$) (Figure 5B).

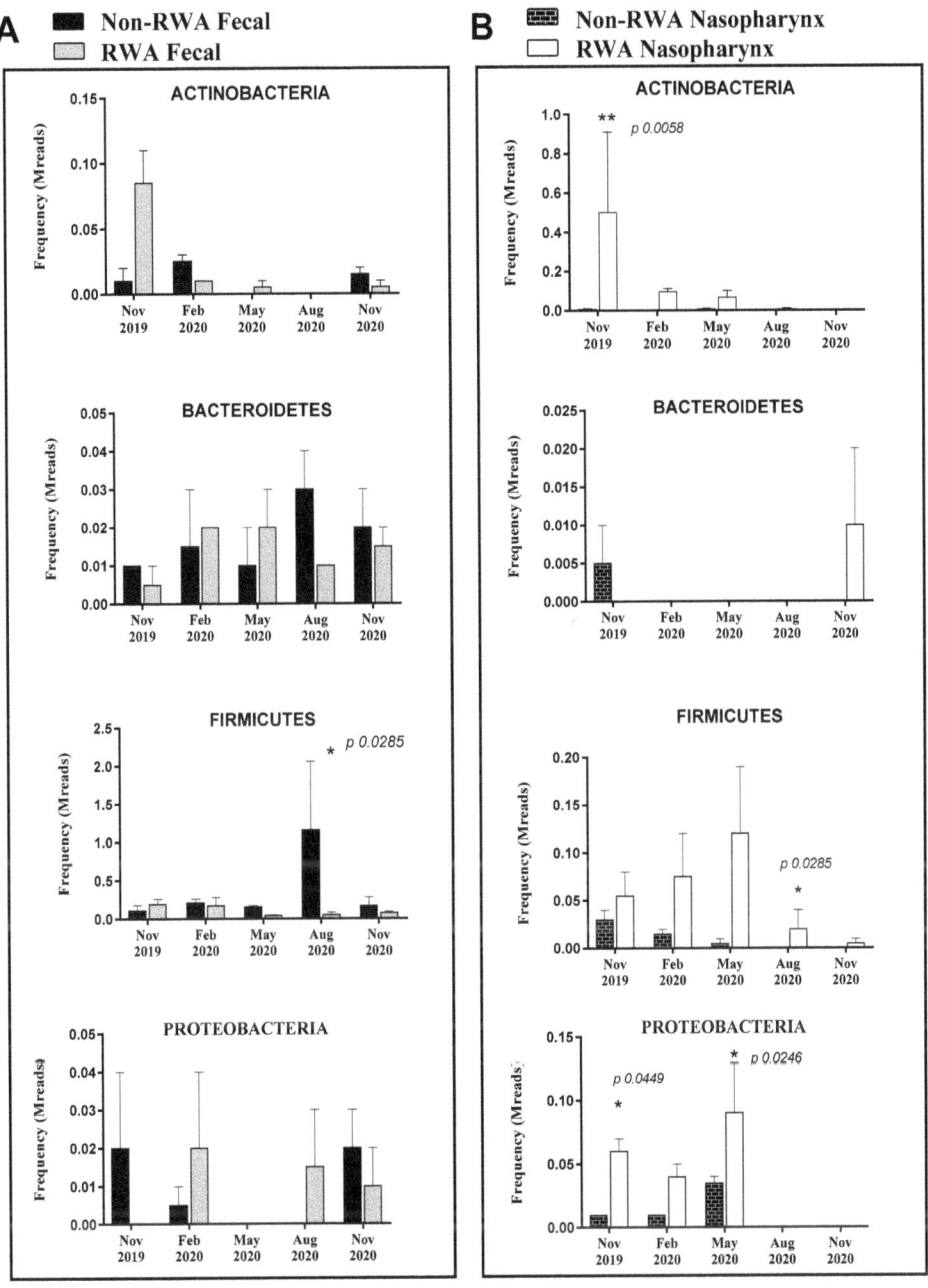

Figure 2. Pathogen prevalence in sow feces (**A**) and sow nasopharynx (**B**) samples. The bars represent the averaged frequency of the pathogens obtained from all bacteriome phyla by extracting the subset of human and/or animal Risk Group 2 species. Two data sets from each type of farm (non-RWA and RWA) were included as biological replicates for statistical analysis. ANOVA 2-way analysis with repeated measures comparing RWA vs. non-RWA with Bonferroni's correction; * $p < 0.05$, ** $p < 0.01$.

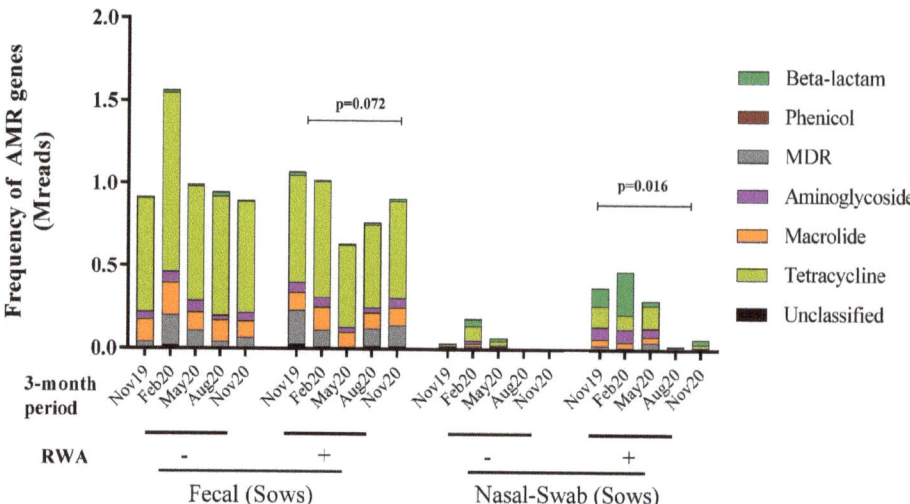

Figure 3. Metagenomic resistome showing the frequency of antibiotic resistance genes (ARGs) clustered into six classes: tetracycline, aminoglycoside, macrolide, phenicol, β-lactam, and multi-drug resistance (MDR) and collected from sow feces and nasal swab samples in non-RWA − (minus sign) and RWA + (plus sign) barns. Two data sets from each type of barn (non-RWA and RWA) were included as biological replicates for PERMANOVA analysis of the non-RWA vs. RWA resistome profiles. The ARG frequency in sow feces in RWA barns was not significantly different ($p = 0.072$) from non-RWA barns (Figures 3 and 4A). The ARG frequency in samples collected from sow nasopharynx was significantly higher ($p = 0.016$) in RWA barns compared to non-RWA barns.

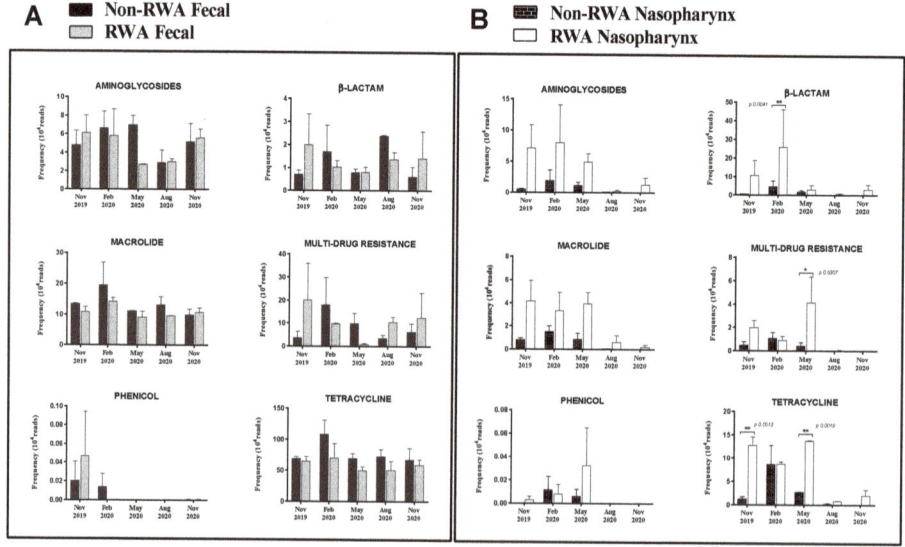

Figure 4. Resistomes from sow feces (**A**) and sow nasopharynx (**B**) in RWA + (plus sign) and non-RWA − (minus sign) barns. The frequency of antibiotic resistance genes (ARG) clustered in six classes: aminoglycoside, β-lactam, macrolide, MDR, phenicol, and tetracycline. Two data sets from each type of barn (non-RWA and RWA) were included as biological replicates for statistical analysis. ANOVA 2-way analysis with repeated measures comparing RWA vs. non-RWA with Bonferroni's correction; * $p < 0.05$, ** $p < 0.01$.

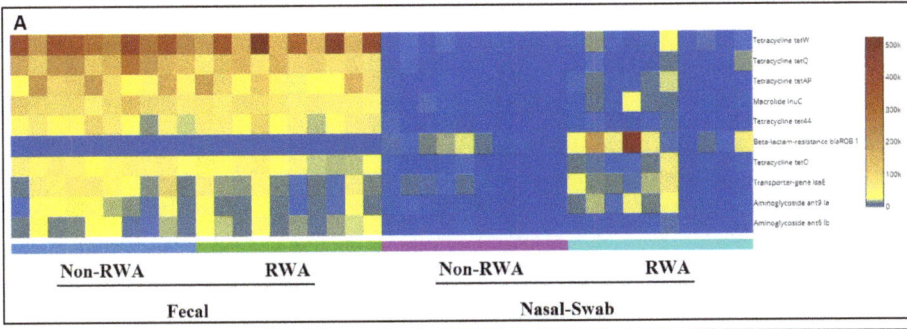
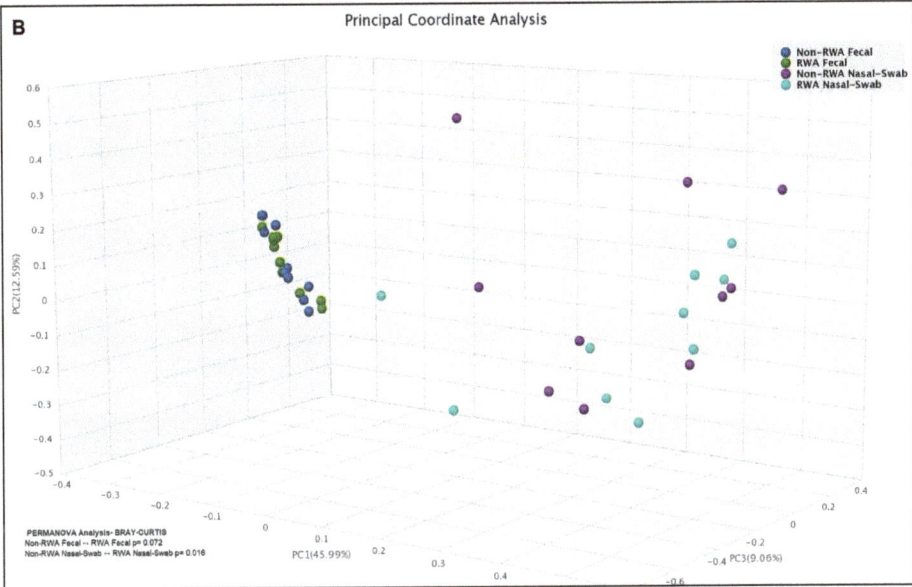

Figure 5. Gene frequency heat map comparative analysis of sow feces and nasal swabs from non-RWA vs. RWA barns, showing the frequencies of the 10 most abundant ARGs (**A**). PCoA and ordination PERMANOVA analysis of the RWA vs. non-RWA resistome profiles from sow feces and nasal swab samples (**B**).

3. Discussion

The impact of antibiotic treatments on the prevalence of pathogens and ARGs in the gut microbiome of piglets and grower-finisher pigs has previously been examined [14–17]; however, limited information is available on the potential differential effects of these treatments on the abundance of pathogens and ARGs in the gut and nasal microbiome of sows. The monitoring of antimicrobial usage in the Canadian swine industry through the Canadian Integrated Program for Antimicrobial Resistance Surveillance (CIPARS) is mainly focused on grower-finisher pigs, with no data on sows available [13]. Similarly, most reports of antimicrobial usage in the United States are mostly focused on nursery and grower-finisher pigs, and data on sows are not well-documented [21]. In Europe, a study conducted by Echtermann et al. [22] involved the monitoring of antimicrobial usage from 71 Swiss non-RWA farrow-to-finish farms in 2017. Based on antimicrobial data expressed in terms of the number of defined daily doses Switzerland (nDDDch) in milligrams per kilogram pig weight, the most prevalent treatment was penicillin (β-lactams), which accounted for 57% of the nDDDch, while tetracyclines were minimal (2%), and antifolates were not reported [22].

These findings contrasted with non-RWA practices in Canadian operations shown in our study, where sows were treated with more antifolates (72% of the cumulative DDDvetCA value) and less β-lactams (1.3%), but consistent with RWA practices (85% β-lactams and no antifolates). These differences could be attributed to a number of factors such as geographic location, animal management, and age of pigs, among others. In non-RWA sows, antifolates were used to treat respiratory impairment and limping symptoms, while β-lactams were administered to sows in participating RWA barns for symptoms related to gestation, as well as infection and injuries (visible swellings). Antifolates are widely used in Canadian swine production; these drugs are antibacterial, immunomodulatory, and chemotherapeutic agents but the mechanism of resistance is poorly documented and is likely linked to inducing efflux multidrug-resistance [23,24]. On the other hand, resistance to β-lactams and tetracyclines have been proven to be globally ubiquitous in pig microbiomes yet still remain in use and clinically valuable [25–27].

In order to assess the impact of the RWA approach on the prevalence of pathogens and ARGs, fecal and nasal swab samples were collected from sows in RWA and non-RWA barns. Analyses of the metagenomes showed increased abundance of pathogenic *Actinobacteria*, *Firmicutes*, and *Proteobacteria* in the nasopharynx microbiome of sows raised under the RWA program relative to non-RWA sows. This could be attributed to the reduced antimicrobial usage of sows in RWA barns, which was about 4.3-fold lower than in non-RWA barns. However, in other studies the impact of antibiotics administration on the nasal microbiota of pigs was variable. In a study by Correa-Fiz et al. [18], the non-RWA practice at early stage of life caused significant increase in the relative abundance of *Campylobacter*, but exhibited a lower relative abundance of other potentially pathogenic bacteria in the nasal microbiota of piglets. Similarly, the administration of antibiotics caused considerable variation in the relative abundance of some pathogenic bacteria in the nasal microbiota of pigs; the variation was dependent on dosing regimen [28], age of pigs [18] and type of antimicrobial treatment [29]. In this study, the decrease in the relative abundance of *Actinobacteria* over time in the nasal microbiota of sows raised under the RWA program could be associated with the stage of growth. In a study by Slifierz et al. [30], only the relative abundance of *Actinobacteria* decreased over time among the bacterial phyla in the nasal microbiota of pigs, and the authors suggested that this temporal shift may have been caused by aging. This decreasing trend, however, was not evident in the nasopharynx samples from non-RWA sows because of their extensive exposure to antibiotic treatments which can disturb the nasal microbiome of pigs [28].

On the other hand, WGS data from the sow gut demonstrated a higher prevalence of pathogenic *Firmicutes* in non-RWA samples than in RWA samples. This is consistent with the findings of Sun et al. [31], where an increase in the abundance of *Firmicutes* in sow fecal samples was observed after the administration of antibiotics. *Firmicutes* was previously found to be the most abundant phylum in the core and variable microbiome of acute diarrheal patients (dysbiosis) and/or a source of ARGs in the infected gut of individuals treated with antibiotics [32]. In addition, the relative abundance of pathogenic bacteria, such as *Clostridium* and *Corynebacterium*, increased in the gut microbiota of finishing pigs administered with lincomycin [15]. This increase, according to the authors, could be due to their antibiotic-resistant properties [15].

In this study, there was no significant difference in the frequency of ARGs detected in the sow feces from RWA and conventional (non-RWA) barns. However, the metagenomics results from the nasal microbiome of sows raised under RWA production exhibited a significant increase in the frequency of resistance genes coding for β-lactams, MDR, and tetracycline compared to non-RWA sows. This could be associated with sows being exposed to higher concentrations of β-lactams and tetracycline in RWA barns relative to non-RWA barns. On the other hand, the impact of the increased usage of these types of antibiotics in RWA barns was not evident in the fecal microbiome of sows, which suggests that the ARGs in the nasal microbiome could be more susceptible to antibiotic exposure than those in the fecal microbiome. In the study by Holman et al. [33] on the impact of antibiotic treatments on the fecal and nasal microbiota of feedlot cattle, antibiotic resistance determinants in the nasal microbiome were more significantly affected by antibiotic treatment than those in the fecal microbiome. To date, information on the correlation between antimicrobial usage and frequency of ARGs in the nasal microbiome of sows is very limited. However, several studies have shown the emergence of a substantial number of antimicrobial resistance determinants in the swine gut microbiome, even in the absence of antimicrobial exposure [16,17,34–36]. For instance, in a study by Looft et al. [35], numerous tetracyclines genes, including *tetB(P)* and *tetQ*, were frequently found in fecal samples from piglets with no antibiotic exposure. Similarly, our present study demonstrated a higher abundance of tetracycline resistance genes *tetW* and *tetQ* in sow fecal samples. The emergence of antimicrobial resistance determinants in swine facilities without direct antimicrobial exposure could be related to the inclusion of high doses of heavy metals such as zinc and copper in swine diets [36–38]. Cross-resistance, as well as co-selection and co-resistance between antimicrobial resistance determinants and heavy metal resistance genes, could potentially explain why antimicrobial resistance genes persist in the pig gut even without prior antimicrobial administration [39,40].

4. Materials and Methods

4.1. Experimental Design and Sample Collection

A 13-month longitudinal study of swine barns that adopted the RWA program, and conventional barns using antibiotics in line with the new regulations (non-RWA), was conducted by collecting fecal and nasopharynx samples from sows at 3-month intervals; these samples were then subjected to whole genome sequencing (WGS) and compared using bioinformatics. During the 13-month period, regular collection of metadata was also conducted, and was comprised of all records of administered antibiotic drugs and illnesses or treatment reasons from the two types (RWA or non-RWA) of participating barns. Table 2 summarizes the type, name, dosages, and routes of administration of antibiotics to sows in RWA and non-RWA barns. Sows in the participating non-RWA barns were fed with wheat/barley-based diets while those in RWA barns had wheat-based and corn-based diets.

Table 2. Type, drug name, dosages, and route of administration of antibiotics to sows in non-RWA and RWA barns.

Barns	Type of Antibiotics	Drug Name	Dosage	Treatment Route [1]
Non-RWA				
	Antifolate	Trimidox (trimethoprim & sulfadoxine)	1 mL/15 kg/day	IV or IM injection
	Tetracycline	Biomycin (Oxytetracycline)	1 mL/10 kg/day	IM or subcutaneous
	β-lactam	Penicillin G	6000 IU per kg (1 mL/50 kg)	IM injection
		Polyflex (ampicillin)	6 mg/kg/day	IM injection
		Excenel (ceftiofur)	3.0 mg/kg/day for 3 days	IM injection
RWA				
	β-lactam	Polyflex (ampicillin)	6 mg/kg/day	IM injection
		Penicillin G	6000 IU per kg (1 mL/50 kg)	IM injection
	Tetracycline	Biomycin (Oxytetracycline)	1 mL/10 kg/day	IM or subcutaneous

[1] IM is intramuscular; IV is intravenous.

A total of five regular animal sampling time points was conducted over the monitoring period. At each time point, fresh fecal samples were collected aseptically from three third-parity sows (approximately 18–22 months old) and stored in sterile 50 mL tubes. The nasal swabs were collected from the same animals by following similar procedures described in the Swab Collection and DNA Preservation System (Norgen Biotek Corp., Thorold, Canada). The nasal swab samples were analyzed to detect potential subsets of respiratory viruses along with other microorganism categories, and their associated antimicrobial resistance genes (ARGs), that may not be well represented in the fecal samples. All samples were stored at 4 °C in a styrofoam container and shipped within 24 h of collection to the laboratory for storage at −80 °C and subsequent analyses. The handling of samples followed the guidelines outlined in the CDC's Biosafety in Microbiological and Biomedical Laboratories (BMBL) manual for Level 1 biologic materials [41].

4.2. Whole Genome Sequencing (WGS) and Sequence Analyses

The total complement of ARGs (the resistome), bacterial diversity, as well as the prevalence of pathogens in the collected samples were identified by random shotgun next-generation sequencing (NGS) using an Illumina HiSeq platform (Omega-Bioservices, Norcross, GA, USA). Sample handling was performed in accordance with the sequencing service procedures and then shipped to Omega-Bioservices for DNA extraction, data quality determination, and NGS. A detailed workflow method of a health metadata-based management approach to compare and quantify WGS data targeting the occurrence of antimicrobial resistance and pathogens in Canadian swine barns was reported previously by the team [40]. DNA extraction from 1 g of sample material, and validation of the purity and yield of the DNA, were carried out using the Mag-Bind Universal Pathogen DNA Kit (Omega Biotek, Inc. Norcross, GA, USA) and Quant-iT™ PicoGreen™ ds DNA System kit (ThermoFisher Scientific, Pittsburgh, PA, USA), respectively. Shotgun NGS libraries were made from DNA using Kapa Biosystems Prep Kit according to manufacturer's instructions (Roche®, KK2103 Pleasanton, CA, USA). Samples corresponding to distinct collection points were run on one lane of a HiSeq4000/X Ten instrument (Illumina, San Diego, CA, USA), generating a total of 100–120 GB of 150-bp paired-end data reads. Each sample generated two FASTQ files (R1 Forward read and R2 Reverse read), producing an average minimum of ~30 million reads (MReads) that were shared through the Illumina BaseSpace Sequence Hub. The sequences were then subjected to quality control (denoising and adaptor trimming) and reported using the MultiQC tool (v1.11 SciLifeLab, Stockholm, Sweden) at https://multiqc.info/, accessed on 9 July 2021 before being uploaded to the platform for metagenomic analysis (CosmosID Inc., Rockville, MD, USA).

4.3. Prevalence of Pathogens and Resistome

A subset of the taxonomic profiles belonging to bacterial pathogens was used to identify the total complement of pathogens (the pathome). As described in a study by Chekabab et al. [14], microbes were classified and identified on the species-, subspecies-, and strain-levels. The relative abundance and frequency of the identified organisms were quantified using GenBook comparators and the GENIUS software implemented within the CosmosID algorithm. This taxonomic profiling included a subset of pathogenic bacteria (the pathome), which was manually assigned to human and animal risk groups (RG2, or RG3).

The ARGs in the microbiome (resistome) were identified and quantified by comparing unassembled sequence reads to CosmosID's curated ARG database. NCBI- RefSeq, PATRIC, M5NR, ENA, DDBJ, CARD, ResFinder, ARDB, and ARG-ANNOT were among the inputs utilized by the ARG database in the platform. These databases contain nearly 4000 distinct ARGs based on percent gene coverage as a function of the gene-specific read frequency in each sample. Using a classification system derived from two antimicrobial resistance pipelines (https://megares.meglab.org/, accessed on 9 July 2021 and https://card.mcmaster.ca/, accessed on 9 July 2021 the resulting ARG profile table was then clustered into 16 drug resistance classes and 7 resistance mechanisms [42].

4.4. Statistical Analysis

Frequency tables with taxa and ARG were subjected to univariate and multivariate analyses for diversity, ordination, and differential frequency. The species richness (Shannon alpha diversity indices and beta diversity distance matrices) was calculated. Two data sets from each type of farm (non-RWA and RWA) were included as biological replicates for statistical analysis.

Principal Coordinate Analysis (PCoA) was performed to cluster the readout frequencies of pathogen species and ARG class in the samples (Bray-Curtis distance matrix; community structure). PERMANOVA analysis was used to identify significantly different readouts. Both PCoA and PERMANOVA analyses were conducted using the CosmosID platform. Individual ARG classes of drug resistance were compared using two-way parametric ANOVA (GraphPad Prism v7.00, San Diego, CA, USA) with non-RWA and RWA as barn groups, and fecal, nasal and time-point repeated measurements as sub-groups.

5. Conclusions

The adoption of RWA measures in sow barns to reduce the total on-farm usage of antibiotics, and consequently to mitigate the emergence of AMR, has caused significant shifts in the diversity and abundance of certain pathogens and ARGs in the gut and nasopharynx microbiome of sows. During the 13-month monitoring period, whole genome sequence analyses revealed that sows raised under the RWA program had a higher frequency of pathogens in the nasopharynx, and a lower frequency of pathogens in the gut relative to sows in conventional non-RWA barns. On the other hand, the reduction of antibiotic usage in RWA barns resulted in an increased abundance of ARGs in sow nasopharynx but had no significant impact on ARG frequency in sow feces. An expanded longitudinal monitoring with more participating non-RWA and RWA barns over a longer timeframe is needed to more definitively validate the correlations and trends observed in this study regarding the impact of reduced antibiotic exposure on the frequency of ARGs and prevalence of pathogens in the gut and nasopharynx microbiome of older animals like sows.

Supplementary Materials: The following supporting information can be downloaded at: https://www.mdpi.com/article/10.3390/antibiotics11091221/s1, Table S1: Pathome-List of pathogens detected in sows feces and nasal-swabs.

Author Contributions: Conceptualization, methodology, experimental design, analyses, and interpretation of the result, A.C.A., S.M.C., B.Z.P. and D.R.K.; writing—original draft preparation, A.C.A. and S.M.C. writing—review and editing, S.M.C., B.Z.P. and D.R.K.; supervision, B.Z.P. and D.R.K.; funding acquisition, B.Z.P. and D.R.K. All authors have read and agreed to the published version of the manuscript.

Funding: Financial support to this project was provided by the Agriculture Development Fund through the Saskatchewan Ministry of Agriculture and the Canada–Saskatchewan Growing Forward 2 bilateral agreement. The work was also partially supported by the Natural Sciences and Engineering Research Council of Canada.

Institutional Review Board Statement: Not applicable. This study involved the collection of samples from pig barns (nasopharynx and fecal samples) and did not involve any sampling from animal organs.

Informed Consent Statement: Not applicable. This study involved the collection of samples from pig barns (nasopharynx and fecal samples) and did not involve any sampling from animal organs.

Data Availability Statement: DNA metagenomics sequencing data are available in Sequence Read Archive (SRA) (https://submit.ncbi.nlm.nih.gov/subs/sra/) with the accessions number PRJNA844237.

Acknowledgments: The authors gratefully acknowledge the financial support provided by the Agriculture Development Fund to this research project through the Saskatchewan Ministry of Agriculture and the Canada–Saskatchewan Growing Forward 2 bilateral agreement. The support provided by the farm owners, management, and production staff and technicians in the participating barns is greatly appreciated. The authors would also like to acknowledge the strategic program funding provided by

Sask Pork, Alberta Pork, Ontario Pork, the Manitoba Pork Council, and the Saskatchewan Agriculture Development Fund.

Conflicts of Interest: The authors declare no conflict of interest. A.C.A., S.M.C. and B.Z.P. declare that the research was conducted in the absence of any commercial or financial relationships that could be construed as a potential conflict of interest. The funders had no role in the design of the study; in the collection, analyses, or interpretation of data; in the writing of the manuscript; or in the decision to publish the results.

References

1. World Health Organization. Antimicrobial Resistance Global Report on Surveillance. 2014. Available online: https://www.who.int/publications/i/item/9789241564748 (accessed on 25 May 2022).
2. Van Boeckel, T.P.; Pires, J.; Silvester, R.; Zhao, C.; Song, J.; Criscuolo, N.G.; Gilbert, M.; Bonhoeffer, S.; Laxminarayan, R. Global trends in antimicrobial resistance in animals in low- and middle-income countries. *Science* **2019**, *365*, eaaw1944. [CrossRef]
3. Public Health Agency of Canada. Canadian Antimicrobial Resistance Surveillance System Report. 2021. Available online: https://www.canada.ca/en/public-health/services/publications (accessed on 10 May 2022).
4. Arnold, C.; Schupbach-Regula, G.; Hirsiger, P.; Malik, J.; Scheer, P.; Sidler, X.; Spring, P.; Perer-Egil, J.; Harisberger, M. Risk factors for oral antimicrobial consumption in Swiss fattening pigs farms—A case-control study. *Porc. Health Manag.* **2016**, *2*, 5. [CrossRef] [PubMed]
5. Public Health Agency of Canada. Canadian Antimicrobial Resistance Surveillance System Report. 2016. Available online: https://www.canada.ca/en/public-health/services/publications (accessed on 13 May 2022).
6. Carmo, L.P.; Schüpbach, G.; Müntener, C.; Alban, L.; Nielsen, L.R.; Magouras, I. Quantification of antimicrobial use in Swiss pigs: Comparison with other Swiss livestock species and with Danish pigs. In Proceedings of the Safe Pork Conference: Epidemiology and Control of Hazards in Pork Production Chain, Porto, Portugal, 7–10 September 2015.
7. Callens, B.; Persoons, D.; Maes, D.; Laanen, M.; Postma, M.; Boyen, F. Prophylactic and metaphylactic antimicrobial use in Belgian fattening pig herds. *Prev. Vet. Med.* **2012**, *106*, 53–62. [CrossRef] [PubMed]
8. Rajić, A.; Reid-Smith, R.; Deckert, A.E.; Dewey, C.E.; McEwen, S.A. Reported antibiotic use in 90 swine farms in Alberta. *Can. Vet. J.* **2006**, *47*, 446–452.
9. Dunlop, R.H.; McEwen, S.A.; Meek, A.H.; Clarke, R.C.; Black, W.D.; Friendship, R.M. Association among antimicrobial drug treatments and antimicrobial resistance of fecal Escherichia coli of swine on 34 farrrow-to-finish farms in Ontario, Canada. *Prev. Vet. Med.* **1998**, *34*, 283–305. [CrossRef]
10. Statistics Canada. Hogs Statistics, Number of Hogs on Farms at End of Semi-Annual Period. 2022. Available online: https://www150.statcan.gc.ca/t1/tbl1/en/tv.action?pid=3210016001 (accessed on 3 May 2022).
11. Cromwell, G.L. Why and how antibiotics are used in swine production. *Anim. Biotechnol.* **2002**, *13*, 7–27. [CrossRef] [PubMed]
12. Arruda, A.G.; Deblais, L.; Hale, V.L.; Madden, C.; Pairis-Garcia, M.; Srivastava, V.; Kathayat, D.; Kumar, A.; Rajashekara, G. A cross-sectional study of the nasal and fecal microbiota of sows from different health status within six commercial swine farms. *PeerJ* **2021**, *9*, e12120. [CrossRef]
13. Canadian Integrated Program for Antimicrobial Resistance Surveillance (CIPARS). Pigs. 2019. Available online: https://www.canada.ca/en/public-health/services/surveillance/canadian-integrated-program-antimicrobial-resistance-surveillance-cipars.html#wb-auto-4 (accessed on 10 May 2022).
14. Chekabab, S.M.; Lawrence, J.R.; Alvarado, A.C.; Predicala, B.Z.; Korber, D.R. Piglet gut and in-barn manure from farms on a raised without antibiotics program display reduced antimicrobial resistance but an increased prevalence of pathogens. *Antibiotics* **2021**, *10*, 1152. [CrossRef]
15. Jo, H.E.; Kwon, M.S.; Whon, T.W.; Kim, D.W.; Yun, M.; Lee, J.; Shin, M.Y.; Kim, S.H.; Choi, H.J. Alteration of gut microbiota after antibiotic exposure in finishing swine. *Front. Microbiol.* **2021**, *12*, 596002. [CrossRef]
16. Zeineldin, M.; Aldridge, B.; Lowe, J. Antimicrobial effects on swine gastrointestinal microbiota and their accompanying antibiotic resistome. *Front. Microbiol.* **2019**, *10*, 1035. [CrossRef]
17. Holman, D.B.; Chénier, M.R. Antimicrobial use in swine production and its effect on the swine gut microbiota and antimicrobial resistance. *Can. J. Microbiol.* **2015**, *61*, 785–798. [CrossRef] [PubMed]
18. Correa-Fiz, F.; Gonçalves dos Santos, J.M.; Illas, F.; Aragon, V. Antimicrobial removal on piglets promotes health and higher bacterial diversity in the nasal microbiota. *Sci. Rep.* **2019**, *10*, 1035. [CrossRef] [PubMed]
19. Man, W.H.; de Steenhuijsen Piters, W.A.; Bogaert, D. The microbiota of the respiratory tract: Gatekeeper to respiratory health. *Nat. Rev. Microbiol.* **2017**, *15*, 259–270. [CrossRef]
20. Canadian Integrated Program. for Antimicrobial Resistance Surveillance (CIPARS) Annual Report. 2016. Available online: https://www.canada.ca/en/public-health/services/surveillance/canadian-integrated-program-antimicrobial-resistance-surveillance-cipars/cipars-reports/2016-annual-report-summary.html (accessed on 10 February 2022).
21. Davies, P.R.; Singer, R.S. Antimicrobial use in wean to market pigs in the United States assessed via voluntary sharing of proprietary data. *Zoonoses Public Health* **2020**, *67*, 6–21. [CrossRef]

22. Echtermann, T.; Muentener, C.; Sidler, X.; Kuemmerlen, D. Antimicrobial usage among different age categories and herd sizes in Swiss farrow-to-finish farms. *Front. Vet. Sci.* **2020**, *7*, 566529. [CrossRef]
23. Visentin, M.; Zhao, R.; Goldman, I.D. The Antifolates. *Hematol. Oncol. Clin. N. Am.* **2012**, *26*, 629–648. [CrossRef]
24. Takemura, Y.; Kobayashi, H.; Miyachi, H. Cellular and molecular mechanisms of resistance to antifolate drugs: New analogues and approaches to overcome the resistance. *Int. J. Hematol.* **1997**, *66*, 459–477. [CrossRef]
25. Bergspica, I.; Kaprou, G.; Alexa, E.A.; Prieto, M.; Alvarez-Ordonez, A. Extended spectrum beta-lactamase (ESBL) producing Escherichia coli in pigs and pork meat in the European Union. *Antibiotics* **2020**, *9*, 678. [CrossRef]
26. Hayer, S.S.; Rovira, A.; Olsen, K.; Johnson, T.J.; Vannucci, F.; Rendahl, A.; Perez, A.; Alvarez, J. Prevalence and trend analysis of antimicrobial resistance in clinical Escherichia coli isolates collected from diseased pigs in the USA between 2006 and 2016. *Transbound. Emerg. Dis.* **2020**, *67*, 1930–1941. [CrossRef]
27. Hayer, S.S.; Rovira, A.; Olsen, K.; Johnson, T.J.; Vannucci, F.; Rendahl, A.; Perez, A.; Alvarez, J. Prevalence and time trend analysis of antimicrobial resistance in respiratory bacterial pathogens collected from diseased pigs in USA between 2006–2016. *Res. Vet. Sci.* **2020**, *128*, 135–144. [CrossRef]
28. Mou, K.T.; Allen, H.K.; Alt, D.P.; Trachsel, J.; Hau, S.J.; Coetzee, J.F.; Holman, D.B.; Kellner, S.; Loving, C.L.; Brockmeier, S.L. Shifts in the nasal microbiota of swine in response to different dosing regimens of oxytetracycline administration. *Vet. Microbiol.* **2019**, *237*, 108386. [CrossRef]
29. Zeineldin, M.; Aldridge, B.; Blair, B.; Kancer, K.; Lowe, J. Microbial shifts in the swine nasal microbiota in response to parenteral antimicrobial administration. *Microb Pathog.* **2018**, *121*, 210–217. [CrossRef] [PubMed]
30. Slifierz, M.J.; Friendship, R.M.; Weese, J.S. Longitudinal study of the early-life fecal and nasal microbiotas of the domestic pig. *BMC Microbiol.* **2015**, *15*, 184. [CrossRef] [PubMed]
31. Sun, J.; Li, L.; Liu, B.; Xia, J.; Liao, X.; Liu, Y. Development of aminoglycoside and β-lactamase resistance among intestinal microbiota of swine treated with lincomycin, chlortetracycline, and amoxicillin. *Front. Microbiol.* **2014**, *5*, 580. [CrossRef]
32. De, R.; Mukhopadhyay, A.K.; Dutta, S. Metagenomic analysis of gut microbiome and resistome of diarrheal fecal samples from Kolkata, India, reveals the core and variable microbiota including signatures of microbial dark matter. *Gut Pathog.* **2020**, *7*, 12–32. [CrossRef]
33. Holman, D.B.; Yang, W.; Alexander, T.W. Antibiotic treatment in feedlot cattle: A longitudinal study of the effect of oxytetracycline and tulathromycin on the fecal and nasopharyngeal microbiota. *Microbiome* **2019**, *7*, 86. [CrossRef] [PubMed]
34. Agga, G.E.; Morgan Scott, H.; Vinasco, J.; Nagaraja, T.G.; Amachawadi, R.G.; Bai, J.; Norby, B.; Renter, D.G.; Dritz, S.S.; Nelssen, J.L.; et al. Effects of chlortetracycline and copper supplementation on the prevalence, distribution, and quantity of antimicrobial resistance genes in the fecal metagenome of weaned pigs. *Prev. Vet. Med.* **2015**, *119*, 179–189. [CrossRef]
35. Looft, T.; Johnson, T.A.; Allen, H.K.; Bayles, D.O.; Alt, D.P.; Stedtfeld, R.D.; Sul, W.J.; Stedtfeld, T.M.; Chai, B.; Cole, J.R.; et al. In-feed antibiotic effects on the swine intestinal microbiome. *Proc. Natl. Acad. Sci. USA* **2012**, *109*, 1691–1696. [CrossRef]
36. Pakpour, S.; Jabaji, S.; Chenier, M.R. Frequency of antibiotic resistance in a swine facility 2.5 years after a ban on antibiotics. *Microb. Ecol.* **2012**, *63*, 41–50. [CrossRef] [PubMed]
37. Stanton, T.B.; Humphrey, S.B.; Stoffregen, W.C. Chlortetracycline-resistant intestinal bacteria in organically raised and feral swine. *Appl. Environ. Microbiol.* **2011**, *77*, 7167–7170. [CrossRef]
38. Mathew, A.G.; Beckmann, M.A.; Saxton, A.M. A comparison of antibiotic resistance in bacteria isolated from swine herds in which antibiotics were used or excluded. *J. Swine Health Prod.* **2001**, *9*, 125–129.
39. Frye, J.G.; Lindsey, R.L.; Meinersmann, R.J.; Berrang, M.E.; Jackson, C.R.; Englen, M.D.; Turpin, J.B.; Fedorka-Cray, P.J. Related antimicrobial resistance genes detected in different bacterial species co-isolated from swine fecal samples. *Foodborne Pathog. Dis.* **2011**, *8*, 663–679. [CrossRef]
40. Baker-Austin, C.; Wright, M.S.; Stepanauskas, R.; McArthur, J.V. Co-selection of antibiotic and metal resistance. *Trends Microbiol.* **2006**, *14*, 176–182. [CrossRef]
41. Centers for Disease Control and Prevention. *Biosafety in Microbiological and Biomedical Laboratories (BMBL)*, 6th ed.; Centers for Disease Control and Prevention: Atlanta, GA, USA, 2018. Available online: https://www.cdc.gov/labs/BMBL.html (accessed on 24 October 2020).
42. Chekabab, S.M.; Lawrence, J.R.; Alvarado, A.C.; Predicala, B.Z.; Korber, D.R. A health metadata-based management approach for comparative analysis of high-throughput genetic sequences for quantifying antimicrobial resistance reduction in Canadian hog barns. *Comput. Struct. Biotechnol. J.* **2020**, *18*, 2629–2638. [CrossRef] [PubMed]

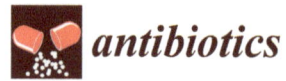

Article

Fecal Carriage of *Escherichia coli* Harboring the *tet*(X4)-IncX1 Plasmid from a Tertiary Class-A Hospital in Beijing, China

Weishuai Zhai [1], Yingxin Tian [2], Dongyan Shao [1], Muchen Zhang [1], Jiyun Li [1], Huangwei Song [1], Chengtao Sun [1], Yang Wang [1], Dejun Liu [1,*] and Ying Zhang [2,*]

[1] Key Laboratory of Animal Antimicrobial Resistance Surveillance, Ministry of Agriculture and Rural Affairs, and Beijing Key Laboratory of Detection Technology for Animal-Derived Food Safety, College of Veterinary Medicine, China Agricultural University, Beijing 100193, China
[2] Department of Laboratory Medicine, the First Medical Centre, Chinese PLA General Hospital, Beijing 100853, China
* Correspondence: liudejun@cau.edu.cn (D.L.); cherryzju@aliyun.com (Y.Z.)

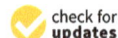

Citation: Zhai, W.; Tian, Y.; Shao, D.; Zhang, M.; Li, J.; Song, H.; Sun, C.; Wang, Y.; Liu, D.; Zhang, Y. Fecal Carriage of *Escherichia coli* Harboring the *tet*(X4)-IncX1 Plasmid from a Tertiary Class-A Hospital in Beijing, China. *Antibiotics* 2022, 11, 1068. https://doi.org/10.3390/antibiotics11081068

Academic Editors: Mitsushige Sugimoto, Anne Farewell and Mehran Monchi

Received: 19 June 2022
Accepted: 3 August 2022
Published: 6 August 2022

Publisher's Note: MDPI stays neutral with regard to jurisdictional claims in published maps and institutional affiliations.

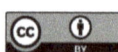

Copyright: © 2022 by the authors. Licensee MDPI, Basel, Switzerland. This article is an open access article distributed under the terms and conditions of the Creative Commons Attribution (CC BY) license (https://creativecommons.org/licenses/by/4.0/).

Abstract: The emergence of the mobile tigecycline-resistance gene, *tet*(X4), poses a significant threat to public health. To investigate the prevalence and genetic characteristics of the *tet*(X4)-positive *Escherichia coli* in humans, 1101 human stool samples were collected from a tertiary class-A hospital in Beijing, China, in 2019. Eight *E. coli* isolates that were positive for *tet*(X4) were identified from clinical departments of oncology (n = 3), hepatology (n = 2), nephrology (n = 1), urology (n = 1), and general surgery (n = 1). They exhibited resistance to multiple antibiotics, including tigecycline, but remained susceptible to meropenem and polymyxin B. A phylogenetic analysis revealed that the clonal spread of four *tet*(X4)-positive *E. coli* from different periods of time or departments existed in this hospital, and three isolates were phylogenetically close to the *tet*(X4)-positive *E. coli* from animals and the environment. All *tet*(X4)-positive *E. coli* isolates contained the IncX1-plasmid replicon. Three isolates successfully transferred their tigecycline resistance to the recipient strain, C600, demonstrating that the plasmid-mediated horizontal gene transfer constitutes another critical mechanism for transmitting *tet*(X4). Notably, all *tet*(X4)-bearing plasmids identified in this study had a high similarity to several plasmids recovered from animal-derived strains. Our findings revealed the importance of both the clonal spread and horizontal gene transfer in the spread of *tet*(X4) within human clinics and between different sources.

Keywords: tigecycline resistance; *tet*(X4); *Escherichia coli*; IncX1; clonal spread

1. Introduction

In recent decades, antimicrobial resistance (AMR) in clinical pathogens has become a significant threat to human health and a major source of concern for microbiologists and clinicians around the world. Tigecycline, the first antibiotic of the glycylcycline class, is considered one of the last antibiotic options for treating clinical infections caused by multi-drug resistance (MDR) Gram-negative bacteria, particularly carbapenem-resistant Enterobacteriaceae (CRE) and carbapenem-resistant *Acinetobacter baumannii* (CRAB) [1]. However, the frequent use of tigecycline promotes the development of tigecycline resistance, which can lead to a clinical treatment failure. Earlier studies found that tigecycline resistance is typically generated by the over-expression of efflux pumps and mutations within the drug-binding site in the ribosome [2], but there have been few reports of a horizontal gene transfer of tigecycline resistance.

The plasmid-carried *tet*(A) mutations can lead to a low-level resistance to tigecycline in *Klebsiella pneumoniae* [3], but it is uncommon. Tet(X), a flavin-dependent monooxygenase that can inactivate tetracyclines, was first described in *Bacteroides fragilis* [4,5]. Tet(X2), an ortholog of Tet(X), was originally isolated from the transposon CTnDOT in *Bacteroides thetaoiotaomicron* [6]. Both *tet*(X) variants are active against the earlier classes of tetracyclines but show limited activity against tigecycline [7]. In 2019, two novel plasmid-encoded mobile tigecycline-resistance genes, tet(X3) and tet(X4), were initially discovered in *A. baumannii* and Enterobacteriaceae isolated from animals, humans, and the environment in multiple provinces of China [8,9]. These two variants confer a high-level resistance to all tetracycline antibiotics, including tigecycline as well as two FDA-approved new antibiotics, eravacycline and omadacycline [8]. Following that discovery, several novel tet(X) variants, tet(X5) [10], tet(X6) [11], tet(X7) to tet(X13) [12], tet(X14) [13], and tet(X15) [14], have been identified in a variety of bacterial species from diverse sources.

Fortunately, most tet(X) variants have only been reported sporadically and cannot be transferred by a plasmid-mediated horizontal gene transfer. However, it should be noted that the tet(X4) gene has gradually become one of the most common plasmid-mediated tigecycline genes in China [15] and has also been identified in more than five countries in Europe and Asia [16,17]. The tet(X4) gene was predominantly found in pigs, pork, and the surrounding environments of pig farms or slaughterhouses but was rare in human health sectors. Unfortunately, the presence of tet(X4) progressively increased in clinical cases [18,19] and in healthy humans [15]. Moreover, a greater concern is that the tet(X4) gene has been sporadically found in coexistence with the mobile colistin gene, mcr-1, [20] or carbapenemase-encoding gene bla_{NDM-5} [21], further limiting the drug options for the treatment of infections caused by these extensively drug-resistant bacterial pathogens. Notably, the rapid spread of the tet(X4) gene between different clinical strains was attributed to horizontal gene transfers within hospitals [18,19], but the clonal transmission of tet(X4) between different sources, particularly animals and humans, cannot be neglected even if it is relatively rare.

In this study, we described the antibiotic-resistance characteristics and molecular epidemiology of the clinical tet(X4)-positive *E. coli* isolates in a Chinese hospital. We further identified that the tet(X4) gene can be transmitted via bacterial clonal spread or horizontal genetic transfer in hospitals. These findings will help us in better understanding the transmission of tet(X4) between animals and humans.

2. Results

2.1. Resistance Genes, Plasmid Replicons, and Virulence Factors

A total of 1101 fresh faeces were collected through a four-month surveillance programme (from June to September) in a tertiary class-A hospital in 2019. Eight tigecycline-resistant isolates that were positive for the tet(X4) gene were identified as *Escherichia coli*. They were isolated from the fecal samples of six male and two female hospitalized patients in June ($n = 1$), August ($n = 5$), and September ($n = 2$), respectively. These patients came from five distinct clinical departments: oncology ($n = 3$), hepatology ($n = 2$), nephrology ($n = 1$), urology ($n = 1$), and general surgery ($n = 1$) (Table S1).

The antimicrobial-susceptibility test revealed that eight tet(X4)-positive *E. coli* isolates displayed resistance to multiple antibiotics, including ampicillin, doxycycline, tigecycline, sulfamethoxazole-trimethoprim, and florfenicol, while still being susceptible to polymyxin B and meropenem (Table S1). In addition, two *E. coli* isolates (YY176 and YY139) were resistant to levofloxacin and ciprofloxacin, but only one isolate, YY176, was also resistant to gentamicin and ceftriaxone. All of the tet(X4)-positive *E. coli* isolates carried the sulphonamide (sul3), trimethoprim (dfrA), phenicol (floR), and tetracycline (tet(A) and tet(X4)) resistance genes and at least one β-lactamase resistance gene (such as bla_{TEM-1A}, bla_{TEM-1B}, $bla_{CTX-M-14}$, and bla_{SHV-12}) (Figure 1), which was basically consistent with the presence of their resistance phenotypes.

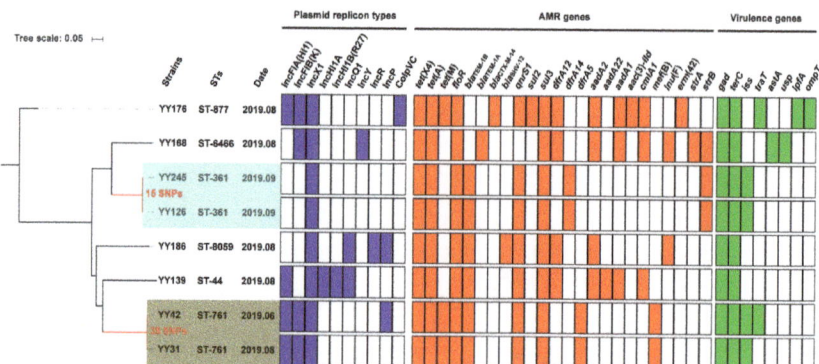

Figure 1. The phylogenetic tree and genomic features of eight *tet*(X4)-positive *E. coli* isolates. On the phylogenetic tree, the light blue and light brown color ranges reflect the two clonal groups. The heatmap in different colors depicts the presence or absence of the plasmid replicon types (blue), antimicrobial-resistance (AMR) genes (red), and virulence genes (green).

The PlasmidFinder analysis of eight isolates identified ten distinct plasmid replicons: IncFIA(HI1), IncFIB(K), IncX1, IncHI1A, IncHI1B(R27), IncQ1, IncY, IncR, IncP, and ColpVC (Figure 1). IncX1 was identified in each of these isolates. In addition, eight virulence genes, including *gad* (n = 8), *terC* (n = 8), *iss* (n = 4), *traT* (n = 2), *astA* (n = 1), *usp* (n = 1), *lpfA* (n = 1), and *ompT* (n = 1), were identified. Only one *E. coli* YY176 isolate exhibited five virulence genes, and the remaining seven isolates possessed two to four virulence genes (Figure 1). Although the presence of virulence genes does not indicate pathogenicity, it still implies a pathogenic potential, which poses a potential threat to human health.

2.2. Genomic Population Structure and the Phylogenetic Context

The MLST analysis revealed that eight *tet*(X4)-carrying isolates had a high degree of genetic diversity and could be classified into six sequence types (STs), including ST8059 (n = 1), ST6466 (n = 1), ST877 (n = 1), ST761 (n = 2), ST361 (n = 2), and ST44 (n = 1) (Figures 1 and 2). Two STs (ST877 and ST761) have already been discovered in animal- and human-derived *tet*(X4)-positive *E. coli* [17,18,22]. The SNP analysis revealed that these isolates shared a total of 65,529 single nucleotide polymorphisms (SNPs), with SNPs ranging from 15 to 49,573 bp between them (Table S2). *E. coli* YY126 and YY245 shared the fewest SNPs (15 SNPs), followed by *E. coli* YY31 and YY42 (39 SNPs), indicating that these strains had a closer genetic relationship. Interestingly, *E. coli* YY126 and YY245 were isolated concurrently, but they originated in separate sections (oncology and hepatology) within the hospital. By contrast, *E. coli* YY31 and YY42 were isolated at separate times from distinct clinical departments in the hospital. These findings suggest that a portion of the *tet*(X4)-positive *E. coli* could be spreading clonally within this hospital.

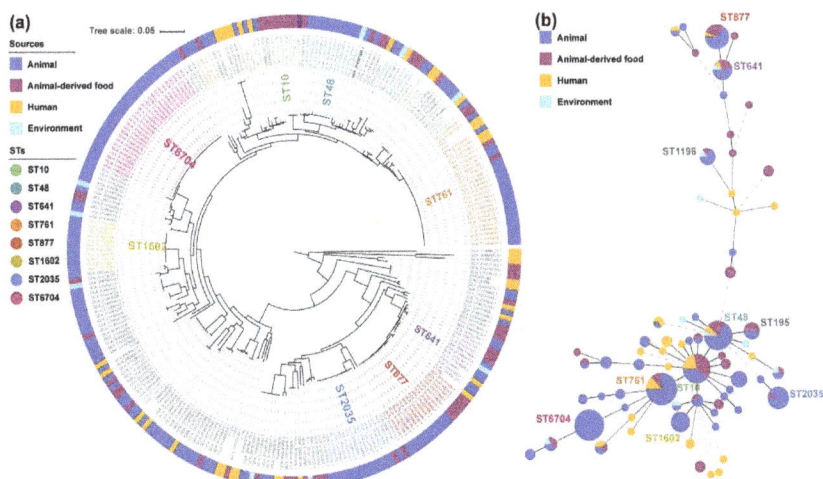

Figure 2. Phylogenetic tree (**a**) and minimum spanning tree (**b**) of 280 *tet*(X4)-positive *E. coli*.

To further explore the potential origin of the eight clinical isolates, a phylogenetic tree was generated using our eight and two-hundred and seventy-two online *tet*(X4)-positive *E. coli* genomes based on a core-genome SNP analysis (Figure 2a), and a minimum spanning tree was constructed using the MLST data (Figure 2b). There were over 70 different STs among the 280 strains, with 8 dominant STs (more than ten strains) accounting for 55% (95% CI, 49.1–60.9%). However, only three STs (ST761, ST877, and ST641) have great potential in the transmission between humans and animals via clonal spread among the eight dominant STs. Most of them were not only obtained from multiple sources but also have a very close evolutionary distance in the individual groups (Figure 2a), especially the previously proved *E. coli* ST761 [23]. In this study, two clonal groups and four non-clonal *E. coli* isolates were located on six separate clades in the phylogenetic tree. Three out of eight isolates belonging to ST761 or ST877 were phylogenetically closely related to the strains from animals and the environment, while the remaining five isolates clustered alone. Therefore, taken as a whole, the transmission of the *tet*(X4) gene in this hospital may be associated with both the clonal spread and horizontal gene transfer.

2.3. Conjugation and the Genetic Environment

The horizontal transmissibility of the *tet*(X4)-bearing plasmid was determined via a conjugation assay. Three isolates, *E. coli* YY42, YY168, and YY186, successfully transferred their tigecycline resistance to the recipient strain, *E. coli* C600, with transfer frequencies ranging from 2.39×10^{-7} to 1.32×10^{-4} (Table S1 and Figure S1), whereas the remaining five strains failed. To better understand the horizontal gene transfer of the *tet*(X4) gene, a third-generation sequencing was performed on *E. coli* YY42, YY168, and YY186 with their transconjugants TCYY42, TCYY168, and TCYY186. However, *E. coli* YY42 and its transconjugant *E. coli* TCYY42 were unable to acquire the entire *tet*(X4)-bearing plasmid sequence due to the multiple tandem repeats of the *tet*(X4)-bearing sequence. Thus, the two genomes were reassembled based on the available long-read data to obtain the complete plasmid sequence. In fact, such tandem repeats are common in the *tet*(X4)-positive strains and frequently result in a failed assembly of the *tet*(X4)-bearing plasmid, as previously described [19,24,25].

We further analysed the genetic context of the *tet*(X4) gene among the eight isolates to observe the possible tandem repeats. The *ISCR2* was detected on the downstream-flanking region of *tet*(X4) in all isolates, but there were several cases of the upstream-flanking region of *tet*(X4) (Figure S2). One such case showed that *ISCR2* was absent or *ISCR2* was terminated by other mobile elements on the upstream-flanking region of tet(X4), which does not affect the normal assembly of the tet(X4)-bearing plasmid. Alternatively, two entire ISCR2 were positioned on both the upstream- and downstream-flanking regions of tet(X4), which could form numerous tandem repeats and ultimately lead to an assembly failure. In short, the presence or absence of the ISCR2 upstream of the tet(X4) gene is a critical determinant of the assembly of the tet(X4)-bearing plasmid. Subsequently, the plasmid analyses of eight isolates using both the hybrid assembly and only-long-read assembly revealed that four tet(X4)-bearing IncX1 plasmids, pYY168, pYY186, YY245, and pYY126_trycycler, with sizes ranging from 40 to 60 kb, were identified in four E. coli isolates; three tet(X4)-bearing IncX1/FIA(HI1)/FIB(K) hybrid plasmids, pYY31, pYY42_trycycler, and pYY176_trycycler, with sizes ranging from 120 to 180 kb, were identified in three E. coli isolates; one 248,932 bp tet(X4)-bearing IncX1/FIA(HI1)/HI1A/HI1B(R27) hybrid plasmid, pYY139, was identified in one isolate.

2.4. The tet(X4)-Carrying IncX1 Plasmid

The analysis of two transferable tet(X4)-carrying IncX1 plasmids showed that pYY168 and pYY186 are composed of three components: a plasmid backbone and two variable regions, including one multidrug-resistance determining region and one conjugative-transfer determining region that contained a VirB family type IV secretion system (T4SS) (Figure 3a,b). The multidrug-resistance determining region of pYY186 possessed six distinct AMR genes, including tet(X4), tet(A), floR, lnu(F), aadA2, and bla_{SHV-12}, but pYY168 lacked bla_{SHV-12}. Through a Blastn alignment, we determined that pYY186 shared 99.97% sequence identity with pYY168 at 83% coverage (Figure 4). Four online IncX1 plasmids from the NCBI database were acquired using pYY186 as a reference query (99% identity and 100% coverage): p1916D6-2 (59,351 bp, accession no. CP046002), pYY76-1-2 (57,105 bp, accession no. CP040929), pHNCF11W-tetX4 (57,104 bp, accession no. CP053047), and p1916D18-1 (59,353 bp, accession no. CP045998) (Figure 4). These plasmids were recovered from four E. coli strains isolated from cows ($n = 1$), chicken ($n = 1$), and swine ($n = 2$). We also found one tet(X4)-bearing plasmid, pEC931_tetX (50,626 bp, accession no. CP049121), from one E. coli strain from a person with a urinary tract infection that shared a 97% identity with 99.97% coverage with pYY168 and an 81% identity with 100% coverage with pYY186. Moreover, another four NCBI-obtained tet(X4)-bearing IncX1 plasmids (accession no. NZ_MN436006, NZ_MN436007, NZ_MT197111, and NZ_MT219821) ranging from 30 to 40 kb in length shared 57% identity and >99.97% coverage with pYY186, but these plasmids lacked the VirB family T4SS, which may result in the functional absence of conjugation (Figure 4). Notably, in the current study, two tet(X4)-bearing IncX1 plasmids, pYY245 and pYY126_trycycler, lacking the conjugation capacity were also devoid of the VirB family T4SS. They were 99.97% identical to two 44,691 bp plasmids, pCD58-3-1(accession no. CP050037) and pCD74-2-2 (accession no. CP050046), recovered from the E. coli strains of a broiler chicken, at 100% coverage, and carried eight AMR genes including tet(X4), tet(A), bla_{TEM-1B}, aph(6)-Id, floR, sul3, qnrS1, and dfrA14 (Figures 3c and S3). The high similarity of the tet(X4)-bearing IncX1 plasmid between animals and humans indicated that the plasmid has achieved a wide distribution among different origins and plays an important role in the transmission of multidrug resistance, including tigecycline resistance.

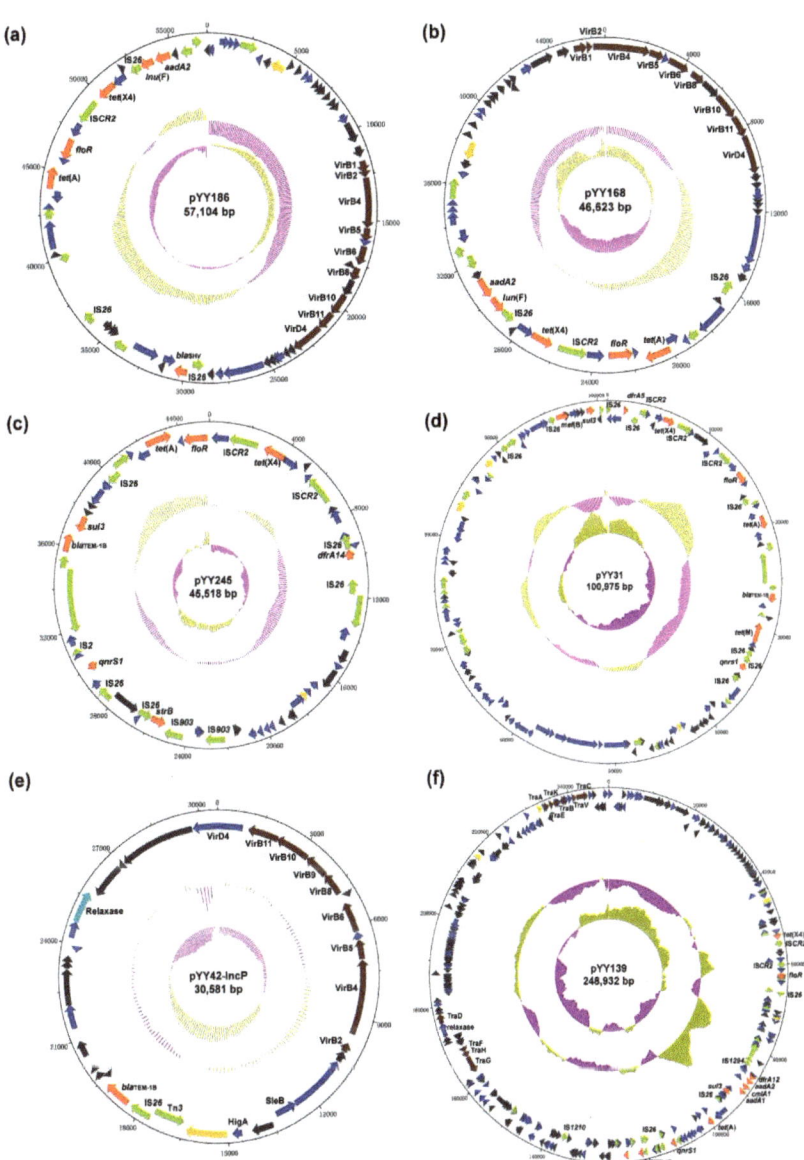

Figure 3. Schematic maps of multiple plasmids. A circular map of pYY186 (**a**), pYY168 (**b**), pYY245 (**c**), pYY31 (**d**), pYY42-IncP (**e**), and pYY139 (**f**). The innermost circle presents the GC-Skew and the middle circle presents the GC content. The gene functions are indicated by arrows with different colors in the outer circle. Red, AMR gene; yellow, replication initiation protein gene; brown, conjugative transfer gene; green, mobile element; dark grey, hypothetical protein gene; navy blue, other functional gene.

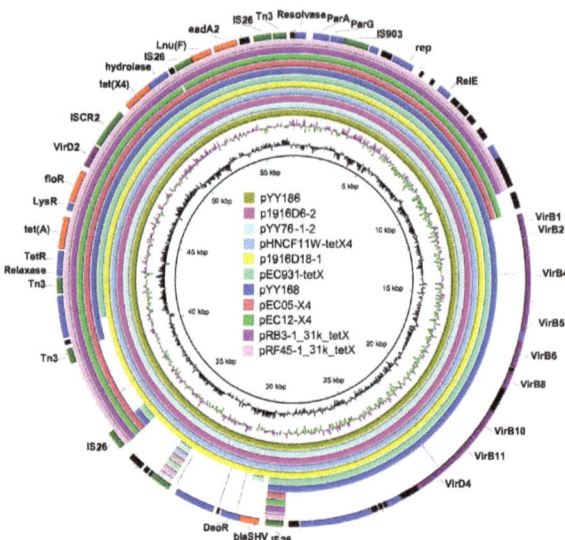

Figure 4. Circular comparison of the *tet*(X4)-bearing IncX1 plasmids with other closely related IncX1 plasmids from the NCBI database. The outermost ring represents the reference IncX1 plasmid pYY186 with its gene positions. Different colors in the outermost ring represent distinct genes: Red represents the resistance gene, purple represents the gene of T4SS, green represents the mobile element, black represents the hypothetical protein, and blue represents other functional genes. The map was constructed using BRIG software.

2.5. The tet(X4)-Carrying IncX1-Containing Hybrid Plasmid

By conducting a Blastn alignment of three IncX1/FIA(HI1)/FIB(K) hybrid plasmids, we established that pYY31 was virtually identical to the long-read assembly plasmid, pYY42_trycycler (>99% identity and 100% coverage) (Figures 3d and S4a), but differed from the long-read assembly plasmid pYY176_trycycler. Using pYY31 as a reference query, more than ten plasmids ranging from 100 to 130 kb recovered from pigs and cattle were retrieved using BLASTn (>99% identity and 100% coverage). These shared a highly similar plasmid backbone and nine AMR genes, including *tet*(X4), *tet*(A), *tet*(M), bla_{TEM-1B}, *mef*(B), *floR*, *sul3*, *qnrS1*, and *dfrA5*. Interestingly, both pYY42_trycycler and pYY31 lacked the conjugative-elements VirB family T4SS, but pYY42_trycycler could be transformed into the recipient strain by conjugation. A further analysis of the full genome sequences revealed the presence of a 30,581 bp IncP plasmid, pYY42-IncP (Figure 3e and Figure S4b), in *E. coli* YY42 and its transconjugants TCYY42, but not in *E. coli* YY31. The plasmid, pYY42-IncP, contained the VirB family T4SS, which may aid in the co-transfer of the plasmid pYY42_trycycler to recipient strains via conjugation. It was 100% identical to a 30,581 bp plasmid, pD72-IncP (accession no. CP035316.1), recovered from an animal-derived *mcr-1*-positive *E. coli* isolate D72 at 100% coverage (Figure S4b). In addition, the long-read assembly plasmid, pYY176_trycycler, was more than 99% identical to four plasmids recovered from the *E. coli* strains of pigs at >87% coverage (Figure S4c). This plasmid carried 11 AMR genes including *tet*(X4), *tet*(A), *tet*(M), *aadA1*, *aadA2*, *floR*, *erm*(42), *cmlA1*, *sul2*, *sul3*, and *dfrA12*. The IncX1/FIA(HI1)/HI1A/HI1B(R27) hybrid plasmid, pYY139 (Figure 3f), was 100% identical to the 219,101 bp plasmid, p1919D3-1 (accession no. CP046004), recovered from an *E. coli* isolate of swine feces, at 89% coverage (Figure S4d). This plasmid carried a multidrug-resistance region that included *tet*(X4), *tet*(A), *aadA1*, *aadA2*, *aadA22*, bla_{TEM-1B}, *qnrS1*, *floR*, *cmlA1*, *sul3*, and *dfrA12*. Overall, these results suggested that the VirB family T4SS played an important role in the transmission of the *tet*(X4)-bearing IncX1 plasmid or IncX1-containing hybrid plasmid.

3. Discussion

Since the plasmid-mediated tigecycline-resistance gene tet(X4) was first described in China in 2019 [8,9], it has been widely detected in animals but sporadically reported in humans. The earliest report revealed that the detection rate of tet(X4)-positive *E. coli* isolates in humans was only 0.07% [8] (4/5485). This proportion increased to 0.73% (8/1101) among clinical tet(X4)-positive *E. coli* isolates in our study. Likewise, some recent studies found that the proportion of clinical tet(X4)-positive *E. coli* in humans increased modestly [15,18], but it was unclear whether the increase was associated with the high prevalence of tet(X4) in animals. Therefore, monitoring their reservoirs and transmission routes is essential, particularly regarding cross-species transmission between animals and humans.

Current epidemiological evidence indicated that the tet(X4) gene was predominantly presented in Enterobacteriaceae, particularly *E. coli* [8,9,15,17,18,26]. Thus, using *E. coli* as a model species for investigating the transmission of tigecycline resistance between diverse sources is preferred. According to a previous study, twelve tet(X4)-positive *E. coli* isolated from the gut microbiota of healthy Singaporeans possessed nine known STs and three untypable STs [17]. In addition, clinical isolates of tet(X4)-positive *E. coli* also exhibited a significant degree of genetic diversity in certain areas of China [18]. Hence, the rapid acquisition and dissemination of tet(X4) are commonly attributed to a horizontal gene transfer via conjugative plasmids and the translocation of the active mobile element, ISCR2 [26,27], rather than to clonal spread. Recently, several dominant clonal types of *E. coli* (such as *E. coli* ST10 and ST48) carrying tet(X4) have been detected in both animals and humans [18,22]; however, the SNP numbers often differ widely between different sources according to the SNP analysis of this study. Notably, unlike these STs, two *E. coli* ST761 isolates in this study shared a close relationship with other tet(X4)-positive *E. coli* ST761 strains isolated from animal-derived samples [23]. We also discovered that one isolate shared a significant degree of genetic similarity with a tet(X4)-positive *E. coli* ST877 strain isolated from pork. These findings suggest that the clonal spread of tet(X4)-positive dominant clonal types across humans and animals poses a great threat to human health.

The IncX-group plasmids, especially IncX3 [28] and IncX4 [29], demonstrated an important role in contributing to the spread of carbapenemase genes and colistin-resistance genes between different strains. Currently, more than eight plasmid-replicon types were observed in the tet(X4)-positive *E. coli* strains [22,24,26]. Of these, IncX1 plasmids have been found in diverse STs of *E. coli* from multiple sources [8,9,15,18,22,24]. All of the tet(X4)-bearing plasmids in this study were IncX1 plasmids or IncX1-containing hybrid plasmids; both groups had a high similarity to several plasmids recovered from animal-derived strains, suggesting a connection of these plasmids between the strains from humans and animals. Notably, the IncX1 plasmid was able to form a hybrid plasmid with other Inc plasmids (e.g., IncF plasmid), which facilitated its survival in a broad range of hosts. Although some IncX1 plasmids have lost the capacity for self-conjugation, their conjugation can occur through a helper plasmid carrying a VirB family T4SS, such as IncP, as observed in this study. Therefore, we propose that IncX1 plasmids or IncX1-containing hybrid plasmids play a significant role in the dissemination of the tet(X4) gene.

4. Materials and Methods

4.1. Sample Collection and Strain Identification

Fresh fecal samples were collected from patients for antibiotic-resistance surveillance at a tertiary class-A hospital in Beijing, China, from June to September 2019 (Table S3). The fresh samples were homogenized in PBS (pH = 7.2). The 100 μL sample of homogenate was then mixed with 10 mL of LB broth (supplemented with 2 mg/L tigecycline) and incubated for 12 h at 37 °C with 200 rpm shaking. Next, the enriched broth was streaked on CHROMagar™ Orientation agar plates with tigecycline (2 mg/L) and incubated at 37 °C for 24 h. Purified colonies were obtained after re-streaking three times on a MacConkey agar plate and were then stored in a Microbank™ (Pro-Lab Diagnostics, Toronto, ON, Canada) at −70 °C. Bacterial species were identified using a MALDI-TOF/MS (Shimadzu,

Kyoto, Japan) and reconfirmed by 16S rRNA gene sequencing. A colony PCR was used to screen *tet*(X)-positive clones using the universal primers, *tet*(X)-F (5′-TGA ACC TGG TAA GAA GAA GTG-3′) and *tet*(X)-R (5′-CAG ACA ATA TCA AAG CAT CCA-3′), and Sanger sequencing was used to confirm all amplicons after PCR amplification.

4.2. Antimicrobial Susceptibility Testing

The minimum inhibitory concentrations (MICs) were determined using the broth microdilution method following the latest guidelines of the Clinical and Laboratory Standards Institute (CLSI) and the European Committee on Antimicrobial Susceptibility Testing (EUCAST). Briefly, all isolates were first streaked onto MHA agar and grown overnight at 37 °C. Then, each isolate was inoculated in 0.9% NaCl to a McFarland standard of 0.5 and was tested for susceptibility to 12 antibiotics using custom-made Sensititre plates (Thermo Fisher Scientific, USA), including ampicillin (AMP), amoxicillin-clavulanate (2:1) (AMC), doxycycline (DOX), tigecycline (TGC), levofloxacin (LVX), ciprofloxacin (CIP), ceftriaxone (CRO), gentamicin (GEN), meropenem (MEM), trimethoprim-sulfamethoxazole (SXT), florfenicol (FFC), and polymyxin B (PB). Finally, all isolates were incubated for 16–20 h at 37 °C. The resistance breakpoints of most antimicrobial drugs were interpreted according to the CLSI guidelines [30], whereas tigecycline MIC was defined by the EUCAST breakpoints [31] for *E. coli*. ATCC25922 was used as a reference strain (quality control).

4.3. Conjugation Assay

The transmission of the *tet*(X4) gene was assessed by performing the conjugation experiment using the filter-mating method with the streptomycin-resistant *E. coli* C600 as the recipient. Briefly, donor and recipient strains were grown overnight and then diluted at 1:100 in fresh LB broth. After a 6 h incubation at 37 °C, the donor and recipient strains were mixed at a 1:3 ratio. The mixtures were subsequently coated on a 0.45 μM microporous composite membrane on a solid medium and incubated at 37 °C for 6 h. Transconjugants were selected on MacConkey agar plates containing 2 mg/L tigecycline with 3000 mg/L of streptomycin and were verified by PCR to confirm the successful transfer. Transfer frequencies were calculated as the number of transconjugants obtained per recipient, as previously described [8].

4.4. Genome Sequencing and Bioinformatics

The whole-genome DNA of all isolates and transconjugants were extracted using a HiPure Bacterial DNA Kit (Magen, Guangzhou, China) following the protocols described by the manufacturer. Samples were sent to Sinobiocore (Beijing, China) for sequencing on the Illumina HiSeq 2500 system with a read length of 150 bp, paired-end. Then, Nanopore libraries were constructed and sequenced on the MinION long-read sequencing platform (Oxford Nanopore Technologies, Oxford, UK). Both Illumina short reads and Oxford Nanopore long reads of each strain were included in a hybrid assembly using a Unicycler (Version 4.0.1, https://github.com/rrwick/Unicycler, accessed on 1 July 2022) [32]. Three plasmids were reassembled using a Trycycler (Version 0.5.3, https://github.com/rrwick/Trycycler, accessed on 1 July 2022) due to the failed assembly of the *tet*(X4)-bearing plasmids caused by multiple tandem repeats [33]. After assembling, medaka (Version 1.4.3, https://github.com/nanoporetech/medaka, accessed on 1 July 2022) and pilon (Version 1.2.4, https://github.com/broadinstitute/pilon, accessed on 1 July 2022) [34] were used to polish the plasmid sequences. Online genomes of *tet*(X4)-carrying *E. coli* were obtained from the NCBI database (Table S4). The AMR determinants, plasmid replicons, and sequence types were identified using a Staramr (Version 0.5.1, https://github.com/phac-nml/staramr, accessed on 1 July 2022) [35] against the ResFinder [36], PlasmidFinder, and MLST databases [37], respectively. Gene prediction and automatic annotation were performed using the RAST service [38]. Putative virulence determinants were identified using VirulenceFinder (version 2.0, https://cge.food.dtu.dk/services/VirulenceFinder, accessed on 1 July 2022) [39]. A minimum spanning tree of all sequence types was constructed in the BioNumerics software (version 7.0, https://www.applied-maths.com/bionumerics, accessed on 1 July 2022) according to correlations among alleles. Phylogenetic trees were performed using the Parsnp (Harvest v1.1.2, https://github.com/marbl/parsnp, accessed on 1 July 2022) and visualized using iTOL (https://itol.embl.de, accessed on 1 July 2022). Plasmid maps were manually annotated using the DNAplotter software [40] and the comparison analysis of multiplex plasmid sequences was performed using a BLAST Ring Image Generator (BRIG, http://brig.sourceforge.net/, accessed on 1 July 2022) [41].

4.5. Statistical Analysis

Data were collected using Microsoft Excel files. A statistical analysis was performed with the IBM SPSS Software, version 25 (IBM SPSS Statistics, Armonk, NY, USA). The confidence interval (CI) reported was at 95%.

5. Conclusions

In conclusion, we characterized the epidemiological and genomic features of *tet*(X4)-positive *E. coli* isolated from the stool of inpatients from a tertiary class-A hospital in China. The clonal spread of the *tet*(X4)-positive isolates indicated the risk of intra-hospital transmission of the *tet*(X4) gene. In addition, although specific origins could not be accurately traced, these strains and plasmids of clinic patient origin showed a strong genetic resemblance to some animal-origin strains, implying a potential risk of transmission between animals and humans. As such, since both the clonal spread and horizontal gene transfer aggravate the spread of the *tet*(X4) gene, the routine surveillance of the *tet*(X) genes is critical for effectively curbing the further transmission of tigecycline-resistance strains between animals and humans.

Supplementary Materials: The following supporting information can be downloaded at: https://www.mdpi.com/article/10.3390/antibiotics11081068/s1, Figure S1: Distribution of antimicrobial-resistance genes and plasmid-replicon types among three *E. coli* isolates and their transconjugants; Figure S2: Characterization of *tet*(X4)-bearing genetic environments in eight isolates; Figure S3: Circular comparison of *tet*(X4)-bearing IncX1 plasmid, pYY245; Figure S4: Circular comparison of four plasmids. Table S1: MICs of eight *tet*(X4)-positive isolates and three transconjugants; Table S2: Pairwise SNP distance matrix for eight *tet*(X4)-positive isolates; Table S3 Information of 1101 fecal samples; Table S4: Information of eight *tet*(X4)-positive *E. coli* and two-hundred and seventy-two online *tet*(X4)-positive *E. coli* genomes.

Author Contributions: Conceptualization: W.Z. and Y.Z.; methodology: W.Z., Y.T., D.S. and J.L.; validation: W.Z., Y.T., D.S. and J.L.; formal analysis: Y.T., M.Z. and H.S.; investigation: W.Z., M.Z. and H.S.; resources: M.Z. and H.S.; writing—original draft preparation: W.Z.; writing—review and editing: Y.W., C.S. and D.L.; visualization: W.Z., D.S. and J.L.; supervision: Y.W. and Y.Z.; project administration: W.Z., M.Z. and H.S.; funding acquisition: C.S., Y.W. and D.L. All authors have read and agreed to the published version of the manuscript.

Funding: This study is supported by the Guangdong Major Project of Basic and Applied Basic Research (No. 2020B0301030007) and the grants from National Natural Science Foundation of China (81991531 and 32002340).

Institutional Review Board Statement: Not applicable.

Informed Consent Statement: Informed consent was not required since we used to-be-discarded stool samples in this study and no personal identifiers, such as names, were collected.

Data Availability Statement: All genome sequences have been deposited in the GenBank database under the BioProject accession number, PRJNA846553. The sequence data of all transconjugants and three only-long-read assembled plasmids were deposited in the figshare database (https://doi.org/10.6084/m9.figshare.20071841, accessed on 1 July 2022) for reference.

Conflicts of Interest: The authors declare no conflict of interest.

References

1. Karageorgopoulos, D.E.; Kelesidis, T.; Kelesidis, I.; Falagas, M.E. Tigecycline for the treatment of multidrug-resistant (including carbapenem-resistant) *Acinetobacter* infections: A review of the scientific evidence. *J. Antimicrob. Chemother.* **2008**, *62*, 45–55. [CrossRef] [PubMed]
2. Sun, Y.; Cai, Y.; Liu, X.; Bai, N.; Liang, B.; Wang, R. The emergence of clinical resistance to tigecycline. *Int. J. Antimicrob. Agents* **2013**, *41*, 110–116. [CrossRef] [PubMed]
3. Yao, H.; Qin, S.; Chen, S.; Shen, J.; Du, X.D. Emergence of carbapenem-resistant hypervirulent *Klebsiella pneumoniae*. *Lancet Infect. Dis.* **2018**, *18*, 25. [CrossRef]
4. Yang, W.; Moore, I.F.; Koteva, K.P.; Bareich, D.C.; Hughes, D.W.; Wright, G.D. TetX is a flavin-dependent monooxygenase conferring resistance to tetracycline antibiotics. *J. Biol. Chem.* **2004**, *279*, 52346–52352. [CrossRef] [PubMed]
5. Speer, B.S.; Bedzyk, L.; Salyers, A.A. Evidence that a novel tetracycline resistance gene found on two *Bacteroides* transposons encodes an NADP-requiring oxidoreductase. *J. Bacteriol.* **1991**, *173*, 176–183. [CrossRef] [PubMed]
6. Whittle, G.; Hund, B.D.; Shoemaker, N.B.; Salyers, A.A. Characterization of the 13-kilobase ermF region of the *Bacteroides* conjugative transposon CTnDOT. *Appl. Environ. Microb.* **2001**, *67*, 3488–3495. [CrossRef]
7. Walkiewicz, K.; Davlieva, M.; Wu, G.; Shamoo, Y. Crystal structure of *Bacteroides thetaiotaomicron* TetX2: A tetracycline degrading monooxygenase at 2.8 A resolution. *Proteins* **2011**, *79*, 2335–2340. [CrossRef] [PubMed]
8. He, T.; Wang, R.; Liu, D.; Walsh, T.R.; Zhang, R.; Lv, Y.; Ke, Y.; Ji, Q.; Wei, R.; Liu, Z.; et al. Emergence of plasmid-mediated high-level tigecycline resistance genes in animals and humans. *Nat. Microbiol.* **2019**, *4*, 1450–1456. [CrossRef]
9. Sun, J.; Chen, C.; Cui, C.Y.; Zhang, Y.; Liu, X.; Cui, Z.H.; Ma, X.Y.; Feng, Y.; Fang, L.X.; Lian, X.L.; et al. Plasmid-encoded *tet*(X) genes that confer high-level tigecycline resistance in *Escherichia coli*. *Nat. Microbiol.* **2019**, *4*, 1457–1464. [CrossRef]
10. Wang, L.; Liu, D.; Lv, Y.; Cui, L.; Li, Y.; Li, T.; Song, H.; Hao, Y.; Shen, J.; Wang, Y.; et al. Novel Plasmid-Mediated *tet*(X5) Gene Conferring Resistance to Tigecycline, Eravacycline, and Omadacycline in a Clinical *Acinetobacter baumannii* Isolate. *Antimicrob. Agents Chemother.* **2019**, *64*, e01326-19. [CrossRef]
11. Liu, D.; Zhai, W.; Song, H.; Fu, Y.; Schwarz, S.; He, T.; Bai, L.; Wang, Y.; Walsh, T.R.; Shen, J. Identification of the novel tigecycline resistance gene *tet*(X6) and its variants in *Myroides*, *Acinetobacter* and *Proteus* of food animal origin. *J. Antimicrob. Chemother.* **2020**, *75*, 1428–1431. [CrossRef] [PubMed]
12. Gasparrini, A.J.; Markley, J.L.; Kumar, H.; Wang, B.; Fang, L.; Irum, S.; Symister, C.T.; Wallace, M.; Burnham, C.D.; Andleeb, S.; et al. Tetracycline-inactivating enzymes from environmental, human commensal, and pathogenic bacteria cause broad-spectrum tetracycline resistance. *Commun. Biol.* **2020**, *3*, 241. [CrossRef] [PubMed]
13. Cheng, Y.; Chen, Y.; Liu, Y.; Guo, Y.; Zhou, Y.; Xiao, T.; Zhang, S.; Xu, H.; Chen, Y.; Shan, T.; et al. Identification of novel tetracycline resistance gene *tet*(X14) and its co-occurrence with *tet*(X2) in a tigecycline-resistant and colistin-resistant *Empedobacter stercoris*. *Emerg. Microbes Infect.* **2020**, *9*, 1843–1852. [CrossRef] [PubMed]
14. Li, R.; Peng, K.; Xiao, X.; Wang, Y.; Wang, Z. Characterization of novel IS*Aba*1-bounded *tet*(X15)-bearing composite transposon Tn6866 in *Acinetobacter variabilis*. *J. Antimicrob. Chemother.* **2021**, *76*, 2481–2483. [CrossRef] [PubMed]
15. Dong, N.; Zeng, Y.; Cai, C.; Sun, C.; Lu, J.; Liu, C.; Zhou, H.; Sun, Q.; Shu, L.; Wang, H.; et al. Prevalence, transmission, and molecular epidemiology of *tet*(X)-positive bacteria among humans, animals, and environmental niches in China: An epidemiological, and genomic-based study. *Sci. Total Environ.* **2021**, *818*, 151767. [CrossRef]
16. Fang, L.X.; Chen, C.; Cui, C.Y.; Li, X.P.; Zhang, Y.; Liao, X.P.; Sun, J.; Liu, Y.H. Emerging High-Level Tigecycline Resistance: Novel Tetracycline Destructases Spread via the Mobile Tet(X). *Bioessays* **2020**, *42*, e2000014. [CrossRef]
17. Ding, Y.; Saw, W.Y.; Tan, L.W.L.; Moong, D.K.N.; Nagarajan, N.; Teo, Y.Y.; Seedorf, H. Emergence of tigecycline- and eravacycline-resistant Tet(X4)-producing Enterobacteriaceae in the gut microbiota of healthy Singaporeans. *J. Antimicrob. Chemother.* **2020**, *75*, 3480–3484. [CrossRef]
18. Cui, C.Y.; Li, X.J.; Chen, C.; Wu, X.T.; He, Q.; Jia, Q.L.; Zhang, X.J.; Lin, Z.Y.; Li, C.; Fang, L.X.; et al. Comprehensive analysis of plasmid-mediated *tet*(X4)-positive *Escherichia coli* isolates from clinical settings revealed a high correlation with animals and environments-derived strains. *Sci. Total Environ.* **2022**, *806*, 150687. [CrossRef]
19. Zhai, W.; Tian, Y.; Lu, M.; Zhang, M.; Song, H.; Fu, Y.; Ma, T.; Sun, C.; Bai, L.; Wang, Y.; et al. Presence of Mobile Tigecycline Resistance Gene *tet*(X4) in Clinical *Klebsiella pneumoniae*. *Microbiol. Spectr.* **2022**, *10*, e0108121. [CrossRef]
20. Ruan, Z.; Jia, H.; Chen, H.; Wu, J.; He, F.; Feng, Y. Co-existence of plasmid-mediated tigecycline and colistin resistance genes *tet*(X4) and *mcr-1* in a community-acquired *Escherichia coli* isolate in China. *J. Antimicrob. Chemother.* **2020**, *75*, 3400–3402. [CrossRef]
21. Sun, H.; Zhai, W.; Fu, Y.; Li, R.; Du, P.; Bai, L. Co-occurrence of plasmid-mediated resistance genes *tet*(X4) and *bla*$_{NDM-5}$ in a multidrug-resistant *Escherichia coli* isolate recovered from chicken in China. *J. Glob. Antimicrob. Resist.* **2021**, *24*, 415–417. [CrossRef] [PubMed]
22. Li, R.C.; Li, Y.; Peng, K.; Yin, Y.; Liu, Y.; He, T.; Bai, L.; Wang, Z.Q. Comprehensive Genomic Investigation of Tigecycline Resistance Gene *tet*(X4)-Bearing Strains Expanding among Different Settings. *Microbiol. Spectr.* **2021**, *9*, e01633-21. [CrossRef] [PubMed]
23. Zhai, W.; Wang, T.; Yang, D.; Zhang, Q.; Liang, X.; Liu, Z.; Sun, C.; Wu, C.; Liu, D.; Wang, Y. Clonal relationship of *tet*(X4)-positive *Escherichia coli* ST761 isolates between animals and humans. *J. Antimicrob. Chemother.* **2022**, *77*, 2153–2157. [CrossRef] [PubMed]
24. Li, R.; Lu, X.; Peng, K.; Liu, Z.; Li, Y.; Liu, Y.; Xiao, X.; Wang, Z. Deciphering the Structural Diversity and Classification of the Mobile Tigecycline Resistance Gene *tet*(X)-Bearing Plasmidome among Bacteria. *mSystems* **2020**, *5*, e00134-20. [CrossRef]

25. Song, H.; Liu, D.; Li, R.; Fu, Y.; Zhai, W.; Liu, X.; He, T.; Wu, C.; Bai, L.; Wang, Y. Polymorphism Existence of Mobile Tigecycline Resistance Gene *tet*(X4) in *Escherichia coli*. *Antimicrob. Agents Chemother.* **2020**, *64*, e01825-19. [CrossRef]
26. Sun, C.T.; Cui, M.Q.; Zhang, S.; Liu, D.J.; Fu, B.; Li, Z.K.; Bai, R.N.; Wang, Y.X.; Wang, H.J.; Song, L.; et al. Genomic epidemiology of animal-derived tigecycline-resistant *Escherichia coli* across China reveals recent endemic plasmid-encoded *tet*(X4) gene. *Commun. Biol.* **2020**, *3*, 412. [CrossRef]
27. Liu, D.; Wang, T.; Shao, D.; Song, H.; Zhai, W.; Sun, C.; Zhang, Y.; Zhang, M.; Fu, Y.; Zhang, R.; et al. Structural diversity of the IS*CR2*-mediated rolling-cycle transferable unit carrying *tet*(X4). *Sci. Total Environ.* **2022**, *826*, 154010. [CrossRef]
28. Zhai, R.; Fu, B.; Shi, X.; Sun, C.; Liu, Z.; Wang, S.; Shen, Z.; Walsh, T.R.; Cai, C.; Wang, Y.; et al. Contaminated in-house environment contributes to the persistence and transmission of NDM-producing bacteria in a Chinese poultry farm. *Environ. Int.* **2020**, *139*, 105715. [CrossRef]
29. Wang, Y.; Tian, G.B.; Zhang, R.; Shen, Y.; Tyrrell, J.M.; Huang, X.; Zhou, H.; Lei, L.; Li, H.Y.; Doi, Y.; et al. Prevalence, risk factors, outcomes, and molecular epidemiology of *mcr-1*-positive Enterobacteriaceae in patients and healthy adults from China: An epidemiological and clinical study. *Lancet Infect. Dis.* **2017**, *17*, 390–399. [CrossRef]
30. CLSI. *Performance Standards for Antimicrobial Susceptibility Testing—Thirtieth Edition: M100*; CLSI: Wayne, PA, USA, 2020.
31. EUCAST. Clinical Breakpoints—Bacteria (v 11.0). Available online: https://www.eucast.org/clinical_breakpoints/ (accessed on 1 July 2021).
32. Wick, R.R.; Judd, L.M.; Gorrie, C.L.; Holt, K.E. Unicycler: Resolving bacterial genome assemblies from short and long sequencing reads. *PLoS Comput. Biol.* **2017**, *13*, e1005595. [CrossRef]
33. Wick, R.R.; Judd, L.M.; Cerdeira, L.T.; Hawkey, J.; Meric, G.; Vezina, B.; Wyres, K.L.; Holt, K.E. Trycycler: Consensus long-read assemblies for bacterial genomes. *Genome Biol.* **2021**, *22*, 266. [CrossRef] [PubMed]
34. Walker, B.J.; Abeel, T.; Shea, T.; Priest, M.; Abouelliel, A.; Sakthikumar, S.; Cuomo, C.A.; Zeng, Q.D.; Wortman, J.; Young, S.K.; et al. Pilon: An Integrated Tool for Comprehensive Microbial Variant Detection and Genome Assembly Improvement. *PLoS ONE* **2014**, *9*, e112963. [CrossRef]
35. Bharat, A.; Petkau, A.; Avery, B.P.; Chen, J.C.; Folster, J.P.; Carson, C.A.; Kearney, A.; Nadon, C.; Mabon, P.; Thiessen, J.; et al. Correlation between Phenotypic and In Silico Detection of Antimicrobial Resistance in *Salmonella enterica* in Canada Using Staramr. *Microorganisms* **2022**, *10*, 292. [CrossRef]
36. Bortolaia, V.; Kaas, R.S.; Ruppe, E.; Roberts, M.C.; Schwarz, S.; Cattoir, V.; Philippon, A.; Allesoe, R.L.; Rebelo, A.R.; Florensa, A.F.; et al. ResFinder 4.0 for predictions of phenotypes from genotypes. *J. Antimicrob. Chemother.* **2020**, *75*, 3491–3500. [CrossRef] [PubMed]
37. Carattoli, A.; Zankari, E.; Garcia-Fernandez, A.; Voldby Larsen, M.; Lund, O.; Villa, L.; Moller Aarestrup, F.; Hasman, H. In silico detection and typing of plasmids using PlasmidFinder and plasmid multilocus sequence typing. *Antimicrob. Agents Chemother.* **2014**, *58*, 3895–3903. [CrossRef]
38. Aziz, R.K.; Bartels, D.; Best, A.A.; DeJongh, M.; Disz, T.; Edwards, R.A.; Formsma, K.; Gerdes, S.; Glass, E.M.; Kubal, M.; et al. The RAST Server: Rapid annotations using subsystems technology. *BMC Genom.* **2008**, *9*, 75. [CrossRef]
39. Malberg Tetzschner, A.M.; Johnson, J.R.; Johnston, B.D.; Lund, O.; Scheutz, F. In Silico Genotyping of *Escherichia coli* Isolates for Extraintestinal Virulence Genes by Use of Whole-Genome Sequencing Data. *J. Clin. Microbiol.* **2020**, *58*, e01269-20. [CrossRef]
40. Carver, T.; Thomson, N.; Bleasby, A.; Berriman, M.; Parkhill, J. DNAPlotter: Circular and linear interactive genome visualization. *Bioinformatics* **2009**, *25*, 119–120. [CrossRef]
41. Alikhan, N.F.; Petty, N.K.; Ben Zakour, N.L.; Beatson, S.A. BLAST Ring Image Generator (BRIG): Simple prokaryote genome comparisons. *BMC Genom.* **2011**, *12*, 402. [CrossRef]

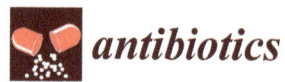

Article

Characterization of bla_{NDM-5}-and $bla_{CTX-M-199}$-Producing ST167 *Escherichia coli* Isolated from Shared Bikes

Qiyan Chen [1,2,†], Zhiyu Zou [1,†], Chang Cai [3], Hui Li [2], Yang Wang [1], Lei Lei [4,*] and Bing Shao [1,2,*]

[1] Beijing Key Laboratory of Detection Technology for Animal-Derived Food Safety, College of Veterinary Medicine, China Agricultural University, Beijing 100193, China; qiyanchen@cau.edu.cn (Q.C.); zouzhiyu@cau.edu.cn (Z.Z.); wangyang@cau.edu.cn (Y.W.)

[2] Beijing Key Laboratory of Diagnostic and Traceability Technologies for Food Poisoning, Beijing Center for Disease Prevention and Control, Beijing 100013, China; lihui@bjcdc.org

[3] College of Arts, Business, Law and Social Sciences, Murdoch University, Perth, WA 6150, Australia; c.cai@murdoch.edu.au

[4] Key Laboratory of Applied Technology on Green-Eco-Healthy Animal Husbandry of Zhejiang Province, Provincial Engineering Research Center for Animal Health Diagnostics & Advanced Technology, Zhejiang International Science and Technology Cooperation Base for Veterinary Medicine and Health Management, China Australia Joint Laboratory for Animal Health Big Data Analytics, College of Animal Science and Technology & College of Veterinary Medicine, Zhejiang A&F University, Hangzhou 311300, China

* Correspondence: leilei910@zafu.edu.cn (L.L.); shaobingch@sina.com (B.S.)

† These authors contributed equally to this work.

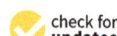

Citation: Chen, Q.; Zou, Z.; Cai, C.; Li, H.; Wang, Y.; Lei, L.; Shao, B. Characterization of bla_{NDM-5}-and $bla_{CTX-M-199}$-Producing ST167 *Escherichia coli* Isolated from Shared Bikes. *Antibiotics* 2022, 11, 1030. https://doi.org/10.3390/antibiotics11081030

Academic Editor: William R. Schwan

Received: 15 June 2022
Accepted: 26 July 2022
Published: 30 July 2022

Publisher's Note: MDPI stays neutral with regard to jurisdictional claims in published maps and institutional affiliations.

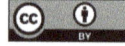

Copyright: © 2022 by the authors. Licensee MDPI, Basel, Switzerland. This article is an open access article distributed under the terms and conditions of the Creative Commons Attribution (CC BY) license (https://creativecommons.org/licenses/by/4.0/).

Abstract: Shared bikes as a public transport provide convenience for short-distance travel. Whilst they also act as a potential vector for antimicrobial resistant (AR) bacteria and antimicrobial resistance genes (ARGs). However, the understanding of the whole genome sequence of AR strains and ARGs-carrying plasmids collected from shared bikes is still lacking. Here, we used the HiSeq platform to sequence and analyze 24 *Escherichia coli* isolated from shared bikes around Metro Stations in Beijing. The isolates from shared bikes showed 14 STs and various genotypes. Two bla_{NDM-5} and $bla_{CTX-M-199}$-producing ST167 *E. coli* have 16 resistance genes, four plasmid types and show >95% of similarities in core genomes compared with the ST167 *E. coli* strains from different origins. The bla_{NDM-5}- or $bla_{CTX-M-199}$-carrying plasmids sequencing by Nanopore were compared to plasmids with bla_{NDM-5}- or $bla_{CTX-M-199}$ originated from humans and animals. These two ST167 *E. coli* show high similarities in core genomes and the plasmid profiles with strains from hospital inpatients and farm animals. Our study indicated that ST167 *E. coli* is retained in diverse environments and carried with various plasmids. The analysis of strains such as ST167 can provide useful information for preventing or controlling the spread of AR bacteria between animals, humans and environments.

Keywords: shared bikes; NDM-5; CTX-M-199; ST167; whole genome analysis

1. Introduction

Shared bikes as a public transport provide more choices and convenience for people's travel. They also act as the last-mile connection between means of transport such as light rail stations or bus stops and people's destinations such as home or the office. Some studies suggest that public transportation such as buses, subways, and taxis can act as a transmission media for bacteria or viruses [1,2], which could cause public health emergencies. Meanwhile, microorganisms on the surface of public transport arouses concern due to the severity of antimicrobial resistance worldwide [3–5]. Previous studies indicated that antimicrobial resistant (AR) Enterobacteriaceae, *Staphylococcus* spp. and *Enterococcus* spp. were already isolated from shared bikes [6–9]. Additionally, various bacteria with antimicrobial resistance genes (ARGs) were found in buses, subways, and aircrafts [1–4].

Several studies showed that both Gram-positive bacteria and Gram-negative bacteria could be isolated from shared bikes. Among them, *Staphylococci* and *Enterococci* were widely distributed in shared bikes around schools, hospitals, metro stations, and from riders, with detection rates of 2.3–12.9% and 0.08–5.5%, respectively [6]. The multiple resistant *Staphylococci* showed diversity in *SCCmec* and sequence type (ST) [8]. Meanwhile, the prevalence of Enterobacteriaceae in shared bikes was 19.7%, which suggested that hospitals might increase the risk of AR Enterobacteriaceae based on the distance from the hospital to the subway station [9]. Wu et al. reported that *Bacillus* was the most abundant bacteria in the shared bicycle bacteria community, and the drug-resistant bacteria in the shared bicycle bacterial community of metro stations, shopping malls, and hospitals showed no significant differences [7].

In recent years, the increasing reports of carbapenem resistance genes have increased the pressure on effective bacterial treatment. ST167 *E. coli* was often reported to carry carbapenem resistance genes such as bla_{KPC-3}, bla_{NDM-5}, and bla_{NDM-1} and was found in various species such as ducks, cattle, and mussels [10–15]. A study on hospitalized neonatal sepsis showed that *E. coli* (34.01%) was one of the main pathogens of neonatal bacteremia, and ST167 was the most prevalent ST [16]. More importantly, ST167 has been reported to spread between companion animals and their owners [12]. The spread of ST167 clones between countries has also been reported [17]. Although characterization of bacteria from shared bikes has attracted widespread attention in recent years, current studies have mainly focused on the prevalence and the phenotypes of strain descriptions in public transportation or the features of isolates themselves. To the best of our knowledge, the whole genome analysis with strains from different locations or biological sources and comparisons of their plasmid profiles are still lacking. *E. coli* is an important representative of Enterobacteriaceae, which can carry a variety of ARGs and has significance for public health safety. Herein, we used the *E. coli* isolates from the shared bikes to investigate the similarities and differences between strains from the shared bikes and other sources to find the relationship of the whole genome sequencing between the *E. coli* isolates from environmental and clinical samples.

2. Results and Discussion

2.1. E. coli Isolates from Shared Bikes

We identified 14 STs among all 24 *E. coli* isolates from shared bikes (14 from Metro Station nearing secondary/tertiary hospitals and ten from non-hospital stations, Supplementary material Table S1), and the ST10 clonal complex (n = 7) were the dominant clonal complex (Figure 1). There is no dominant ST or clonal complex related to hospitals, although ST10, ST48, and ST167 found in this study were the most prevalent STs in hospitals [18–20].

The phylogenetic tree analysis showed that the 24 *E. coli* strains from shared bikes had different profiles. The number of ARGs in each of the strains ranged from one to sixteen, and plasmid types ranged from zero to five (Table S1). The resistance phenotypes showed that some strains (such as 770, 776) which have a higher number of resistance genes exhibited more resistance to antimicrobial agents than other strains. However, the number of strains exhibiting resistance phenotype mismatch the number of ARGs. Some strains showed high similarity in one small clade, for instance, 26, 25, 31 and 769, 780. Almost all AR strains have resistance genes of aminoglycosides, quinolones, sulfonamides, tetracyclines and beta-lactams. Despite most strains (66.7%) from hospital-related stations have resistance gene to different kinds of antimicrobial agents, there is no significant difference between multidrug resistance (MDR) *E. coli* from hospital-related stations and non-hospital stations ($p > 0.05$). The two strains (770 and 776) collected, respectively, from hospital-related stations and non-hospital stations carried the maximum number of resistance genes and plasmid types of all strains and showed >95% similarities in core genomes with the same sequence type ST167 (Figure 2).

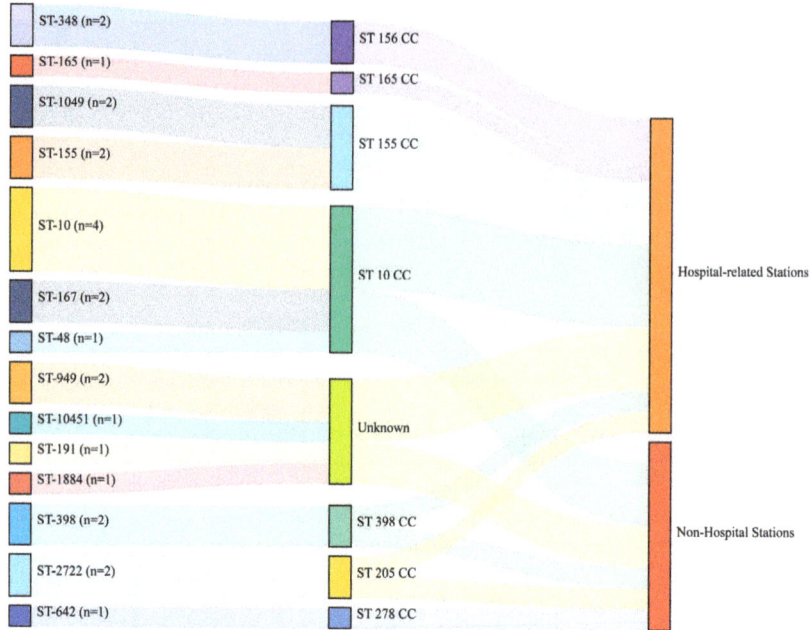

Figure 1. The distribution of STs from 24 *E. coli* in shared bikes. (CC: clonal complex, hospital-related stations represent Metro Stations nearing secondary/tertiary hospitals).

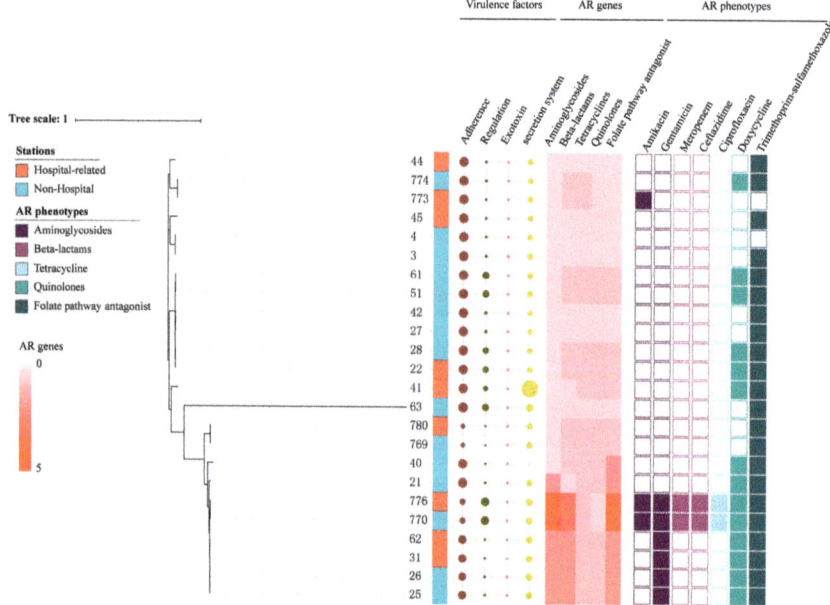

Figure 2. The phylogenetic tree of 24 *E. coli* from shared bikes. (The size of circles represents the number of virulence factors. The color of the heatmap indicated the number of resistance genes found in different antibiotic classes. Different colors were used to distinguish AR phenotypes of each antibiotic class).

Furthermore, these two strains carried bla_{NDM-5} and $bla_{CTX-M-199}$, and another 14 resistance genes including aminoglycoside resistance genes *aadA2*, *aadA5*, *aph(3″)-Ib*, *aph(6)-Id*, *rmtB* beta-lactam resistance genes bla_{EC-15} and bla_{TEM-1}, phenicol resistance gene *floR*, macrolide resistance gene *mph*(A), tetracycline resistance gene *tet*(A), sulfonamide resistance genes *sulI*, *sulII*, trimethoprim resistant genes *dfrA12* and *dfrA17*. In addition, the comparison of virulence factors between hospital-related and non-hospital stations showed no significant difference ($p > 0.05$). ST167 is one of the epidemic STs in *E. coli* that carried ARGs, especially β-lactamase genes [21]. Previous studies indicated that ARGs-carrying ST167 *E. coli* were isolated from humans, food animals, companion animals and environments [10,15,22,23]. Until now, ST167 *E. coli* were found in countries and districts across five continents, such as China, Tunisia, Switzerland, Italy, Finland, Canada, Brazil, and Tanzania [22–28]. The ST167 *E. coli* carrying the bla_{NDM} gene were previously identified in hospitals, livestock farms, poultry farms, and the environment [10,15,23,25,29]. Growing evidence indicated that the public environment is of increasing concern as a reservoir for the transmission of MDR bacteria and genes. However, unlike strains from farm environments, the AR bacteria strains from public transportation mean that they can be transferred between individual populations due to personnel movement.

2.2. Comparison of Core Genome with ST167 E. coli from Different Origins

Due to the high prevalence of ST167 *E. coli* in the world, we would like to compare the profiles of ST167 *E. coli* from shared bikes and from other origins (Supplementary material Table S2). A total of 404 ST167 *E. coli* from the NCBI database were selected for comparative analysis with two *E. coli* from shared bikes. These strains were collected from human (n = 370), food animals (n = 11), companion animals (n = 15), environment (n = 8) samples (Figure 3) from 35 countries or districts (Supplementary material Figure S1). More than half of strains carried bla_{NDM} (n = 288) and bla_{CTX-M} gene (n = 272). bla_{NDM-5} were the most prevalent NDM type (n = 254) but $bla_{CTX-M-199}$ were found on only one strain. The phylogenetic tree indicated that all ST167 *E. coli* strains exhibited various characterizations in the core genome and have 21~11,206 single nucleotide polymorphisms (SNPs) compared to strains from shared bikes. The two ST167 *E. coli* from shared bikes show high similarity (SNPs < 50) with 33 strains (Pink color range in the Figure 3) from samples of human (n = 18), dogs (n = 12), cats (n = 1), chicken (n = 1) as well as environment (n = 1). The human samples were identified from Bangladesh (n = 1), the United Kingdom (n = 7), China (n = 6), Switzerland (n = 1), Italy (n = 2) and the United States (n = 1). The dog strains were originated from Switzerland (n = 2) and the United States (n = 10). Other strains were collected from a cat in Italy, a chicken in China and an environmental source from the United States. All strains were collected from 2015 to 2021, while 32 of these strains carried bla_{NDM-5}.

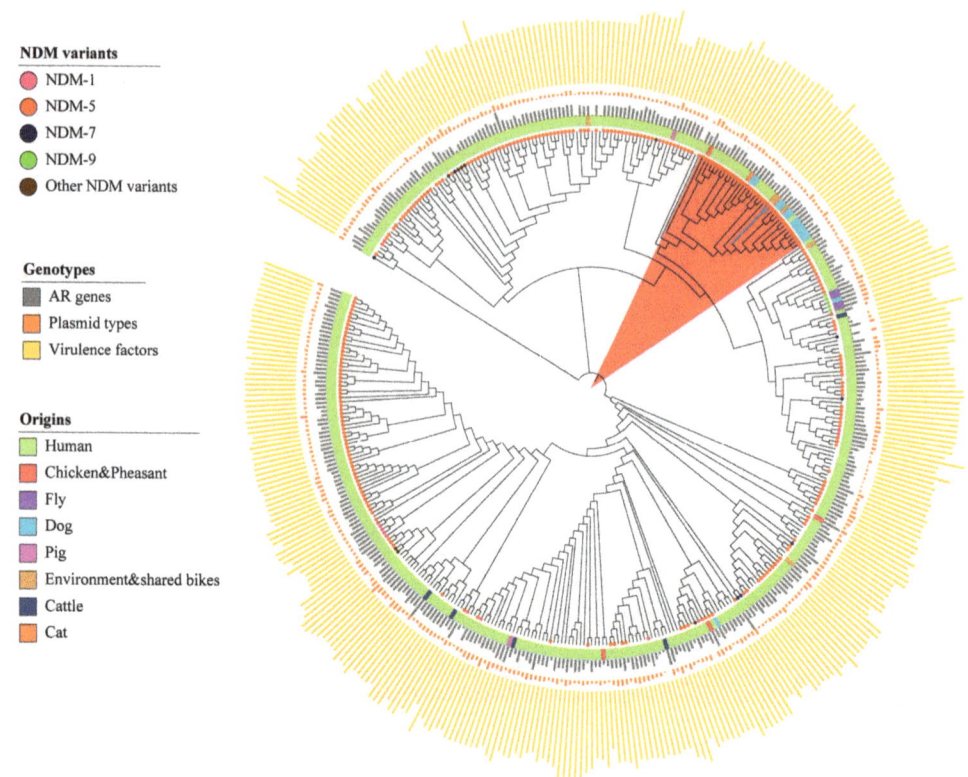

Figure 3. The core genome phylogenetic tree of ST167 *E. coli* from humans, animals and the environment. (The blue branches are the strains from shared bikes, the length of the bar represents the number of ARGs/Plasmid types/Virulence factors. The circles attached to the leaves represent the NDM variants).

2.3. Comparison of Plasmid Profiles with ST167 E. coli from Different Origins

Illumina and Nanopore sequencing of bla_{NDM-5} or $bla_{CTX-M-199}$-carrying isolates indicated that bla_{NDM-5} and $bla_{CTX-M-199}$ were located on a ~98.5 kb IncFII plasmid and a ~113 kb IncFII plasmid, respectively. From the NCBI database, we downloaded nine plasmids that have the highest coverage and identities in sequences with bla_{NDM-5}- or $bla_{CTX-M-199}$-carrying plasmid of shared bikes (Supplementary material Table S3). Nine bla_{NDM-5}-carrying plasmids belong to strains from patients in China (n = 3), Japan (n = 1), Tanzania (n = 1), Myanmar (n = 2) and Switzerland (n = 1), and from chicken meat in Laos (n = 1). Plasmid pNDM-EC16-50 in one *E. coli* strain from China showed >90% coverage and highest identifies with the bla_{NDM-5}-carrying plasmid of shared bikes (Figure 4a). Nine $bla_{CTX-M-199}$-carrying plasmids belong to strains from human (n = 3), chicken (n = 1), goose (n = 1) in China, humans in the United States (n = 1), Japan (n = 1), and Lebanon (n = 1), and water samples from India (n = 1). The nucleotide sequence of the $bla_{CTX-M-199}$-carrying plasmid of shared bikes displayed the highest similarity with *E. coli* strain L100 plasmid pL100-3 and *E. coli* plasmid J-8 plasmid pCTX from goose and chicken in China (Figure 4b). According to the information of NCBI, we download the isolates that carried these similar plasmids (bla_{NDM-5} or $bla_{CTX-M-199}$) and identified the ST of these isolates (except nine plasmids without the whole genome of isolates upload). The results showed that three bla_{NDM-5} plasmids were from ST167 *E. coli* of human origin, the other three plasmids were from non-ST167 *E. coli*, and three $bla_{CTX-M-199}$ plasmids were from ST10

E. coli of human origin, ST148, ST156 *E. coli* of food animal origin. The results of the plasmid profiles comparison indicated that maybe some bacteria carrying plasmids with ARGs from patients and farm animals are possible to persist in the environment and further plasmid conjugative transfer to the bacteria of environments. Moreover, ST167 can acquire plasmids easily from other STs, which makes plasmids with ARGs commonly available.

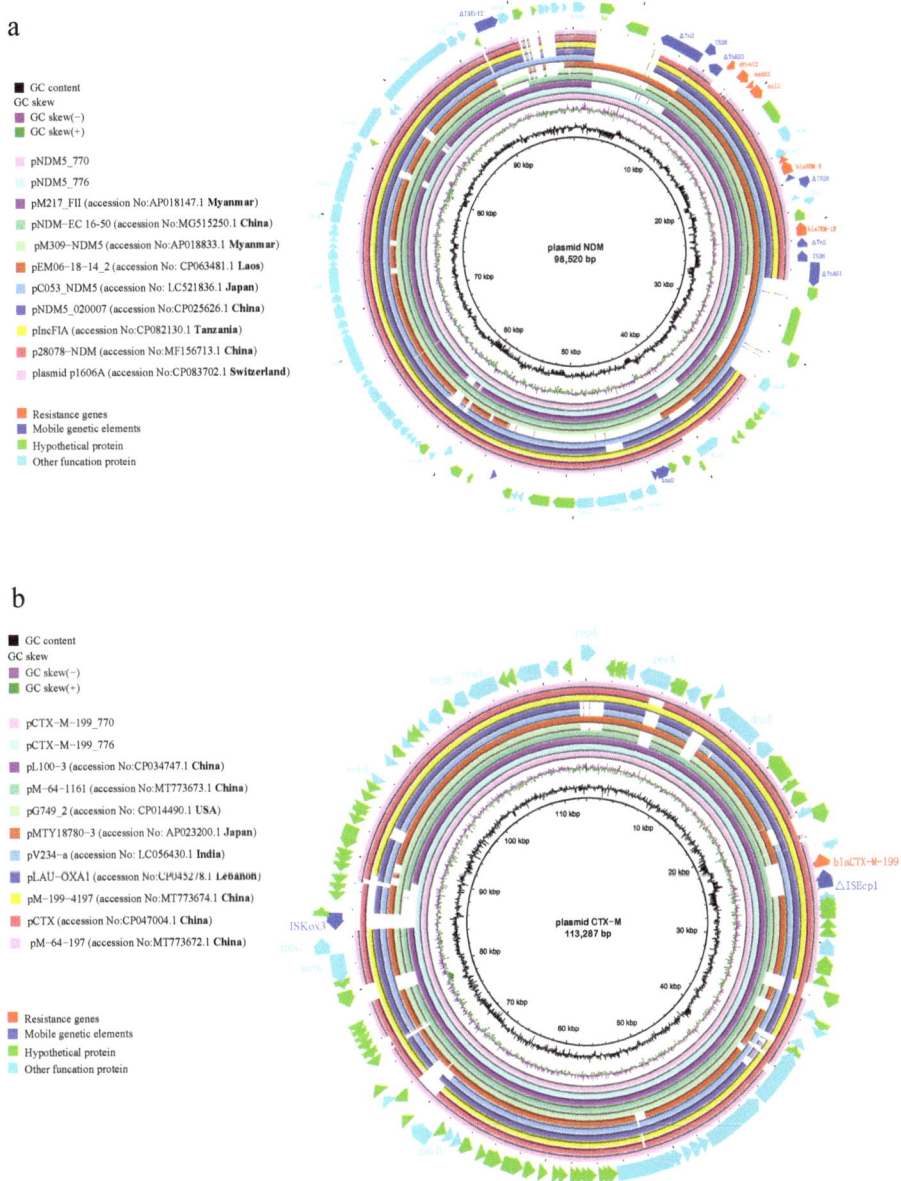

Figure 4. The plasmid profiles of (**a**) bla_{NDM-5} and (**b**) $bla_{CTX-M-199}$. (The reference sequences were bla_{NDM-5}- or $bla_{CTX-M-199}$-carrying plasmid of shared bikes. The shade of circles represents the number of identities, the blank means sequences were not consistent with the reference).

The plasmid analysis of ST167 *E. coli* from shared bikes showed that ST167 might be an important strain for plasmid-borne ARGs across different origins. Furthermore, combined with the results of the phylogenetic tree, the strains which have good environmental adaptability can increase the possibility of plasmid transfer between different bacteria which enhances the dissemination of ARGs among animals, humans and the environment, and threaten public health. Researchers are also concerned about the AR bacteria and gene transmission via the environment [30–32]. Furthermore, these strains increased the difficulty of AR control. However, not only can ST167 act as the vector but also some other prevalent strains can play the same role as ST167, so the control of prevalent strains requires substantial concern.

We found a high similarity of strains from the shared bikes and other origins, which means that some well-adapted isolates can persist in different environments. Many studies proved that AR bacteria isolated from the same environment are convergence in molecular profile because the environment has prevalent AR bacteria and genes [33]. However, now some prevalent STs such as ST131, ST167 and ST 10 *E. coli* which have good environmental adaptability with ARGs can be a potential reservoir of ARGs in the environment [13]. Moreover, ST 167 *E. coli* carried important resistant genes, such as bla_{NDM}, $mcr-1$, bla_{CTX-M} [33], which are stable in the environment and pose a threat to public health. The flow of population further accelerates ARGs spread to diverse environments or different species, which adds pressure to control antimicrobial resistance. Therefore, the dominant host of ARGs like ST 167 in the environment should be concerned and focused on.

3. Materials and Methods

3.1. Bacterial Isolates, Whole Genome Sequencing

A total of 444 Enterobacteriaceae were isolated from shared bikes in the previous study and *E. coli* was the species that exhibited more drug resistance than others [9]. Therefore, *E. coli* was chosen for further analysis. A total of 28 *E. coli* strains were isolated from samples in the previous study, excluding 4 from stations outside the fifth Ring Road of Beijing; finally, 24 *E. coli* isolates were collected. Genomic DNA was extracted using a HiPure Bacterial DNA Kit. DNA libraries were prepared and sequenced with HiSeq PE150. Two bla_{NDM-5} and $bla_{CTX-M-199}$-producing *E. coli* were sequenced with Nanopore to obtain the complete plasmids. The sequences were assembled by SPAdes and Unicycler.

3.2. Assembled Data of ST167 E. coli from Different Sources

We searched all *E. coli* available in the NCBI database which were collected from January 2014 to December 2021 and downloaded those. We only selected assembled data of whole genome sequencing. Furthermore, we reorganized the detailed information related to the assembled data we downloaded and excluded strains without information on the host. All genomes were confirmed the ST using MLST. Additionally, only *E. coli* with ST167 were chosen for the following analysis.

3.3. Genomic Analysis of Sequenced and Collected E. coli Strains

ARGs and plasmid incompatibility groups were determined using the database (resfinder, plasmidfinder) from the Center for Epidemiology (http://www.genomicepidemiology.org/, accessed on 12 February 2022). According to the mechanism of resistance classified ARGs in different antibiotic classes. MLST was confirmed using MLST in the Center for Epidemiology and database from public databases for molecular typing and microbial genome diversity (https://pubmlst.org/, accessed on 23 February 2022). The Sankey diagram of the ST clonal complex was performed using plug-in components of Excel named EasyShu. Virulence genes were identified using the VFDB database and virulencefinder of Center for Epidemiology. The criteria of different groups of virulence genes in accordance with VFDB. The tests were used for the comparison of the number of virulence factors from hospital-related Stations and non-hospital Stations. Core genomes were extracted using Snippy [34]. Core genome phylogenetic trees were constructed using Snippy and Fasttree [35]. Phylogenetic tree of the core genomes with ARGs, plasmid types, stations and phenotypes displayed with iTOL [36]. Genes in the plasmids were annotated using PATRIC and NCBI. The comparison of plasmid profiles was performed using BLAST and BRIG. The reference plasmid was annotated using the DNAplotter.

4. Conclusions

ST167 *E. coli* found on shared bikes showed high similarities with strains from patients and food-producing animals, and the plasmids also showed high identities with those from humans and animals in this study. These AR bacteria may originate from hospitals or farms. Vectors such as shared bikes may contribute to the dissemination of these AR bacteria in the environment. Furthermore, the persistence of these AR bacteria in the environment challenges the control of AR bacteria and ARGs. In the future, we need to take measures to assess the risk of AR bacteria in the environment and cut off transmission.

Supplementary Materials: The following supporting information can be downloaded at: https://www.mdpi.com/article/10.3390/antibiotics11081030/s1, Figure S1. Number of ST 167 *E. coli* from different countries or districts. Table S1. The information of *E. coli* collected from shared bikes. Table S2. The information of ST167 *E. coli* of NCBI database. Table S3. The information of plasmids compared with bla_{NDM-5} and $bla_{CTX-M-199}$-carrying plasmids from shared bikes.

Author Contributions: Conceptualization, B.S., Y.W. and L.L.; Methodology, Q.C., Z.Z. and L.L.; Validation, Q.C., Z.Z. and L.L.; Formal Analysis, L.L. and Q.C.; Data Curation, Q.C., H.L. and L.L.; Writing—Original Draft Preparation, Q.C., Z.Z. and L.L.; Writing—Review & Editing, Y.W., B.S. and C.C.; Visualization, Q.C., Z.Z. and L.L. All authors have read and agreed to the published version of the manuscript.

Funding: This study was supported by the grants from the National Natural Science Foundation of China (81861138051, 81991535, 32141002) and Beijing Natural Science Foundation (6222017).

Institutional Review Board Statement: Not applicable.

Informed Consent Statement: Not applicable.

Data Availability Statement: The data and material information used and analyzed in the current study are available from the corresponding author upon reasonable requests.

Conflicts of Interest: The authors declare no conflict of interest.

References

1. Shen, C.; Feng, S.; Chen, H.; Dai, M.; Paterson, D.L.; Zheng, X.; Wu, X.; Zhong, L.L.; Liu, Y.; Xia, Y.; et al. Transmission of *mcr-1*-producing multidrug-resistant Enterobacteriaceae in public transportation in Guangzhou, China. *Clin. Infect. Dis.* **2018**, *67* (Suppl. 2), S217–S224. [CrossRef] [PubMed]
2. Peng, Y.; Ou, Q.; Lin, D.; Xu, P.; Li, Y.; Ye, X.; Zhou, J.; Yao, Z. Metro system in Guangzhou as a hazardous reservoir of methicillin-resistant Staphylococci: Findings from a point-prevalence molecular epidemiologic study. *Sci. Rep.* **2015**, *5*, 16087. [CrossRef] [PubMed]
3. Mendes, Â.; Martins da Costa, P.; Rego, D.; Beça, N.; Alves, C.; Moreira, T.; Conceição, T.; Aires-de-Sousa, M. Contamination of public transports by *Staphylococcus aureus* and its carriage by biomedical students: Point-prevalence, related risk factors and molecular characterization of methicillin-resistant strains. *Public Health* **2015**, *129*, 1125–1131. [CrossRef]
4. Lutz, J.K.; van Balen, J.; Crawford, J.M.; Wilkins, J.R., 3rd; Lee, J.; Nava-Hoet, R.C.; Hoet, A.E. Methicillin-resistant *Staphylococcus aureus* in public transportation vehicles (buses): Another piece to the epidemiologic puzzle. *Am. J. Infect. Control* **2014**, *42*, 1285–1290. [CrossRef] [PubMed]
5. Conceição, T.; Diamantino, F.; Coelho, C.; de Lencastre, H.; Aires-de-Sousa, M. Contamination of public buses with MRSA in Lisbon, Portugal: A possible transmission route of major MRSA clones within the community. *PLoS ONE* **2013**, *8*, e77812. [CrossRef]
6. Wu, Y.; Xie, J.; Li, J.; Zhao, J.; Qiao, S.; Li, Y.; Zeng, J. Shared bicycle microbial community: A potential antibiotic-resistant bacteria warehouse. *Folia Microbiol.* **2021**, *66*, 49–58. [CrossRef] [PubMed]
7. Gu, J.; Xie, X.J.; Liu, J.X.; Shui, J.R.; Zhang, H.Y.; Feng, G.Y.; Liu, X.Y.; Li, L.C.; Lan, Q.W.; Jin, Q.H.; et al. Prevalence and transmission of antimicrobial-resistant Staphylococci and Enterococci from shared bicycles in Chengdu, China. *Sci. Total Environ.* **2020**, *738*, 139735. [CrossRef]

8. Xu, Z.; Liu, S.; Chen, L.; Liu, Y.; Tan, L.; Shen, J.; Zhang, W. Antimicrobial resistance and molecular characterization of methicillin-resistant coagulase-negative *Staphylococci* from public shared bicycles in Tianjin, China. *J. Glob. Antimicrob. Resist.* **2019**, *19*, 231–235. [CrossRef]
9. Zou, Z.Y.; Lei, L.; Chen, Q.Y.; Wang, Y.Q.; Cai, C.; Li, W.Q.; Zhang, Z.; Shao, B.; Wang, Y. Prevalence and dissemination risk of antimicrobial-resistant Enterobacteriaceae from shared bikes in Beijing, China. *Environ. Int.* **2019**, *132*, 105119. [CrossRef] [PubMed]
10. Mani, Y.; Mansour, W.; Mammeri, H.; Denamur, E.; Saras, E.; Boujâafar, N.; Bouallègue, O.; Madec, J.Y.; Haenni, M. KPC-3-producing ST167 *Escherichia coli* from mussels bought at a retail market in Tunisia. *J. Antimicrob. Chemother.* **2017**, *72*, 2403–2404. [CrossRef]
11. Huang, J.L.; Jianjun Zhu, J.J.; Gong, D.J.; Wu, L.; Zhu, Y.Z.; Hu, L.Q. Whole genome sequence of EC16, a bla_{NDM-5}-, $bla_{CTX-M-55}$-, and *fosA3*-coproducing *Escherichia coli* ST167 clinical isolate from China. *J. Glob. Antimicrob. Resist.* **2022**, *29*, 296–298. [CrossRef] [PubMed]
12. Grönthal, T.; Österblad, M.; Eklund, M.; Jalava, J.; Nykäsenoja, S.; Pekkanen, K.; Rantala, M. Sharing more than friendship—transmission of NDM-5 ST167 and CTX-M-9 ST69 *Escherichia coli* between dogs and humans in a family, Finland, 2015. *Eurosurveillance* **2018**, *23*, 1700497. [CrossRef] [PubMed]
13. Zhang, X.; Lou, D.; Xu, Y.; Shang, Y.; Li, D.; Huang, X.; Li, Y.; Hu, L.; Wang, L.; Yu, F. First identification of coexistence of bla_{NDM-1} and bla_{CMY-42} among *Escherichia coli* ST167 clinical isolates. *BMC Microbiol.* **2013**, *13*, 282. [CrossRef]
14. Wang, M.G.; Zhang, R.M.; Wang, L.L.; Sun, R.Y.; Bai, S.C.; Han, L.; Fang, L.X.; Sun, J.; Liu, Y.H.; Liao, X.P. Molecular epidemiology of carbapenemase-producing *Escherichia coli* from duck farms in south-east coastal China. *J. Antimicrob. Chemother.* **2021**, *76*, 322–329. [CrossRef] [PubMed]
15. He, W.Y.; Zhang, X.X.; Gao, G.L.; Gao, M.Y.; Zhong, F.G.; Lv, L.C.; Cai, Z.P.; Si, X.F.; Yang, J.; Liu, J.H. Clonal spread of *Escherichia coli* O101: H9-ST10 and O101: H9-ST167 strains carrying *fosA3* and $bla_{CTX-M-14}$ among diarrheal calves in a Chinese farm, with Australian *Chroicocephalus* as the possible origin of *E. coli* O101: H9-ST10. *Zool. Res.* **2021**, *42*, 461–468. [CrossRef]
16. Zou, H.; Jia, X.; He, X.; Su, Y.; Zhou, L.; Shen, Y.; Sheng, C.; Liao, A.; Li, C.; Li, Q. Emerging treat of multidrug resistant pathogens from neonatal sepsis. *Front. Cell. Infect. Microbiol.* **2021**, *11*, 694093. [CrossRef] [PubMed]
17. Chakraborty, T.; Sadek, M.; Yao, Y.; Imirzalioglu, C.; Stephan, R.; Poirel, L.; Nordmann, P. Cross-border emergence of *Escherichia coli* producing the carbapenemase NDM-5 in Switzerland and Germany. *J. Clin. Microbiol.* **2021**, *59*, e02238-20. [CrossRef]
18. Cantón, R.; Gijón, D.; Ruiz-Garbajosa, P. Antimicrobial resistance in ICUs: An update in the light of the COVID-19 pandemic. *Curr. Opin. Crit. Care* **2020**, *26*, 433–441. [CrossRef]
19. Xu, L.; Wang, P.; Cheng, J.; Qin, S.; Xie, W. Characterization of a novel bla_{NDM-5}-harboring IncFII plasmid and an *mcr-1*-bearing IncI2 plasmid in a single *Escherichia coli* ST167 clinical isolate. *Infect. Drug Resist.* **2019**, *12*, 511–519. [CrossRef]
20. Chen, Y.; Chen, X.; Zheng, S.; Yu, F.; Kong, H.; Yang, Q.; Cui, D.; Chen, N.; Lou, B.; Li, X.; et al. Serotypes, genotypes and antimicrobial resistance patterns of human diarrhoeagenic *Escherichia coli* isolates circulating in southeastern China. *Clin. Microbiol. Infect.* **2014**, *20*, 52–58. [CrossRef]
21. Garcia-Fernandez, A.; Villa, L.; Bibbolino, G.; Bressan, A.; Trancassini, M.; Pietropaolo, V.; Venditti, M.; Antonelli, G.; Carattoli, A. Novel insights and features of the NDM-5-producing *Escherichia coli* sequence type 167 high-risk clone. *mSphere* **2020**, *5*, e00269-20. [CrossRef] [PubMed]
22. Alba, P.; Taddei, R.; Cordaro, G.; Fontana, M.C.; Toschi, E.; Gaibani, P.; Marani, I.; Giacomi, A.; Diaconu, E.L.; Iurescia, M.; et al. Carbapenemase IncF-borne bla_{NDM-5} gene in the *E. coli* ST167 high-risk clone from canine clinical infection, Italy. *Vet. Microbiol.* **2021**, *256*, 109045. [CrossRef] [PubMed]
23. Dziri, R.; Klibi, N.; Alonso, C.A.; Jouini, A.; Ben Said, L.; Chairat, S.; Bellaaj, R.; Boudabous, A.; Ben Slama, K.; Torres, C. Detection of CTX-M-15-producing *Escherichia coli* isolates of lineages ST131-B2 and ST167-A in environmental samples of a Tunisian hospital. *Microb. Drug Resist.* **2016**, *22*, 399–403. [CrossRef] [PubMed]
24. Santos Tufic-Garutti, S.D.; de Araújo Longo, L.G.; Fontana, H.; Garutti, L.H.G.; de Carvalho Girão, V.B.; Fuga, B.; Lincopan, N.; de Pinho Rodrigues, K.M.; Moreira, B.M. OXA-181 carbapenemase carried on an IncX3 plasmid in high-risk *Escherichia coli* ST167 isolated from a traveler returning from Sub-Saharan Africa to Brazil. *Diagn. Microbiol. Infect. Dis.* **2022**, *102*, 115570. [CrossRef]
25. Baloch, Z.; Lv, L.; Yi, L.; Wan, M.; Aslam, B.; Yang, J.; Liu, J.H. Emergence of almost identical F36: A-:B32 plasmids carrying bla_{NDM-5} and *qepA* in *Escherichia coli* from both Pakistan and Canada. *Infect. Drug Resist.* **2019**, *12*, 3981–3985. [CrossRef] [PubMed]
26. Huang, Y.; Yu, X.; Xie, M.; Wang, X.; Liao, K.; Xue, W.; Chan, E.W.; Zhang, R.; Chen, S. Widespread dissemination of carbapenem-resistant *Escherichia coli* sequence type 167 strains harboring bla_{NDM-5} in clinical settings in China. *Antimicrob. Agents Chemother.* **2016**, *60*, 4364–4368. [CrossRef] [PubMed]
27. Nukui, Y.; Ayibieke, A.; Taniguchi, M.; Aiso, Y.; Shibuya, Y.; Sonobe, K.; Nakajima, J.; Kanehira, S.; Hadano, Y.; Tohda, S.; et al. Whole-genome analysis of EC129, an NDM-5-, CTX-M-14-, OXA-10- and MCR-1-co-producing *Escherichia coli* ST167 strain isolated from Japan. *J. Glob. Antimicrob. Resist.* **2019**, *18*, 148–150. [CrossRef] [PubMed]
28. Peterhans, S.; Stevens, M.J.A.; Nüesch-Inderbinen, M.; Schmitt, S.; Stephan, R.; Zurfluh, K. First report of a bla_{NDM-5}-harbouring *Escherichia coli* ST167 isolated from a wound infection in a dog in Switzerland. *J. Glob. Antimicrob. Resist.* **2018**, *15*, 226–227. [CrossRef]

29. Sánchez-Benito, R.; Iglesias, M.R.; Quijada, N.M.; Campos, M.J.; Ugarte-Ruiz, M.; Hernández, M.; Pazos, C.; Rodríguez-Lázaro, D.; Garduño, E.; Domínguez, L.; et al. *Escherichia coli* ST167 carrying plasmid mobilisable *mcr-1* and *bla*$_{CTX-M-15}$ resistance determinants isolated from a human respiratory infection. *Int. J. Antimicrob. Agents* **2017**, *50*, 285–286. [CrossRef] [PubMed]
30. Yang, Y.; Liu, Z.; Xing, S.; Liao, X. The correlation between antibiotic resistance gene abundance and microbial community resistance in pig farm wastewater and surrounding rivers. *Ecotoxicol. Environ. Saf.* **2019**, *182*, 109452. [CrossRef]
31. Jamborova, I.; Johnston, B.D.; Papousek, I.; Kachlikova, K.; Micenkova, L.; Clabots, C.; Skalova, A.; Chudejova, K.; Dolejska, M.; Literak, I.; et al. Extensive genetic commonality among wildlife, wastewater, community, and nosocomial isolates of *Escherichia coli* sequence type 131 (H30R1 and H30Rx subclones) that carry *bla*$_{CTX-M-27}$ or *bla*$_{CTX-M-15}$. *Antimicrob. Agents Chemother.* **2018**, *62*, e00519-18. [CrossRef] [PubMed]
32. Shen, Y.; Xu, C.; Sun, Q.; Schwarz, S.; Ou, Y.; Yang, L.; Huang, Z.; Eichhorn, I.; Walsh, T.R.; Wang, Y.; et al. Prevalence and genetic analysis of *mcr-3*-positive *Aeromonas* species from humans, retail meat, and environmental water samples. *Antimicrob. Agents Chemother.* **2018**, *62*, e00404-18. [CrossRef] [PubMed]
33. Li, J.; Bi, Z.; Ma, S.; Chen, B.; Cai, C.; He, J.; Schwarz, S.; Sun, C.; Zhou, Y.; Yin, J.; et al. Inter-host transmission of carbapenemase-producing *Escherichia coli* among humans and backyard animals. *Environ. Health Perspect.* **2019**, *127*, 107009. [CrossRef]
34. Seemann T Snippy: Fast Bacterial Variant Calling from NGS Reads. Available online: https://github.com/tseemann/snippy (accessed on 30 December 2018).
35. Price, M.N.; Dehal, P.S.; Arkin, A.P. FastTree: Computing large minimum evolution trees with profiles instead of a distance matrix. *Mol. Biol. Evol.* **2009**, *26*, 1641–1650. [CrossRef] [PubMed]
36. Letunic, I.; Bork, P. Interactive Tree of Life (iTOL) v4: Recent updates and new developments. *Nucleic Acids Res.* **2019**, *47*, W256–W259. [CrossRef]

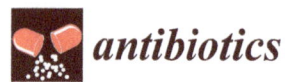

Article

Global Spread of MCR-Producing *Salmonella enterica* Isolates

Zengfeng Zhang, Xiaorong Tian and Chunlei Shi *

MOST-USDA Joint Research Center for Food Safety, School of Agriculture and Biology, and State Key Laboratory of Microbial Metabolism, Shanghai Jiao Tong University, Shanghai 200240, China; zhangzengfeng118@163.com (Z.Z.); tianxr@sjtu.edu.cn (X.T.)
* Correspondence: clshi@sjtu.edu.cn

Abstract: Colistin resistance in bacteria has become a significant threat to food safety and public health, and its development was mainly attributed to the plasmid-mediated *mcr* genes. This study aimed to determine the global prevalence and molecular characteristics of *mcr*-producing *Salmonella enterica* isolates. A total of 2279 *mcr*-producing *Salmonella* genomes were obtained from the public database, which were disseminated in 37 countries from five continents worldwide, including Asia, Europe, America, Australia, and Africa. Human samples (39.5%; 900/2279) were the predominant sources of *mcr*-producing *Salmonella* isolates, followed by foods (32.6%), animals (13.7%), and environment (4.4%). Furthermore, 80 *Salmonella* serotypes were identified, and Typhimurium and 1,4,[5],12:i:- were the predominant serotypes, accounting for 18.3% and 18.7%, respectively. Twenty *mcr* variants were identified, and the most common ones were *mcr-9.1* (65.2%) and *mcr-1.1* (24.4%). Carbapenems-resistance gene bla_{NDM-1} and tigecycline-resistance gene *tet*(X4) were identified in one isolate, respectively. Phylogenetic results indicated that *mcr*-producing *Salmonella* fell into nine lineages (Lineages I-IX), and *Salmonella* Typhimurium, 1,4,[5],12:i:- and 4,[5],12:i:- isolates from different countries were mixed in Lineages I, II and III, suggesting that international spread occurred. These findings underline further challenges for the spread of *Salmonella*-bearing *mcr* genes.

Keywords: *Salmonella*; *mcr* genes; phylogenetic analysis

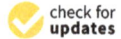

Citation: Zhang, Z.; Tian, X.; Shi, C. Global Spread of MCR-Producing *Salmonella enterica* Isolates. *Antibiotics* **2022**, *11*, 998. https://doi.org/10.3390/antibiotics11080998

Academic Editors: Yongning Wu and Zhenling Zeng

Received: 2 June 2022
Accepted: 22 July 2022
Published: 25 July 2022

Publisher's Note: MDPI stays neutral with regard to jurisdictional claims in published maps and institutional affiliations.

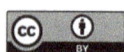

Copyright: © 2022 by the authors. Licensee MDPI, Basel, Switzerland. This article is an open access article distributed under the terms and conditions of the Creative Commons Attribution (CC BY) license (https:// creativecommons.org/licenses/by/ 4.0/).

1. Introduction

Colistin was considered the last resort drug in the treatment for multidrug-resistant (MDR) and even carbapenem-resistant Gram-negative bacteria. Colistin-resistant bacteria have spread across Asia, Africa, Europe, North America, South America, and Oceania [1–3]. The colistin resistance in bacteria was previously reported to result from mutations in chromosomes [4]. Until 2015, the novel plasmid-borne colistin resistance gene *mcr-1* was firstly reported in an *Escherichia coli* isolate [5]. MCR-1 is a phosphoethanolamine (pEtN) transferase that is able to modify the phosphate groups in lipid A [5], the catalysis of which could be offered mainly by *mcr-1* from plasmids but also encoded by chromosome in the *Enterobacteriaceae* family [6].

Among countries with *mcr*-producing *Salmonella enterica* isolates, China was the most frequent one, and countries in Europe harbored a wide diversity of *mcr* variants [1]. The *mcr* gene was frequently identified in animal- and human-borne *Salmonella enterica* isolates [1]. Among more than 2600 *Salmonella* serotypes, *Salmonella* Typhimurium was the top serovar to carry the *mcr* genes [1]. Besides *Salmonella*, *Escherichia coli*, *Klebsiella Pneumoniae*, *Klebsiella oxytoca*, *Cronobacter sakazakii*, *Kluyvera ascorbata*, *Shigella sonnei*, *Citrobacter freundii*, *Citrobacter braakii*, *Raoultella ornithinolytica*, *Proteus mirabilis*, *Aeromonas*, *Moraxella*, and *Enterobacter* species were also found to be *mcr*-producing Gram-negative bacteria [3]. Furthermore, the *mcr* genes were widely distributed in various sample sources, including humans, animals, animal-origin foods, and environment [3].

Currently, a variety of *mcr* genes, including *mcr-1* to *-10*, have been reported in bacteria [6]. Furthermore, *mcr* genes were also found to co-exist with carbapenem resistance genes such as bla_{VIM-1}, bla_{NDM-5}, and bla_{NDM-9} [7–9]. Hence, the quick spread of plasmid-mediated *mcr* genes poses a significant threat to public health, requiring global surveillance.

Here, we characterized the global distribution of *mcr*-positive *Salmonella* using a data set of 2279 *Salmonella* genomes from humans, foods, animals, and environment. *Salmonella* serotypes, *mcr* variants, and phylogenomic characteristics were further analyzed.

2. Results
2.1. Widely Spread of mcr-Producing Salmonella Enterica in the Global and Sources Analysis

Currently, a total of 2279 *mcr*-producing *Salmonella* genomes are available in the NCBI database. It was found that these *mcr*-producing *Salmonella* isolates had spread in 37 countries on five continents, including Asia, Europe, America, Australia, and Africa (Figure 1A). The top six countries are the United States (*n* = 1187), China (*n* = 256), United Kingdom (*n* = 211), Germany (*n* = 184), Australia (*n* = 79), and Canada (*n* = 28) (Figure 1A).

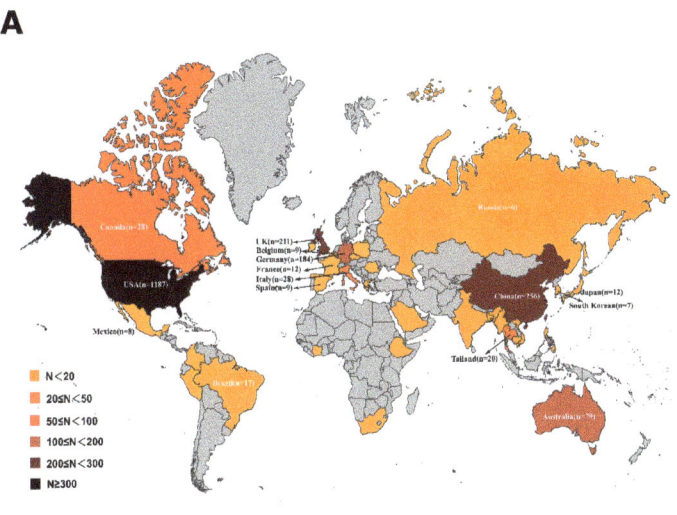

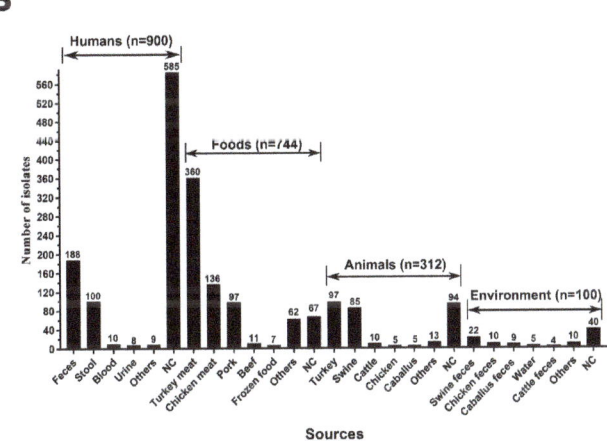

Figure 1. Global spread of MCR-producing *Salmonella enterica* isolates (**A**) and sources analysis (**B**).

In this study, human samples (39.5%; 900/2279) were the predominant sources of *mcr*-producing *Salmonella* isolates (Figure 1B). It was further demonstrated that human samples were mainly composed of feces (*n* = 188), stool (*n* = 100), blood (*n* = 10), and urine (*n* = 8). A total of 744 (32.6%) isolates were recovered from foods. Turkey meats (*n* = 360) accounted for the largest portion, and then chicken meat (*n* = 136), pork (*n* = 97), beef (*n* = 11), and frozen foods (*n* = 7) (Figure 1B), which suggested that turkey meats were the main dissemination vehicle of *mcr*-producing *Salmonella* isolates. A total of 312 (13.7%) isolates were recovered from animals. Turkey (*n* = 97) accounted for the largest portion, and then swine (*n* = 85), cattle (*n* = 10), chicken (*n* = 5), and caballus (*n* = 5). In addition, 100 (4.4%) isolates were recovered from the environment, such as swine feces (*n* = 22), chicken feces (*n* = 10), caballus feces (*n* = 9), water (*n* = 5), and cattle feces (*n* = 4).

2.2. Typhimurium and 1,4,[5],12:i:- Were the Main Serotypes Carrying mcr Genes in Salmonella

We collected and analyzed *Salmonella* serotypes in these 2279 isolates, and the missing serotypes information in some isolates was compensated by the predicted results from SeqSero 1.2 software (UGA College of Agricultural and Environmental Sciences food science, Athens, GA, USA). A total of 80 *Salmonella* serotypes were identified among these *Salmonella* isolates. Typhimurium and 1,4,[5],12:i:- were the predominant serotypes, accounting for 18.3% and 18.7%, respectively (Figure 2A). Other serotypes were Saintpaul (12.4%), Heidelberg (9.1%), 4,[5],12:i:- (5.5%), Agona (4.1%), Paratyphi B var. d-tartrate+ (3.9%), Schwarzengrund (2.0%), Senftenberg (1.7%), Enteritidis (1.5%), Montevideo (1.5%), Mbandaka (1.4%), Cubana (1.2%), Ouakam (1.0%), Infantis (1.0%), Kentucky (0.9%), Thompson (0.9%), Anatum (0.9%), and Java (0.9%) (Figure 2A).

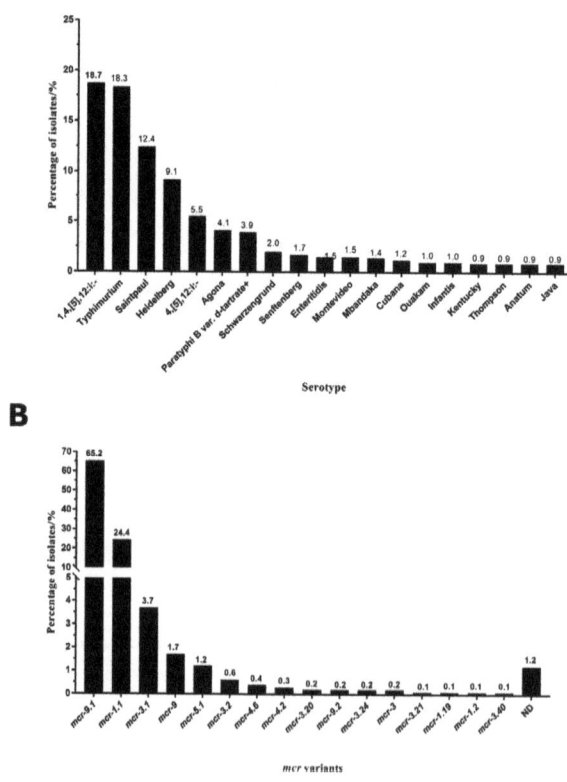

Figure 2. The distribution of the serotypes (**A**) and *mcr* variants (**B**) in MCR-producing *Salmonella*.

It was found that the prevalent *mcr*-producing *Salmonella* serotypes varied in different countries (Figure 3A). In the United States, the most common *Salmonella* serotype was Saintpaul (21.4%), followed by Heidelberg (14.2%), 1,4,[5],12:i:- (12.7%), 4,[5],12:i:- (8.3%), Agona (5.9%), Schwarzengrund (3.0%), and Typhimurium (2.7%) (Figure 3A). In China, the most frequently identified *Salmonella* serotype was 1,4,[5],12:i:- (45.7%), followed by Typhimurium (38.7%), Anatum (3.5%), Thompson (2.0%), Goldcoast (2.0%), Indiana (1.2%), and Albany (1.2%). In the United Kingdom, the most common *Salmonella* serotype was Typhimurium (40.8%), followed by 1,4,[5],12:i:- (20.9%), Java (8.1%), Mbandaka (3.8%), Enteritidis (2.8%), Bovismorbificans (1.9%), and Choleraesuis (1.9%). In the Germany, the most frequently identified *Salmonella* serotype was Paratyphi B var. d-tartrate+ (45.7%), followed by Typhimurium (11.4%), 1,4,[5],12:i:- (10.9%), Paratyphi B (7.1%), Infantis (4.9%), Saintpaul (3.3%), and Ohio (3.3%). In Australia, the most common *Salmonella* serotype was Typhimurium (59.5%), followed by 1,4,[5],12:i:- (29.1%), Enteritidis (5.1%), Senftenberg (3.8%), and Havana (1.3%). In Canada, the most frequently identified *Salmonella* serotype was Heidelberg (50.0%), followed by 4,[5],12:i:- (14.3%), 1,4,[5],12:i:- (10.7%), Albany (7.1%), Typhimurium (7.1%), and Agona (3.6%).

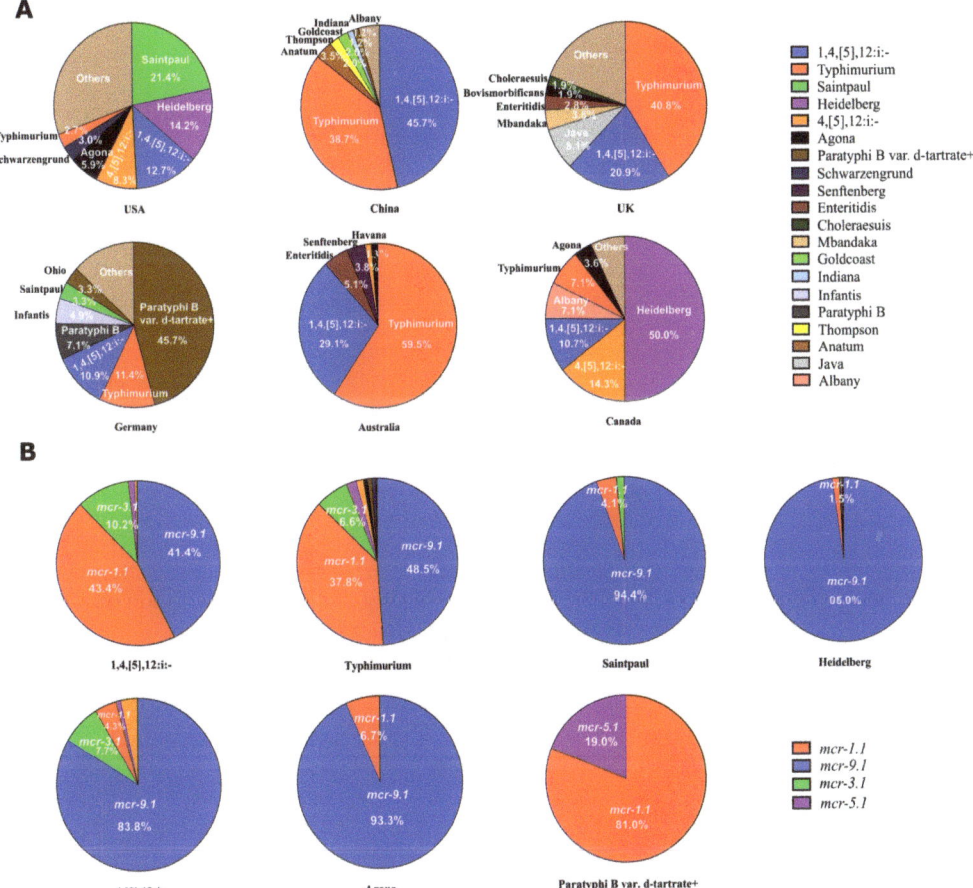

Figure 3. (**A**) The distribution of *mcr*-positive *Salmonella* serotypes in the USA, China, UK, Germany, Australia, and Canada. (**B**) The distribution of *mcr* variants in serotypes 1,4,[5],12:i:-, Typhimurium, Saintpaul, Heidelberg, 4,[5],12:i:-, Agona, and Paratyphi B var. d-tartrate+.

2.3. mcr-9.1 and mcr-1.1 Were the Dominant Variants in Salmonella

We identified the *mcr* variants from genomes through ResFinder 4.1 (Lyngby, Denmark). A total of 20 *mcr* variants were identified, and the most common variant was *mcr-9.1*, accounting for 65.2% (Figure 2B). Other *mcr* variants were *mcr-1.1* (24.4%), *mcr-3.1* (3.7%), *mcr-9* (1.7%), *mcr-5.1* (1.2%), *mcr-3.2* (0.6%), *mcr-4.6* (0.4%), *mcr-4.2* (0.3%), *mcr-3.20* (0.2%), *mcr-9.2* (0.2%), *mcr-3.24* (0.2%), *mcr-3* (0.2%), *mcr-3.21* (0.1%), *mcr-1.19* (0.1%), *mcr-1.2* (0.1%), and *mcr-3.40* (0.1%). The difference of *mcr* variant sequences could be found in Supplementary Materials. The partial or incomplete *mcr* genes could not be confirmed to a specific subtype, which were defined as not determined (ND) in Figure 2B, accounting for 1.2%.

Then, we analyzed the prevalence of *mcr* variants in the top seven *Salmonella* serotypes (1,4,[5],12:i:-, Typhimurium, Saintpaul, Heidelberg, 4,[5],12:i:-, Agona, and Paratyphi B var. d-tartrate+). It was found that *mcr-9.1* was the most common variant in these serotypes except for 1,4,[5],12:i:- (Figure 3B). Gene *mcr-1.1* (43.4%) was the most frequently identified variant in *Salmonella* 1,4,[5],12:i:-, followed by *mcr-9.1* (41.4%), and *mcr-3.1* (10.2%). Gene *mcr-9.1* (48.5%) was the most common variant in *Salmonella* Typhimurium, followed by *mcr-1.1* (37.8%), and *mcr-3.1* (6.6%). Gene *mcr-9.1* (94.4%) was the most frequently identified variant in *Salmonella* Saintpaul, and then *mcr-1.1* (4.1%). Gene *mcr-9.1* (95.9%) was the most common variant in *Salmonella* Heidelberg, and then *mcr-1.1* (1.5%). Gene *mcr-9.1* (83.8%) was the most frequently identified variant in *Salmonella* 4,[5],12:i:-, followed by *mcr-3.1* (7.7%), and *mcr-1.1* (4.3%). Gene *mcr-9.1* (93.3%) was the most common variant in *Salmonella* Agona, and then *mcr-1.1* (6.7%). Gene *mcr-1.1* (81.0%) was the most frequently identified variant in *Salmonella* Paratyphi B var. d-tartrate+, and then *mcr-5.1* (19.0%).

2.4. Antimicrobial Resistance (AMR) Genotypes in mcr-Producing Salmonella Isolates

A total of 68 acquired AMR genes were found in these *mcr*-producing *Salmonella* isolates (Table 1). Carbapenems-resistance gene bla_{NDM-1} was identified in one isolate. It was noted that a tigecycline-resistance gene *tet*(X4) was identified in one isolate. Furthermore, a total of 8 bla_{CTX-M} variants were identified, $bla_{CTX-M-14}$ (6.0%) of which were the most common one, followed by $bla_{CTX-M-9}$ (4.8%), $bla_{CTX-M-55}$ (3.9%), $bla_{CTX-M-15}$ (0.8%), $bla_{CTX-M-65}$ (0.6%), $bla_{CTX-M-3}$ (0.6%), $bla_{CTX-M-2}$ (0.2%), and $bla_{CTX-M-130}$ (0.1%). Gene *mph*(A) (5.0%) was the most common macrolides-resistance gene, then *erm*(B) (0.4%), *mef*(B) (0.3%), and *erm*(42) (0.2%). Fosfomycin-resistance gene *fos*A7 and *fos*A3 accounted for 14.3% and 6.0%, respectively. Gene *qnr*B2 (9.4%) was the most common plasmid-mediated quinolones-resistance (PMQR) gene, followed by *oqx*AB (7.9%), *qnr*S1 (7.0%), *qnr*B19 (2.6%), *qnr*B4 (1.4%), and *qnr*S2 (0.4%). Tetracycline-resistance genes *tet*(B) (48.2%), *tet*(A) (25.4%), *tet*(D) (16.1%), *tet*(M) (3.1%), and *tet*(C) (1.5%) were identified. Mutations in genes associated with AMR from genomes were also identified. It was found that *gyr*A_D87G (5.6%) was the most common mutation, followed by *gyr*A_D87N (4.3%), *gyr*A_S83Y (2.5%), *gyr*A_S83F (2.5%), *par*C_S80I (0.5%), and *par*C_S80R (0.2%). In addition, *gyr*A_G81C and *par*E_S458P were identified in one isolate, respectively.

Table 1. AMR genotypes in *mcr*-producing *Salmonella* isolates.

Antibiotic Resistance Determinants		Numbers	Ratio/%
Carbapenems	bla_{NDM-1}	1	0.0
Tigecycline	*tet*(X4)	1	0.0
Aminoglycosides	*dfr*A12	232	10.2
-	*dfr*A14	42	1.8
-	*dfr*A17	21	0.9
-	*dfr*A16	59	2.6
-	*dfr*A19	382	16.8

Table 1. Cont.

Antibiotic Resistance Determinants		Numbers	Ratio/%
-	dfrA23	19	0.8
-	dfrA5	35	1.5
-	dfrA1	212	9.3
-	aph(6)-Id	1023	44.9
-	aph(3″)-Ib	1143	50.2
-	aph(3′)-Ia	685	30.1
-	aph(4)-Ia	246	10.8
-	aadA2	931	40.9
-	aadA1	1063	46.6
-	aadA22	15	0.7
-	aadA5	35	1.5
-	aac(6′)-IIc	357	15.7
-	aac(6′)-Ib-cr5	85	3.7
-	aac(3)-IId	129	5.7
-	aac(3)-IVa	212	9.3
-	aac(3)-IIe	12	0.5
-	aac(3)-IIg	160	7.0
β-Lactamase	$bla_{CTX-M-14}$	136	6.0
-	$bla_{CTX-M-55}$	90	3.9
-	$bla_{CTX-M-65}$	14	0.6
-	$bla_{CTX-M-15}$	19	0.8
-	$bla_{CTX-M-3}$	13	0.6
-	$bla_{CTX-M-9}$	109	4.8
-	$bla_{CTX-M-130}$	3	0.1
-	$bla_{CTX-M-2}$	4	0.2
-	bla_{CMY-2}	46	2.0
-	bla_{CMY-16}	1	0.0
-	bla_{TEM}	1315	57.7
-	bla_{SHV-12}	307	13.5
-	bla_{DHA-1}	33	1.4
-	bla_{OXA-1}	115	5.0
-	bla_{OXA-10}	3	0.1
Rifampicin	arr-3	86	3.8
Chloramphenicol	cmlA1	292	12.8
-	catB3	76	3.3
-	catA2	296	13.0
Macrolides	mph(A)	113	5.0
-	mef(B)	7	0.3
-	erm(B)	10	0.4
-	erm(42)	5	0.2
Fosfomycin	fosA7	326	14.3
-	fosA3	137	6.0
-	fosA4	1	0.0
Florfenicol	floR	480	21.1
Lincomycin	lnu(F)	64	2.8
-	lnu(G)	8	0.4
Sulfonamide	sul3	334	14.7
-	sul2	1220	53.5
-	sul1	1184	52.0
Tetracyclines	tet(A)	578	25.4
-	tet(M)	71	3.1
-	tet(B)	1099	48.2
-	tet(C)	34	1.5
-	tet(D)	368	16.1

Table 1. Cont.

Antibiotic Resistance Determinants		Numbers	Ratio/%
Quinolones	qnrS1	160	7.0
-	oqxA	180	7.9
-	oqxB	181	7.9
-	qnrS2	10	0.4
-	qnrB4	32	1.4
-	qnrB19	60	2.6
-	qnrB2	214	9.4
AMR mutations	gyrA_D87G	128	5.6
-	gyrA_S83Y	58	2.5
-	gyrA_D87N	98	4.3
-	gyrA_G81C	1	0.0
-	gyrA_S83F	57	2.5
-	parC_S80I	12	0.5
-	parC_S80R	5	0.2
-	parE_S458P	1	0.0

2.5. Phylogenomic Analysis of mcr-Producing Salmonella

To provide the evolutionary characteristics of *mcr*-producing *Salmonella*, we compared 2145 genomes of different *Salmonella* serotypes from different countries. A total of 25,735 core SNPs were identified to construct a maximum likelihood tree (Figure 4). The evolutionary strategy was based on serotypes. Currently, among 2145 isolates, the gene *mcr* (*mcr-5.1*) could be traced back to a *Salmonella* Typhimurium isolate in 1985, which was recovered from *Bos taurus* in Japan. It was found that Typhimurium and 1,4,[5],12:i:- as well as the close serotypes such as Saintpaul, Heidelberg and 4,[5],12:i:- were the main serotypes carrying *mcr* genes in *Salmonella* (Figure 4). The *Salmonella* Typhimurium, 1,4,[5],12:i:- and 4,[5],12:i:- isolates were distributed in Lineages I, II, and III. The phylogenetic tree showed that Lineages I and II were mixed clusters, suggesting their close genetic relationship. Lineage I was mainly composed of *Salmonella* 4,[5],12:i:- and 1,4,[5],12:i:- isolates. Lineage II was mainly composed of *Salmonella* 1,4,[5],12:i:- as well as some *Salmonella* 4,[5],12:i:- and *Salmonella* Typhimurium isolates. Lineage III was almost composed of *Salmonella* Typhimurium isolates. Furthermore, *Salmonella* Typhimurium isolates from the United Kingdom and Australia in Lineage III were divided into two sub-clades, respectively. It was found that most isolates of Lineage II were from China, but the base isolates were recovered from Germany, suggesting that *mcr*-producing *Salmonella* 1,4,[5],12:i:- isolates might be introduced into China from Germany. Similar results were also found in Lineage IV. Lineage IV was composed of *Salmonella* Saintpaul isolates from the USA, and their evolutionary path implied that a major introduction might occur in the USA from Germany and then nationwide spread. Indeed, the predominant serotype carrying *mcr* genes in Germany was *Salmonella* Paratyphi B var. d-tartrate+, which could be found in Lineage VI. We also found that isolates from Lineages I, II, V, VII, VIII, and IX were mostly isolated after 2013, but those from Lineages IV and VI were mainly isolated from 2002 to 2013. In addition, isolates from different sources shared a close genetic relationship, which suggested that clonal spread occurred. For example, most isolates of Lineage II were recovered from humans but also clustered with some isolates from animals. Similar results were also found in isolates of Lineages I and III.

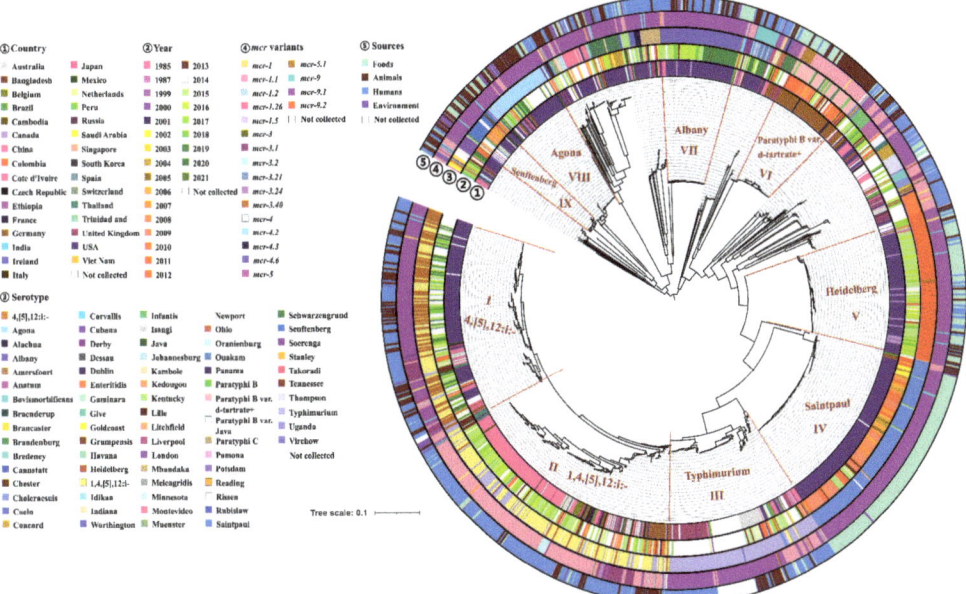

Figure 4. Phylogenetic tree of 2145 *Salmonella* genomes from different countries. Circles ①–⑤ denote countries, years, serotypes, *mcr* variants, and sources, respectively. The detailed information in circles ①–⑤ using various colors shown in the key.

3. Discussion

Colistin had been considered a therapeutic drug and feed additive for animals since the early 1980s and was approved for clinical treatment of human beings in 2017 in China [10,11]. In a previous study, *mcr-1*-producing *E. coli* isolates were able to transfer from animals to humans through the chicken production chain [12]. *E. coli*, *E. cloacae*, *Salmonella* spp., and *K. pneumonia* were reported to be the dominant *mcr-1*-producing bacteria members [1,5,11,13]. China's government has banned colistin as a feed additive to prevent colistin resistance in clinics, and then the drug production decreased markedly from 27,170 tons in 2015 to 2,497 tons in 2018, and the corresponding sale also decreased from USD 71.5 million in 2015 to USD 8.0 million in 2018 in China [14]. Furthermore, the median relative abundance of *mcr-1* per 16S RNA in *E. coli* from animals and humans decreased significantly from 0.0009 in 2017 to 0.0002 in 2018 [14]. Therefore, the ban on colistin in animal farming causes a significant decrease in *mcr-1* of *E. coli* isolates from animals and humans.

The emergence of plasmid-borne *mcr* genes has attracted significant attention worldwide [3,5]. In a previous study about the prevalence of *mcr*-producing bacterial isolates, it was found that a significant increase occurred in 2009 [3]. The chicken-borne *mcr-1*-producing *E. coli* isolates increased from 5.2% in 2009 to 30.0% in 2014 [15]. In a retrospective survey from China, the earliest chicken-borne *mcr-1*-producing *E. coli* isolate was found in the 1980s, which corresponded to the start use of colistin in animal husbandry as a feed additive [15]. In this study, the earliest emergence of *mcr* was identified from a *Salmonella* Typhimurium isolate from *Bos taurus* in 1985 (Japan, *mcr-5.1*), and the earliest *mcr* gene from humans was identified in a *Salmonella* 1,4,[5],12:i:- isolate in 2001 (the USA, *mcr-9.1*). Up to 1 January 2022, a total of 2279 *mcr*-positive *Salmonella* genomes were available from the NCBI database and were widely spread in 37 countries. Therefore, it was necessary to monitor the prevalence of *mcr-1* in *Salmonella* to evaluate its burden on human health.

In this study, 80 *Salmonella* serotypes were identified to be carrying *mcr* genes, among which Typhimurium (18.3%) and 1,4,[5],12:i:- (18.7%) were the predominant ones. *S.*

Typhimurium and 1,4,[5],12:i:- generally exhibited high-level prevalence and strong MDR features and spread worldwide [16]. Furthermore, the top three *mcr* variants in both Typhimurium and 1,4,[5],12:i:- were *mcr-1.1*, *mcr-9.1*, and *mcr-3.1*. Typhimurium and 1,4,[5],12:i:- were the predominant serotypes carrying *mcr* genes in China, the UK, and Australia. Furthermore, the phylogenetic relationship of *S*. Typhimurium and 1,4,[5],12:i:- isolates from these three countries was close, suggesting the possibility of the international spread among them. Unlike China, 1,4,[5],12:i:- (12.7%) was the third serotype carrying *mcr* genes in the USA, lower than Saintpaul (21.4%) and Heidelberg (14.2%). In Germany, Paratyphi B var. d-tartrate+ was the predominant serotype carrying *mcr* genes, and the top 2 *mcr* variants were *mcr-1.1* and *mcr-5.1*. Therefore, the prevalence of *Salmonella* serotypes and their *mcr* variants showed a wide variety in different geographical regions.

Here are some limitations of this study. First, the numerous genomes used in this study were associated with the development of sequencing technology. The genome information used was hard to represent the real prevalence of *mcr*-producing isolates. Second, the majority of the *mcr*-producing *Salmonella* genomes originated from the United States, China, the United Kingdom, and Germany, but data were limited from other countries. Therefore, the above limitations would bias the deduced results.

In conclusion, our study highlighted that *mcr*-producing *Salmonella* isolates have spread in five continents (Asia, Europe, America, Australia, and Africa) globally. Typhimurium and 1,4,[5],12:i:- were the predominant serotypes carrying *mcr* genes in *Salmonella*, and *mcr-9.1* and *mcr-1.1* were the predominant variants. The spread of such various *mcr* variants is of great concern for food safety and public health, and it is urgent to enhance surveillance and control the spread of *mcr* genes among *Salmonella*.

4. Materials and Methods

4.1. Salmonella Genomes Collected

We searched two important words, "*mcr*" and "*Salmonella*", in the public NCBI database on 1 January 2022. A total of 2279 *Salmonella* isolates were positive for *mcr* genes, and the detailed information of isolates, including years, countries, host, and serotypes, were then downloaded. However, 2145 out of 2279 genomes were available because the rest had not been released. These genomes were used for phylogenetic analysis to explore the implied spread of MCR-producing *Salmonella* worldwide.

4.2. The Identification of mcr Variants and Serotypes

The genomes used were further to identify the variant types of *mcr* genes through ResFinder (https://cge.cbs.dtu.dk/services/ResFinder/, accessed on 1 June 2022). *Salmonella* serotypes were available from the uploaded information, and the serotypes that were not submitted by the uploader were predicted by SeqSero 1.2 (https://cge.cbs.dtu.dk/services/SeqSero/, accessed on 1 June 2022).

4.3. Phylogenetic Analysis

A total of 2145 *Salmonella* genomes from different countries were used for phylogenetic analysis. Single-nucleotide polymorphisms (SNPs) were extracted using Snippy (https://github.com/tseemann/snippy, accessed on 1 June 2022) to generate core genomic alignment. Gubbins [17] was then used to identify and remove recombination regions using an algorithm that iteratively identifies loci containing elevated densities of base substitutions, and then resulting pairwise SNP differences were calculated. The core SNP alignment was used to generate a maximum-likelihood phylogeny using RAxML v8.1.23 (Karlsruhe, Germany) [18] with the GTR nucleotide substitution model. The display, annotation, and management of phylogenetic trees were performed by the ITOL tool [19]. The antibiotic resistance genes in all genomes were identified by ResFinder 4.1 (Lyngby, Denmark) [20].

4.4. Data Analysis

The bar and circle charts used to analyze the prevalence of *mcr* serotypes were generated with GraphPad Prism 7 software (San Diego, California, CA, USA). The world map marked with the distribution of *mcr*-positive *Salmonella* was drawn by Inkscape 0.92 (New York, NY, USA).

Supplementary Materials: The following supporting information can be downloaded at: https://www.mdpi.com/article/10.3390/antibiotics11080998/s1, Comparison of *mcr* variant sequences from *Salmonella* (.fas profile).

Author Contributions: Conceptualization, Z.Z.; methodology, Z.Z. and X.T.; validation, Z.Z.; investigation, Z.Z.; data curation, Z.Z.; writing—original draft preparation, Z.Z.; writing—review and editing, Z.Z. and C.S.; supervision, C.S.; project administration, C.S.; funding acquisition, C.S. All authors have read and agreed to the published version of the manuscript.

Funding: This research was funded by the Shanghai Agriculture Applied Technology Development Program, China (grant number 2020-02-08-00-08-F01487) and the National Natural Science Foundation of China (grant number 31972169).

Data Availability Statement: Not applicable.

Conflicts of Interest: The authors declare no conflict of interest.

References

1. Portes, A.B.; Rodrigues, G.; Leitão, M.P.; Ferrari, R.; Conte Junior, C.A.; Panzenhagen, P. Global Distribution of Plasmid-Mediated Colistin Resistance *Mcr* Gene in *Salmonella*: A Systematic Review. *J. Appl. Microbiol.* **2022**, *132*, 872–889. [CrossRef]
2. Wang, R.; van Dorp, L.; Shaw, L.P.; Bradley, P.; Wang, Q.; Wang, X.; Jin, L.; Zhang, Q.; Liu, Y.; Rieux, A.; et al. The Global Distribution and Spread of the Mobilized Colistin Resistance Gene *Mcr-1*. *Nat. Commun.* **2018**, *9*, 1179. [CrossRef] [PubMed]
3. Nang, S.C.; Li, J.; Velkov, T. The Rise and Spread of *Mcr* Plasmid-Mediated Polymyxin Resistance. *Crit. Rev. Microbiol.* **2019**, *45*, 131–161. [CrossRef] [PubMed]
4. Olaitan, A.O.; Morand, S.; Rolain, J.-M. Mechanisms of Polymyxin Resistance: Acquired and Intrinsic Resistance in Bacteria. *Front. Microbiol.* **2014**, *5*, 643. [CrossRef] [PubMed]
5. Liu, Y.-Y.; Wang, Y.; Walsh, T.R.; Yi, L.-X.; Zhang, R.; Spencer, J.; Doi, Y.; Tian, G.; Dong, B.; Huang, X.; et al. Emergence of Plasmid-Mediated Colistin Resistance Mechanism MCR-1 in Animals and Human Beings in China: A Microbiological and Molecular Biological Study. *Lancet Infect. Dis.* **2016**, *16*, 161–168. [CrossRef]
6. Hussein, N.H.; AL-Kadmy, I.M.S.; Taha, B.M.; Hussein, J.D. Mobilized Colistin Resistance (*Mcr*) Genes from 1 to 10: A Comprehensive Review. *Mol. Biol. Rep.* **2021**, *48*, 2897–2907. [CrossRef]
7. Poirel, L.; Kieffer, N.; Liassine, N.; Thanh, D.; Nordmann, P. Plasmid-Mediated Carbapenem and Colistin Resistance in a Clinical Isolate of *Escherichia coli*. *Lancet Infect. Dis.* **2016**, *16*, 281. [CrossRef]
8. Du, H.; Chen, L.; Tang, Y.-W.; Kreiswirth, B.N. Emergence of the *Mcr-1* Colistin Resistance Gene in Carbapenem-Resistant Enterobacteriaceae. *Lancet Infect. Dis.* **2016**, *16*, 287–288. [CrossRef]
9. Yao, X.; Doi, Y.; Zeng, L.; Lv, L.; Liu, J.-H. Carbapenem-Resistant and Colistin-Resistant *Escherichia coli* Co-Producing NDM-9 and MCR-1. *Lancet Infect. Dis.* **2016**, *16*, 288–289. [CrossRef]
10. Shen, Y.; Zhou, H.; Xu, J.; Wang, Y.; Zhang, Q.; Walsh, T.R.; Shao, B.; Wu, C.; Hu, Y.; Yang, L.; et al. Anthropogenic and Environmental Factors Associated with High Incidence of *Mcr-1* Carriage in Humans across China. *Nat. Microbiol.* **2018**, *3*, 1054–1062. [CrossRef]
11. Wang, Y.; Tian, G.-B.; Zhang, R.; Shen, Y.; Tyrrell, J.M.; Huang, X.; Zhou, H.; Lei, L.; Li, H.-Y.; Doi, Y.; et al. Prevalence, Risk Factors, Outcomes, and Molecular Epidemiology of *Mcr-1*-Positive *Enterobacteriaceae* in Patients and Healthy Adults from China: An Epidemiological and Clinical Study. *Lancet Infect. Dis.* **2017**, *17*, 390–399. [CrossRef]
12. Wang, Y.; Zhang, R.; Li, J.; Wu, Z.; Yin, W.; Schwarz, S.; Tyrrell, J.M.; Zheng, Y.; Wang, S.; Shen, Z.; et al. Comprehensive Resistome Analysis Reveals the Prevalence of NDM and MCR-1 in Chinese Poultry Production. *Nat. Microbiol.* **2017**, *2*, 16260. [CrossRef] [PubMed]
13. Quan, J.; Li, X.; Chen, Y.; Jiang, Y.; Zhou, Z.; Zhang, H.; Sun, L.; Ruan, Z.; Feng, Y.; Akova, M.; et al. Prevalence of *Mcr-1* in *Escherichia coli* and *Klebsiella Pneumoniae* Recovered from Bloodstream Infections in China: A Multicentre Longitudinal Study. *Lancet Infect. Dis.* **2017**, *17*, 400–410. [CrossRef]
14. Wang, Y.; Xu, C.; Zhang, R.; Chen, Y.; Shen, Y.; Hu, F.; Liu, D.; Lu, J.; Guo, Y.; Xia, X.; et al. Changes in Colistin Resistance and *Mcr-1* Abundance in *Escherichia coli* of Animal and Human Origins Following the Ban of Colistin-Positive Additives in China: An Epidemiological Comparative Study. *Lancet Infect. Dis.* **2020**, *20*, 1161–1171. [CrossRef]
15. Shen, Z.; Wang, Y.; Shen, Y.; Shen, J.; Wu, C. Early Emergence of *Mcr-1* in *Escherichia coli* from Food-Producing Animals. *Lancet Infect. Dis.* **2016**, *16*, 293. [CrossRef]

16. Sun, H.; Wan, Y.; Du, P.; Bai, L. The Epidemiology of Monophasic *Salmonella* Typhimurium. *Foodborne Pathog. Dis.* **2020**, *17*, 87–97. [CrossRef]
17. Croucher, N.J.; Page, A.J.; Connor, T.R.; Delaney, A.J.; Keane, J.A.; Bentley, S.D.; Parkhill, J.; Harris, S.R. Rapid Phylogenetic Analysis of Large Samples of Recombinant Bacterial Whole Genome Sequences Using Gubbins. *Nucleic Acids Res.* **2015**, *43*, e15. [CrossRef]
18. Stamatakis, A. RAxML Version 8: A Tool for Phylogenetic Analysis and Post-Analysis of Large Phylogenies. *Bioinformatics* **2014**, *30*, 1312–1313. [CrossRef]
19. Letunic, I.; Bork, P. Interactive Tree Of Life (ITOL) v4: Recent Updates and New Developments. *Nucleic Acids Res.* **2019**, *47*, W256–W259. [CrossRef]
20. Bortolaia, V.; Kaas, R.S.; Ruppe, E.; Roberts, M.C.; Schwarz, S.; Cattoir, V.; Philippon, A.; Allesoe, R.L.; Rebelo, A.R.; Florensa, A.F.; et al. ResFinder 4.0 for Predictions of Phenotypes from Genotypes. *J. Antimicrob. Chemother.* **2020**, *75*, 3491–3500. [CrossRef] [PubMed]

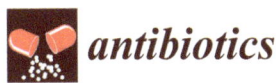

Article

Identification of Mobile Colistin Resistance Gene *mcr-10* in Disinfectant and Antibiotic Resistant *Escherichia coli* from Disinfected Tableware

Senlin Zhang [1], Honghu Sun [2], Guangjie Lao [3], Zhiwei Zhou [3], Zhuochong Liu [3], Jiong Cai [2] and Qun Sun [1,3,*]

1. College of Biomass Science and Engineering, Sichuan University, Chengdu 610064, China; zslforest@gmail.com
2. Irradiation Preservation Key Laboratory of Sichuan Province, Chengdu Institute of Food Inspection, Chengdu 611135, China; sunhonghu901@hotmail.com (H.S.); caijiongcj@gmail.com (J.C.)
3. Key Laboratory of Bio-Resource and Eco-Environment of the Ministry of Education, College of Life Sciences, Sichuan University, Chengdu 610064, China; laoguangjie@stu.scu.edu.cn (G.L.); zhouzhiwei@stu.scu.edu.cn (Z.Z.); liuzhuochong_hmc@stu.scu.edu.cn (Z.L.)
* Correspondence: qunsun@scu.edu.cn; Tel.: +86-28-85418810

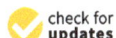

Citation: Zhang, S.; Sun, H.; Lao, G.; Zhou, Z.; Liu, Z.; Cai, J.; Sun, Q. Identification of Mobile Colistin Resistance Gene *mcr-10* in Disinfectant and Antibiotic Resistant *Escherichia coli* from Disinfected Tableware. *Antibiotics* 2022, 11, 883. https://doi.org/10.3390/antibiotics11070883

Academic Editor: William R. Schwan

Received: 25 May 2022
Accepted: 27 June 2022
Published: 1 July 2022

Publisher's Note: MDPI stays neutral with regard to jurisdictional claims in published maps and institutional affiliations.

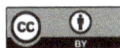

Copyright: © 2022 by the authors. Licensee MDPI, Basel, Switzerland. This article is an open access article distributed under the terms and conditions of the Creative Commons Attribution (CC BY) license (https://creativecommons.org/licenses/by/4.0/).

Abstract: The widespread escalation of bacterial resistance threatens the safety of the food chain. To investigate the resistance characteristics of *E. coli* strains isolated from disinfected tableware against both disinfectants and antibiotics, 311 disinfected tableware samples, including 54 chopsticks, 32 dinner plates, 61 bowls, 11 cups, and three spoons were collected in Chengdu, Sichuan Province, China to screen for disinfectant- (benzalkonium chloride and cetylpyridinium chloride) and tigecycline-resistant isolates, which were then subjected to antimicrobial susceptibility testing and whole genome sequencing (WGS). The coliform-positive detection rate was 51.8% (161/311) and among 161 coliform-positive samples, eight *E. coli* strains were multidrug-resistant to benzalkonium chloride, cetylpyridinium chloride, ampicillin, and tigecycline. Notably, a recently described mobile colistin resistance gene *mcr-10* present on the novel IncFIB-type plasmid of *E. coli* EC2641 screened was able to successfully transform the resistance. Global phylogenetic analysis revealed *E. coli* EC2641 clustered together with two clinically disinfectant- and colistin-multidrug-resistant *E. coli* strains from the US. This is the first report of *mcr-10*-bearing *E. coli* detected in disinfected tableware, suggesting that continuous monitoring of resistance genes in the catering industry is essential to understand and respond to the transmission of antibiotic resistance genes from the environment and food to humans and clinics.

Keywords: disinfectant resistance; colistin; multidrug resistance; *mcr-10*; plasmid; *E. coli*

1. Introduction

The development of antimicrobial resistance (AMR) has led to difficulties in the clinical treatment of serious bacterial infections. In response to global efforts to reduce AMR by minimizing antibiotic use, biocides (e.g., disinfectant and preservative) have increasingly been used as an important component of infection control [1], especially during the COVID-19 pandemic [2]. These biocides, including quaternary ammonium disinfectant, aldehydes, alcohols, phenols, bisphenols, and halogenic compounds, are currently considered the first line of defense against foodborne pathogens in hospitals or food processing facilities due to the versatility and efficiency of their chemical active ingredients [3]. Among them, quaternary ammonium disinfectant is non-corrosive and non-irritating, with low toxicity and high antimicrobial efficacy over a wide pH range, making them a widely used surface disinfectant and cleaning agent in food processing and production environments [4]. Benzalkonium chloride (BAC) and cetylpyridinium chloride (CPC), the most commonly used members of quaternary ammonium disinfectant, have broad-spectrum (i.e., bacteria, algae, fungi, and viruses) antimicrobial activity [5]. As a result, they are widely used as a surface disinfectant in food processing lines (e.g., poultry facilities, cleaning, and sanitizing facilities), dairy/agricultural environments, health care facilities, and home oral care [6,7].

However, this raises questions about the possible role of quaternary ammonium disinfectants in promoting the development of antimicrobial resistance, particularly multidrug resistance to antimicrobials. The epidemiological relationship between antibiotic resistance and higher MIC values of quaternary ammonium disinfectant in clinical *E. coli* isolates has been confirmed [8]. Recent studies have shown that BAC exposure can induce antibiotic resistance through multiple genetic mechanisms, including the coexistence of BAC and antibiotic resistance genes on the same mobile DNA molecule, mutations in the *pmrB* (colistin resistance) gene, and the overexpression of efflux pump genes [9]. Russell et al. mentioned that the frequent use of CPC could likewise result in bacterial resistance [10]. The use of quaternary ammonium disinfectant in food production and processing environments may not be as effective as expected, which provides selection pressure for strains with acquired resistance to other antimicrobial agents [11].

Resistance to most antimicrobials and a lack of novel antimicrobials against Gram-negative bacteria can lead to the reuse of older antibiotics. For example, colistin (polymyxin E), a cationic polypeptide antibiotic, was one of the first antibiotics to have a significant effect against Gram-negative bacteria [12]. It binds to the negatively charged lipopolysaccharide (LPS) of the outer membrane of Gram-negative bacteria, leading to membrane rupture and ultimately to cell death. Colistin and tigecycline are considered to be the remedy and last line of defense for serious bacterial infections [13,14]. Unfortunately, mobile colistin resistance genes (*mcr-1* to *mcr-10*) and tigecycline resistance genes (*tetX* to *tetX6*) carried by plasmids have recently been found to be horizontally transmitted with plasmids; the emergence of these genes accelerates the fall of the last line of defense against antibiotics [15,16]. Of the ten *mcr* gene variants, *mcr-1* is common in more than forty countries on six continents [17]. *mcr-10* is a novel allele, first isolated in ascites from a patient in China in 2020, and has been identified in animals, humans, and the environment [16,18,19]. However, little attention has been paid to *mcr-10* resistant isolates from disinfected tableware environments. Potentially, this is an important route of *mcr-10* transmission from the environment and food to healthy humans.

Previous studies on the multidrug resistance of bacterial disinfectants and antibiotics have mainly focused on hospital clinical infectious bacteria and rarely on multidrug resistance of foodborne bacteria to disinfectant and antibiotic. Additionally, studies on foodborne bacteria in tableware have mostly focused on the evaluation of disinfection effects, and few studies have been conducted on disinfectant- and antibiotic-resistant strains. Meanwhile, *E. coli*, as an important opportunistic pathogen among foodborne bacteria, is one of the common outbreak factors of foodborne diseases in China. Therefore, monitoring multidrug resistance to disinfectant and antibiotic in *E. coli* from disinfected tableware in the catering industry is important to understand the spread of resistance genes in foodborne bacteria and to regulate sanitization practices. This study aimed to monitor resistant *E. coli* to commonly used disinfectants and the last antibiotic in disinfected tableware to understand their resistance characteristics.

2. Results

2.1. Strain Identification and Antimicrobial Susceptibility

In our study, a total of 161 coliform-positive disinfected tableware samples were detected from 311 tableware samples, with a detection rate of 51.8%. From the 161 coliform-positive disinfected tableware samples, eight isolates of quaternary ammonium disinfectant and tigecycline resistance were detected. They were identified as *E. coli* by API-20E biochemical identification and whole genome sequencing. For all eight isolates, resistance to tigecycline, benzalkonium chloride, and cetylpyridinium chloride was detected, with the MIC values recorded of 2, 16, and 8 μg/mL, respectively. The majority (6/8) exhibited resistance to multiple antimicrobial agents other than meropenem (Table 1). Ampicillin resistance ($n = 8$) and tetracycline resistance ($n = 6$) were commonly detected in 6/8 quaternary ammonium disinfectant resistant isolates, followed by cefoxitin ($n = 2$), ceftriaxone sodium ($n = 2$), and chloramphenicol ($n = 2$). In addition, resistance phenotypes to colistin and polymyxin B were observed in isolates EC2639 and EC2641. All eight *E. coli* strains exhibited multidrug resistance characteristics, with TGC-AMP-TET-BAC-CPC being the most frequently observed resistance profile. Multilocus sequence typing (MLST) showed that eight strains were identified in seven ST types: ST2795, ST1571, ST4537, ST218, ST3907, ST3076, and ST5783.

Table 1. MIC profile of multidrug-resistant *E. coli* isolates.

Isolate ID	MIC (µg/mL)										
	TGC	MEM	AMP	CST	PME	FOX	CRO	CHL	TET	BAC	CPC
EC740	2	0.06	≥256	1	1	2	<0.6	16	8	16	8
EC799	2	0.03	32	2	1	2	<0.6	32	32	16	8
EC875	2	0.03	128	1	1	8	<0.6	256	256	16	8
EC2299	2	0.06	≥256	1	0.5	4	≥32	8	128	16	8
EC2639	2	0.03	256	8	4	4	<0.6	8	16	16	8
EC2641	2	0.12	32	4	4	4	<0.6	16	16	16	8
EC2783	2	0.06	≥256	0.5	0.5	4	≥32	16	128	16	8
SY3705	2	0.03	32	2	2	16	<0.6	8	4	16	8

Abbreviation: CRO, ceftriaxone; MEM, meropenem; AMP, ampicillin; FOX, cefoxitin; CHL, chloramphenicol; PMB, polymyxin B; CST, colistin; TGC, tigecycline; TET, tetracycline; BAC, benzalkonium chloride; CPC, cetylpyridinium chloride. The data in bold represent resistance.

2.2. ARG Characterization of Multidrug-Resistant Positive E. coli

In silico analysis showed that all strains contained the *mdf* (A) gene, a multidrug efflux pump gene with broad spectrum specificity that mediates antibiotic resistance to erythromycin, tetracycline, rifampin, kanamycin, chloramphenicol and ciprofloxacin, in addition to resistance to quaternary ammonium disinfectants [20]. Additionally, most (7/8) isolates carried *formA*, a gene resistant to formaldehyde (preservative) (Table 2) [21]. The quinolone resistance gene *qnrS1*, β-lactam resistance-associated genes bla_{TEM-1A}, bla_{ZEG-1}, bla_{OXA-10}, and bla_{MIR-2}, third-generation cephalosporins resistance-related gene $bla_{CTX-M-55}$, aminoglycoside resistance-related genes *strB* and *aadA1*, tetracycline resistance gene *tet* (A), trimethoprim resistance-related gene *dfrA14* and sulfonamide resistance-related gene *sul2* were detected in 2 (25.0%), 8 (100.0%), 1 (12.5%), 2 (25.0%), 2 (25.0%), 2 (25.0%), and 1 (12.5%) of these isolates, respectively. It was worth noting that the recently described mobile colistin resistance gene *mcr-10* was identified in the isolate EC2641. No mobile tigecycline resistance genes (*tet* variants) were found. The plasmid replicon results showed that all strains had 1–5 plasmid replicon types, with IncFIB-type plasmids being the most common type, followed by IncY, IncFIA, and Col440I.

Table 2. Characteristics of quaternary ammonium disinfectant and antibiotic multidrug-resistant *E. coli* isolated from disinfected tableware samples.

Isolate	Plasmid Replicons	Serotype	STs	Antimicrobial Resistance Profile	Resistance Determinants Identified Based on WGS
EC740	Col156	O104: H27	ST2795	TGC-AMP-BAC-CPC	*mdf* (A), bla_{ZEG-1}, *formA*
EC799	Col440I, IncFIA (HI1), IncFIB (K), IncY	O81: H9	ST1571	TGC-AMP-CHL-TET-BAC-CPC	*mdf* (A), bla_{ZEG-1}, *formA*
EC875	IncFIB (K)	OND: H16	ST4537	TGC-AMP-CHL-TET-BAC-CPC	*aadA1, mdf* (A), bla_{OXA-10}, *qnrS1, dfrA14, cmlA1, floR, ARR-2, tet* (A), *formA*, bla_{MIR-2}
EC2299	IncY	O159: H34	ST218	TGC-AMP-CRO-TET-BAC-CPC	*mdf* (A), bla_{ZEG-1}, *formA*
EC2639	Col440I, Col156, IncR	O155: H27	ST2795	TGC-AMP-CST-PME-TET-BAC-CPC	*mdf* (A), bla_{ZEG-1}, *formA*
EC2641	Col440I, FIA (pBK30683), IncFIB (K), IncHI1A, IncHI1B (R27)	O112ab: H9	ST3907	TGC-AMP-CST-PME-TET-BAC-CPC	*mdf* (A), *mcr-10*, bla_{ZEG-1}, *formA*
EC2783	IncFIA, IncFIB (AP001918), IncFIC (FII), IncI1-I (Alpha), IncX9	O128ac: H34	ST3076	TGC-AMP-CST-PME-TET-BAC-CPC	$bla_{CTX-M-55}$, bla_{TEM-1B}, *qnrS1, tet* (A), sit_{ABCD}, *strB, dfrA14, mdf* (A), *sul2*
SY3705	IncFIB (K), IncFII, IncY	O83: H19	ST5783	TGC-AMP-BAC-CPC	*mdf* (A), bla_{ZEG-1}, *formA*

Abbreviation: CRO, ceftriaxone; AMP, ampicillin; CHL, chloramphenicol; PMB, polymyxin B; CST, colistin; TGC, tigecycline; TET, tetracycline; BAC, benzalkonium chloride; CPC, cetylpyridinium chloride. OND, O-antigen not detected.

2.3. Genetic Characterization of Colistin-Resistant E. coli EC2641

Long-read whole genome sequencing of *E. coli* EC2641 yielded 1.93 clean gigabytes, second generation short read length whole genome sequencing yielded 1.204 GB of clean sequence, mixed assembly of second- and third-generation sequencing data, screening to one complete chromosome sequence and two complete plasmid sequences. The sizes were 4.74 Mb, 129.9 kb, and 198.3 kb, with G + C contents of 50.9, 51, and 48.55%, respectively. Among them, the mobile colistin resistance gene *mcr-10* was located on the lncFIB (K)-type plasmid of size 123.9 kb and no other resistance genes were found on this plasmid. In addition, the acquired resistance gene *mdf* (A), bla_{ZEG-1}, and *formA* were found in the chromosomal DNA of this strain. The MLST typing database and serotype database were queried and the strain EC2641 was identified as ST3907 and O112ab:H9. Virulence factor predictions indicated that the isolate encodes a uropathogenic specific protein USP and is an *E. coli* causing urinary tract infections.

2.4. Conjugation of mcr-10 among E. coli Isolate EC2641 under Laboratory Conditions

Conjugation experiments showed that the colistin resistance gene *mcr-10* was able to transfer into the recipient bacterium J53 with a conjugation frequency of 5.03×10^{-4}. The *mcr-10* gene could be detected by PCR (Figure S1) in both the parental strains and their transconjugants. In the case of the transconjugants, colistin MIC values were re-evaluated and found to be a 4-fold (0.5 μg/mL to 2 μg/mL) increase compared to the recipient bacterium J53.

To understand the origin of the plasmid carrying *mcr-10* in *E. coli* EC2641, a sequence comparison of plasmid pMCR_10_2641 was performed on NCBI. The results of the five plasmids with the highest similarity were characterized (Table S1). The most closely related plasmid to pMCR_10_2641 was the unnamed plasmid from *E. coli* strain A1_180 (GenBank Accession Number NZ_CP040383.1), with 45.34% coverage and up to 99.99% nucleotide identity. *E. coli* strain A1_180 was isolated from seagull feces from mudflats in Anchorage, the USA in 2016. A comparison of the pMCR_10_2641 plasmid sequence with the top five plasmid sequences of similarity revealed that the *xerC-mcr-10* structure is unique to pMCR_10_2641 (Figure 1). A genomic island (GI) of 8.7 kb in size was identified at 4.5 kb upstream of *mcr-10*, which had eight open reading frames (ORF) encoding the type 3 fimbriae of bacterium.

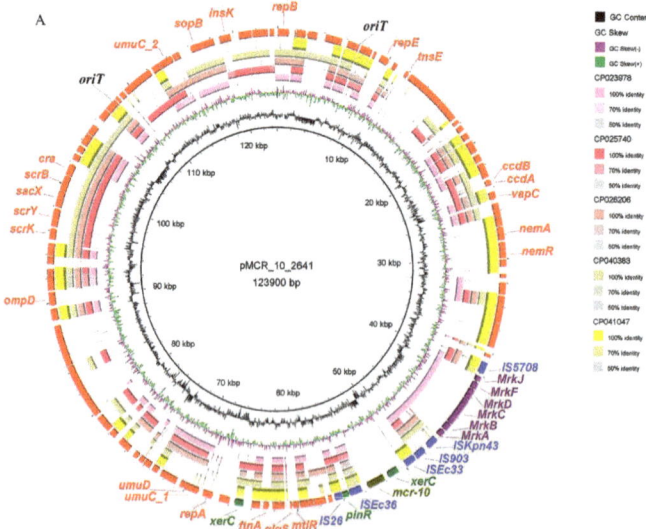

Figure 1. *Cont.*

B

```
1......5......10......15......20......25......30......35......40......45......50......55......60
AGGTTATTGCTACTTAATGCCGATAACGACTCAGGCTTTGAGGTTTTTTTATACGGTTCA

CATTTCGTTAGCAAGGTCAGGGTTTTTTGATAAAATTCTGGTTAGTTTGGTTAAAAAGTG

TTACAAGTATGGGTAATGGCTGAAAGGTTAGTTTTAAGGTTCAAAGCGGCAGTATTAAAA

TTCCAAAAGTTACTTTTCATCCTTCAGAATCCAGACCTTAATTTCATGTAGAAGATTCGT

ACAATTGTATTGGCGCAAGGACAATCCGCACATGTCAGAATCAGA
```

Figure 1. Genetic structural characterization of the antimicrobial resistance plasmid pMCR_10_2641. (**A**) Comparison of pMCR_10_2641 with the five highest matched plasmids in the NCBI reference database. The out-layer (red color) represents the plasmid pMCR_10_2641 in this study, which was used as the reference plasmid for a sequence comparison. Green arrows in the outer circle indicate integrons, blue arrows indicate various insertion sequences, and purple arrows indicate complete virulence islands. Colistin resistance gene *mcr-10* is highlighted by the olive. The arrow direction indicates the direction of transcription. The graph was generated by BRIG v0.95. (**B**) Schematic of the origin of the transfer sites (*oriT*) structure. The red font indicates the conserved nick region; The purple arrow is a pair of inverted repeats (IRs).

No genes associated with the bacterial type IV secretion system (T4SS) and relaxase gene mediating conjugative transfer were identified in the plasmid pMCR_10_2641. However, the plasmid had two 285 bp origin of transfer sites (*oriT*). Another plasmid with a size 198.3 Kb in this strain, p2641_2, was found to carry a locus encoding a protein related to the bacterial type IV secretion system. Combined with the results of the conjugative experiments (Figure S1), plasmid pMCR_10_2641 was shown to be a novel non-self-transmissible mobile plasmid that may mediate the mobilization of the colistin resistance gene *mcr-10* by the helper plasmid p2641_2.

2.5. Genetic Characterization of mcr-10 Carrying Plasmids

To understand the horizontal transfer mechanism of *mcr-10*, the genetic environment of *mcr-10* was characterized by local covariance analysis (Figure 2). The six *mcr-10*-bearing plasmid sequences, including pMCR_10_2641, were isolated in this study and the remaining five plasmids were from animals (n = 1), hospital wastewater (n = 2), and clinical samples (n = 2). Among them, pMCR10_090065 is the first isolated and reported to harbor *mcr-10* gene. Compared to the recently described genetic environment of *mcr-10*, our *mcr-10* was linked to the upstream *xerC* gene, except that IS*Ec36* was interrupted by the insertion sequence IS*kos1*Δ in plasmid pMCR10_090065, and the downstream formed a conserved *xerC-mcr-10-*IS*Ec36* structure with the insertion sequence IS*Ec36*.

To further understand the origin of *mcr-10* in *E. coli* non-self-mobilizable plasmids, a comparative analysis of plasmid sequences carrying *mcr-10* reported by NCBI and articles was performed (Figure 3). A total of 20 complete plasmids sequences carrying *mcr-10* were retrieved on NCBI (Table S2), including *Enterobacter roggenkampii* (30%, 6/20), *Raoultella ornithinolytica* (10%, 2/20), *Enterobacter cloacae* (15%, 3/20), *Cronobacter sakazakii* (5%, 1/20), *Citrobacter freundii* (5%, 1/20), *Enterobacter hormaechei* (5%, 1/20), *Enterobacter kobei* (5%, 1/20), *Enterobacter asburiae* (5%, 1/20), *Enterobacter* sp. (10%, 2/20), and *Klebsiella quasipneumoniae* (10%, 2/20), which demonstrated its wide host range. Typing of these plasmids revealed a smaller range of host plasmids for *mcr-10*, concentrated in three plasmid replicon types, IncFIB (n = 12), IncFIA (n = 2), and IncFII (n = 4). Structural comparisons of plasmids carrying *mcr-10* revealed the insertion sequence IS*903* upstream of *xerC-mcr-10*, which is immediately downstream of the mobile element IS*Ec36* (except for individual plasmids where this position is interrupted).

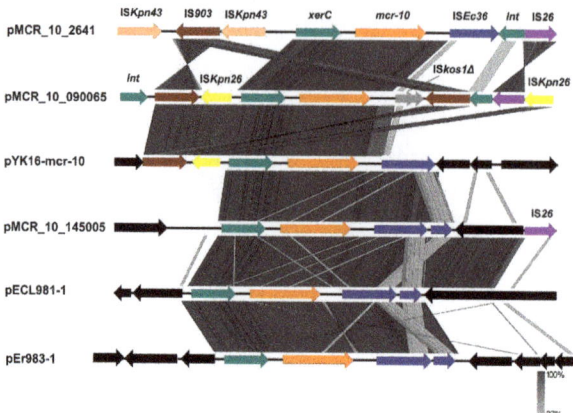

Figure 2. Comparison with the recently reported genetic environment of *mcr-10*. pMCR_10_2641 is the plasmid isolated for this study, pMCR_10_090065 the first plasmid identified and reported for *mcr-10* [18], pMCR_10_145005 plasmid was obtained from the stool samples of healthy volunteers in Chengdu [22], pYK-*mcr-10* is the most recent plasmid isolated from animal sources [23], pECL981-1 and pEr983-1 are the most recent plasmids isolated from hospital wastewater [19]. Orange arrows represent the drug resistance gene *mcr-10*, dark cyan arrows indicate site-specific recombinase-encoding genes (integrons), black arrows indicate other functional genes, and the remaining colored arrows represent the corresponding insertion sequences or mobile progenitors. The graph was generated by easyfig v2.2.5.

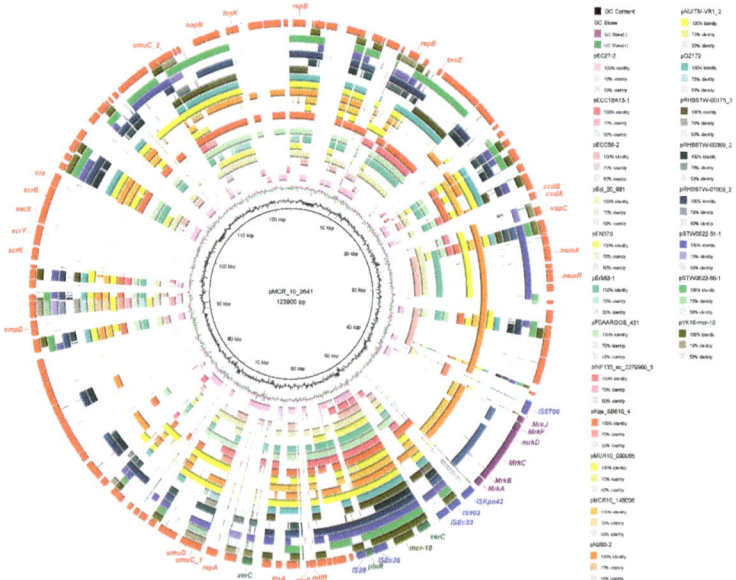

Figure 3. DNA alignment of *mcr-10*-containing plasmids. The out-layer (red color) represents the plasmid pMCR_10_2641 in this study, which was used as the reference plasmid for sequence comparison. Green arrows in the outer circle indicate integrons, blue arrows indicate various insertion sequences, and purple arrows indicate complete virulence islands. Colistin resistance gene *mcr-10* is highlighted by the olive. The arrow direction indicates the direction of transcription. The graph was generated by BRIG v0.95.

2.6. Upregulation of mcr-10 Expression at Subinhibitory Concentrations of Colistin

To understand whether *mcr-10* expression is inducible in the original strain, four drug stresses were selected to investigate the expression characteristics of *mcr-10* (Figure S2). The relative expression of this gene was significantly upregulated 2-fold in 2 µg/mL (1/2 MIC) colistin ($p < 0.001$), and no significant changes were observed after the disinfectants benzalkonium chloride (1/2 MIC, 8 µg/mL) and cetylpyridinium chloride (1/2 MIC, 4 µg/mL) disinfectant stresses. *mcr-10* was upregulated 1.5-fold after IPTG induction. Two disinfectants, benzalkonium chloride and cetylpyridinium chloride, did not affect the expression of the mobile colistin resistance gene *mcr-10*. The results of the induction assay showed that the *mcr-10* gene could be specifically induced by colistin in *E. coli* EC2641. It was shown that the original host of *mcr-10*, *E. coli* EC2641 can adapt rapidly under colistin stress.

2.7. Global Phylogenetic Analysis of E. coli Carrying the mcr Variant

Core SNP-based phylogenetic analysis was performed to determine the epidemiological relevance of the isolate EC2641 to publicly available *E. coli* isolates ($n = 208$) that have the *mcr* gene in the NCBI database (Table S3). Isolate EC2641 was clustered with two clinical isolates (ST32) from the United States carrying the disinfectant resistance gene *qacE*. Our isolate EC2641 was clustered into a large evolutionary branch including humans (clinical), animals, the environment, and food ($n = 141$) from various countries (USA, Germany, Czech Republic, Egypt, Canada, Australia, Vietnam, and China) that exhibit global epidemiological characteristics (Figure 4).

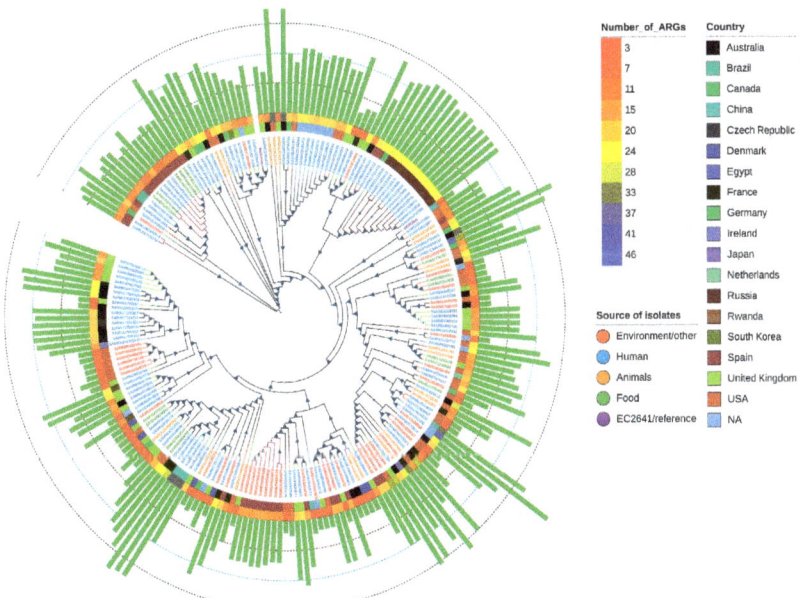

Figure 4. Global phylogenetic analysis of *E. coli* carrying the *mcr* variant. The isolate sequences were compared to the *E. coli* reference genome ATCC25922 by snippy and core SNP comparisons were generated. Maximum likelihood phylogenetic trees were constructed using RAxML-NG. The size of the blue triangle represents the size of the bootstrap value (ranging from 0–100). The label color indicates the source of isolation of the strain; the first circle from the inside is the country information of the isolate, and the second circle is the information of the number abundance of ARGs.

3. Discussion

We used the resistance profile of *E. coli* to quaternary ammonium disinfectants and the last antibiotic to indirectly assess the risk of potential resistance transmission of coliform bacteria in disinfected tableware. Our data suggest that the detection of coliform in disinfected tableware is of concern, which may involve the latent presence of multiple pathogenic bacteria. Consistent with previous studies on disinfectant-resistant *E. coli* isolated from hospitals [8], the *E. coli* we isolated also exhibited multidrug resistance. The identification of multidrug-resistant *E. coli* to tigecycline and colistin in our study suggests that this may pose risks and challenges for our last resort antibiotics. Although no mobile tigecycline resistance genes (*tet* variants) were found in our study, these eight *E. coli* strains still exhibited tigecycline resistance, which poses a concern for last resort antibiotic therapy. Bacterial efflux pumps were the main mechanism of tigecycline resistance before it was found that mobile tigecycline resistance genes were located in plasmid-mediated bacterial resistance. For example, previous studies have shown that mutations in the *adeS* gene can lead to the overexpression of the AdeABC efflux pump, resulting in the decreased susceptibility of *A. baumannii* to tigecycline [24–26]. Antibiotics and disinfectants have different bactericidal effects on bacteria and are used in different settings, but bacteria have a similar response strategy to disinfectants and antibiotics, namely the bacterial efflux pump mechanism [10]. Additionally, the mechanism of tigecycline resistance in *E. coli* isolated in this study requires further experimental confirmation.

Most disinfectant resistance genes are carried by chromosomes that are usually part of the bacterial efflux pump system, including the resistance-nodulation-division (RND) superfamily, the main promoter superfamily (MFS), the multidrug and toxic compound extrusion (MATE) family, small multidrug resistance (SMR) family, and the ATP binding cassette (ABC) super family [27]. A previous study on disinfectant resistance in *E. coli* isolated from retail meat in Sichuan, China, found that the most frequent disinfectant resistance genes were *ydgE/ydgF*, *mdf* (A), and *sugE* located on chromosomes [11]. Zhou et al. identified the chromosomally encoded quaternary ammonium disinfectant resistance gene *mdf* (A) exhibiting the highest prevalence in *E. coli* isolated from retail meat in the United States [28]. Few disinfectant resistance genes located in mobile elements were found. This is consistent with the detection of the quaternary ammonium disinfectant resistance gene *mdf* (A) in our *E. coli* (100%, 8/8). Multilocus sequence typing (MLST) showed that *mdf* (A) was identified in seven STs, suggesting that its presence in *E. coli* is widespread and may provide a genetic advantage for the spread of AMR bacteria.

Since the first report of the colistin resistance gene *mcr-1* in 2015 [29], *mcr* variants have been widely identified in various species of different origins worldwide. Nine *mcr* homologs (*mcr-2* to *mcr-10*) have been identified [18]. Plasmid-mediated *mcr* genes have spread worldwide and pose a high threat to public health networks. Currently, the novel colistin resistance gene variant *mcr-10* gene has been recently monitored in animals, healthy humans (clinical), hospital wastewater, and raw milk [16,19,22,23]. Genetic structural characterization of the antimicrobial resistance plasmid pMCR_10_2641 indicated that the plasmid we identified carrying the antimicrobial resistance gene *mcr-10* is a probable novel plasmid. The resistance gene *mcr-10* is adjacent to a virulence island carrying locus encoding the type 3 fimbriae system of *Klebsiella pneumoniae* (*mrkABCDFJ*), allowing the host to attach to surfaces and form biofilms to resist the action of disinfectants and antibiotics, which are associated with virulence in *Enterobacteriaceae* [30,31]. Importantly, we report for the first time that a strain of *E. coli* carrying *mrc-10* is multidrug-resistant to disinfectants and antibiotics isolated from disinfected tableware in Chengdu, China, which not only expands the source range of *mcr-10* but also suggests that the spread of the novel colistin resistance gene *mcr-10* is implicated in humans.

It is generally believed that nonconjugative plasmids cannot be transferred horizontally to the recipient bacterium, yet this ignores the role of other plasmids carrying binding modules generated in the original strain. Xu et al. demonstrated that *Klebsiella pneumoniae* can transfer nonconjugative virulence plasmids (containing *oriT* sites) and conjugative plasmids under conditions that reduce extracellular polysaccharides or use *E. coli* as an intermediate strain [32]. Consistent with previous studies, the *mcr-10*-bearing plasmid we identified lacked a binding module and is not self-transmissible, but our experimental results suggest that *mcr-10* may be transferred horizontally into the recipient bacteria via a type IV secretion system carried by the helper plasmid. This helper plasmid employs the *oriT* of the mobilized plasmid to accomplish mobilization, which is consistent with a previous study [33].

Unlike the plasmid preference of *mcr-1* (IncI2, IncX4) [34], *mcr-10* prefers lncFIB-type plasmids. The *mcr-10*-bearing IncFIB-type plasmid pMCR_10_2641 is an antimicrobial resistant and virulence co-existing plasmid, which may have important implications for clinical treatment. In fact, IncFIB-type plasmids usually carry multiple resistance genes, and a recent study reported a novel resistance gene cluster *tnfxB1-tmexCD1-toprJ1* located in an IncFIB-type plasmid carrying multiple resistance genes (*strAB*, *armA*, *aph(3')- ia*, *qnrB4*, *sul1*, *mphA*, *mphE*, *msrE*, and *bla*$_{dha1}$) [35]. Despite the structural diversity of *mcr-10*-bearing plasmids, the genetic environment of *mcr-10* is generally the same, mostly composed of elements such as *xerC*, IS26, IS903, and IS*Ec36*. Unusually, the plasmid pMCR_10_2641 in this study is inserted immediately after the sequence IS*Ec36* with a serine site-specific recombinase encoding gene *pinR*. *xerC* and *pinR* are tyrosine site-specific recombinant genes and serine site-specific recombinant genes, respectively, both of which are integrons. *xerC*-type tyrosine recombinase can mediate the transfer of its surrounding carbapenem resistance gene *bla*$_{NMC}$ through site-specific recombination [36], but it is unclear whether the integrin *pinR* has a mobilizing effect on *mcr-10*. The covariance results suggest that *mcr-10* is in the midst of a complex insertion sequence with mobile elements and that the *xerC-mcr-10*-IS *Ec36* structure may be an important structure leading to the horizontal transfer of *mcr-10*. The genetic environment of *mcr-10* in all six plasmids highlights the importance of the insertion element IS*Ec36* in this genetic structure, and the results combined with plasmid comparisons suggest that the insertion sequences IS*903* and IS*Ec36* may be closely associated with *xerC*-mediated specific recombination. The conserved genetic environment and transferability between different bacterial hosts may lead to the widespread availability of *mcr-10* containing colistin-resistant isolates from different sources.

In fact, little is known about whether the transcription of resistance genes can be affected by disinfectant exposure and thus lead to antibiotic resistance [37,38]. In the present study, we confirmed no significant change in *mcr-10* expression under disinfectant stress, suggesting that *mcr-10* transcription may not be affected under disinfectant stress. Furthermore, induction with IPTG did not result in significant changes in *mcr-10* expression, which is consistent with previous studies in which the MIC of colistin remained unchanged [18]. The expression of *mcr-10* was significantly upregulated 2-fold in *E. coli* EC2641 under colistin stress, which was similar to the observations of Xu et al. in *E. roggenkampii* [19], and also indicates that *mcr-10* is functional for the host to cope with the selective pressure of colistin. Disinfectant exposure plays an important role in promoting the development of antibiotic resistance. It has been shown that bactericides used for disinfection can enhance antibiotic resistance in Gram-negative bacteria; for example, *Burkholderia lata* developed resistance to ceftazidime, imipenem, and ciprofloxacin after exposure to low concentrations of benzalkonium chloride and was found to be associated with significant upregulation of outer membrane proteins and ABC transporter proteins [39]. In cells adapted to benzalkonium chloride, new resistance was most frequently found to ampicillin (eight species), cefotaxime (six species), and sulfamethoxazole (three species), some of them with relevance for healthcare-associated infections such as *Enterobacter cloacae* or *E. coli* [40]. In *A. baumannii* ATCC17978, BAC increased the MIC of several aminoglycoside antibiotics (kanamycin, tobramycin, streptomycin, gentamicin, and amikacin) [41].

Global phylogenetic analysis showed that *mcr*-bearing *E. coli* exhibited a global epidemic profile (USA, Germany, Czech Republic, Egypt, Canada, Australia, Egypt, Vietnam, and China, etc.) and our isolate EC2641 was clustered with 141 *E. coli* from different sources including humans, the environmental, food and animals, supporting the direct/indirect transmission between humans and animals and the environment, which is consistent with the recent global concept of spreading mobilized colistin resistance genes from the environment to humans [16,42,43]. It is worth noting that *E. coli* EC2641 showed a close evolutionary relationship with two *E. coli* (ST 32) strains from the USA clinically carrying the *mcr-9* and quaternary ammonium disinfectant resistance gene *qacE*. In early studies, *E. coli* ST32 was isolated from the feces and hides of cattle in the United States [44], indicating that ST32 is not host-specific and is readily transmitted from animals to humans. We reasonably speculate that disinfectant-resistant bacteria may be important vectors of globally important antimicrobial resistance gene mobilization. The use of disinfectants in environmental disinfection has exploded since the COVID-19 epidemic, and monitoring of the multidrug resistance of such disinfectants with other antibiotics (e.g., tigecycline, colistin, imipenem, and meropenem) warrants further study. We emphasize the importance of disinfectants in the development and spread of bacterial antibiotic resistance.

4. Materials and Methods

4.1. Bacterial Isolation and Species Identification

This study was carried out during the period between June 2019 and December 2020. A total of 311 disinfected tableware samples were collected from 119 restaurants (using chemical disinfectant) in Chengdu, China. The fast test paper for coliform of tableware (NANJING SAN-AI, Nanjing, China) wet with sterile phosphate-buffered saline were used to sample the collected tableware samples, following the sampling principle of tableware surface in oral and food contact. Coliform detection sheets were placed in a 37 °C incubator for overnight culture. When the paper turned yellow or showed red spots on a yellow background, it was judged to be positive for coliform. Coliform were collected from positive paper with wet sterile cotton swabs for further analysis.

The wet swabs of coliform-positive samples were enriched in 30 mL of buffered peptone water (BPW, Oxoid, Hampshire, UK) and incubated overnight at 37 °C. Benzalkonium chloride, cetylpyridinium chloride, and tigecycline were used for the isolation of antibiotic and disinfectant resistant bacteria. Briefly, the overnight incubated culture was treated with benzalkonium chloride and cetylpyridinium chloride at a final concentration of 2000 µg/mL for 30 min at room temperature, and then screened for tigecycline resistant *E. coli* on the CHROMagar^{TM} Orientation plate (CHROMagar^{TM}, Paris, France) containing 2 µg/mL tigecycline. Further strain identification was determined by API-20E biochemical testing and whole genome sequencing.

4.2. In Vitro Antimicrobial Susceptibility Testing

The broth dilution method was used for determining the minimum inhibitory concentration (MIC) of polymyxin B, colistin, tigecycline, ceftazidime, ceftriaxone, meropenem, ampicillin, chloramphenicol, cetylpyridinium chloride, and benzalkonium chloride. Resistance to polymyxin B, colistin, and tigecycline was determined according to the European Committee on Antimicrobial Resistance Testing (EUCAST). Clinical breakpoints (https://eucast.org/clinical_breakpoints/, accessed on 5 October 2021) and minimum inhibitory concentrations (MICs) for benzalkonium chloride and cetylpyridinium chloride MICs higher than those of standard strain *E. coli* ATCC 25922 were considered as resistant. Resistance to the other antibiotics was interpreted according to the CLSI instructions [45], with *E. coli* ATCC 25922 used as quality control strains.

4.3. Transconjugation Assay

Transconjugation assay was performed according to a previously described method [15]. The transferability of *mcr-10* in *E. coli* EC2641 was determined by the filtration membrane method. Briefly, *E. coli* J53 (resistant to sodium azide) was the recipient strain, and strain EC2641 (carrying *mcr-10*) was the donor strain in this study. Firstly, the donor and recipient were cultured in LB medium to logarithmic phase, and then the donor and recipient were mixed and inoculated on 0.22 filter membrane in the ratio of 1:3 and cultured overnight at 37 °C. Putative transconjugants were screened in LB agar medium containing 150 µg/mL sodium azide and 2 µg/mL colistin, and the successful transconjugants were identified by PCR amplification of the target gene (*mcr-10*) [18].

4.4. Induced Expression, RNA Extraction, Real-Time Reverse Transcription PCR (RT–PCR)

For induction assays, isolate EC2641 was grown in LB without antibiotic until OD600 = 0.5. Overnight culture of the bacteria was diluted in fresh LB broth (1:100, *v/v*) with final colistin concentration of 2 μg/mL, benzalkonium chloride concentration of 4 μg/mL, cetylpyridine chloride concentration of 4 μg/mL, and IPTG concentration of 1 mmol/L [18]. The antibiotic-free medium was used as the control. The culture was incubated at 37 °C for 10–12 h and harvested by centrifugation at 4 °C. RNA was extracted using a small amount of the total RNA extraction kit (TIANMO BIO, Beijing, China) according to the manufacturer's instructions, followed by genomic DNA elimination and cDNA synthesis using the PrimeScript™ RT Reagent Kit with gDNA Eraser (Takara Bio USA, San Jose, CA, USA). gDNA removal was confirmed using PCR. RNA size, integrity and total amount were determined using a BioDrop μLite+ (Biochrom, Cambridge, UK).

The primers used for RT-qPCR were designed using Primer Premier 6.0 (Table S4). The amplification efficiency of all primer pairs was tested using standard dilution procedures. RT-qPCR analysis was conducted on a QuantStudio™ 3 Real-Time system with SYBR green fluorescence dye. The *16s* gene was used as a reference control for normalization. The relative differences in gene expression were calculated as a fold change using the formula $2^{-\Delta\Delta CT}$ [19].

4.5. DNA Extraction, Whole-Genome Sequencing

A single colony of *E. coli* isolates was selected and cultured in LB medium at 37 °C. Genomic DNA was extracted using a Gentra Puregene Yeat/Bact.Kit (Qiagen, Chatsworth, CA, USA). The harvested DNA was detected by the agarose gel electrophoresis and quantified by a Qubit® 2.0 Fluorometer (Thermo Scientific, Waltham, MA, USA). According to the manufacturer's instructions, the harvested DNA was subjected to WGS on the Illumina NovaSeq 6000 system (Illumina, San Diego, CA, USA), which generated 150-bp paired-end reads from a library with an average insert size of 350 bp. The *E. coli* EC2641 was further sequenced by a Nanopore PromethION platform (Nanopore, Oxford, UK) following a 10-Kbp library protocol.

4.6. Sequence Assembly, Annotation and Bioinformatic Analysis

For each isolate, >550 Mbp high-quality clean paired-end reads were obtained and de novo assembled using SPAdes v.3.9.0 [46]. In addition, the *E. coli* EC2641 hybrid assembly of short Illumina reads and long PromethION reads was performed using Unicycler v0.4.8 [47]. Then, we compared the reads to the assembled sequence, counted the distribution of sequencing depth, distinguished whether the assembled sequence was a chromosomal sequence or a plasmid sequence according to sequence length and alignment, and checked whether it is a circular genome.

The prokka version 1.14.6 with default parameters was used to call the blast+ to search for a small core set of well-characterized proteins and the Hidden Markov Model (HMM) to identify coding regions to accomplish rapid annotation of bacterial genomes and plasmid sequences [48]. Serotypes, sequence types, virulence genes, and antimicrobial resistance genes were identified using SerotypeFinder version 2.0.1, Multi-Locus Sequence Typing (MLST) version 2.0.4, VirulenceFinder version 2.0.3, and ResFinder version 4.0.1 from the Center for Genomic Epidemiology (CGE) [49]. Genes with 80% identity and greater than 90% coverage were considered present, and genes with coverage between 40% and 90% were considered present but partial genes. The IslandPath-DIOMB version 0.2 was used to predict GIs based on both the detection of dinucleotide bias in eight genes or more and the identification of a mobility gene in the same region [50].

The annotated GBK files were uploaded to the online tool oriTfinder to identify the classification of plasmids (conjugated, mobilizable, and non-mobilizable) by using the integration of the profile HMM-based relaxase gene search module with a BLAST-based *oriT* sequence search module [51]. The plasmid replicon genotype and insertion sequence (IS) elements of the plasmid were identified using PlasmidFinder version 2.0.1 and

ISfinder [52,53], replicons and IS with 80% identity and greater than 90% coverage were considered present, and replicons with coverage between 40% and 90% were considered present but partial replicons. All plasmid sequences carrying *mcr-10* were searched on NCBI. BLAST Ring Image Generator (BRIG) and Easyfig v2.2.5 were used for comparative analysis of plasmids and generation of physical maps [54,55]. The above bioinformatics analysis tools used default parameters if not otherwise specified.

4.7. Phylogenetic Analysis

Phylogenetic analysis based on single nucleotide polymorphisms (SNPs) was performed for the *E. coli* isolate EC2641 carrying *mcr-10* gene. Our isolate EC2641 was compared to the publicly available genomes of *E. coli* in the NCBI database, updated on January 14th, 2022, that carried a variant of the *mcr* gene ($n = 208$). Isolates were mapped to the reference *E. coli* complete genome ATCC25922 (CP032085.1) for all the collected *mcr*-carrying isolates. Metadata for the selected *E. coli* sequences from NCBI were collected (Table S2). SNPs variant calling were determined using Snippy v4.6.0 (https://github.com/tseemann/snippy, accessed on 15 January 2022) and the output files were combined into a core SNPs alignment using Snippy core. Maximum likelihood phylogenetic trees were then generated from SNPs alignment using RAxML-NG [56] and the trees were visualized with iTOL [57].

4.8. Accession Numbers

WGS data of all eight isolates, including two complete plasmid sequences of *E. coli* EC2641, were deposited in GenBank database (accession no. PRJNA818460).

4.9. Statistical Analysis

Statistical analysis was performed by the modular Student *t*-test using Prism 9 software (GraphPad Software, San Diego, CA, USA). Results are shown as the mean ± SD of the three individual test results. *p*-values < 0.05 were considered statistically significant.

5. Conclusions

In summary, we recovered eight strains of quaternary ammonium disinfectant- and antibiotic-resistant *E. coli* in disinfected tableware and characterized their resistance profile and the prevalence of the recently identified colistin resistance gene *mcr-10* in *E. coli* isolates. The non-self-transmissible novel plasmid carrying *mcr-10* identified in this study was mobilized by a helper plasmid, highlighting the potential widespread ability of *mcr-10* to the environment and humans. To achieve the "One Health" strategy for humans, the characterization and spread of bacterial resistance in the sanitized environment associated with the food industry should be continuously monitored. Therefore, monitoring the multidrug resistance profile of disinfectants and antibiotics in tableware can be an important reference for preventing and controlling the spread of resistance genes.

Supplementary Materials: The following supporting information can be downloaded at: https://www.mdpi.com/article/10.3390/antibiotics11070883/s1, Table S1: Information of plasmids with the five highest matched plasmids to pMCR_10_2641 in NCBI. Table S2: Plasmids carrying *mcr-10* gene on NCBI. Table S3: Details of Global 208 strains of *mcr*-bearing *E. coli*. Table S4: The PT-qPCR oligonucleotide primer sequences used in this study. Figure S1: Agarose gel electrophoresis of the *mcr-10* PCR product from DNA extracts of the transconjugants. Figure S2: Relative expression of the resistance gene *mcr-10* in *E. coli* EC2641 (the original host of *mcr-10* gene) under colistin, benzalkonium chloride, Cetylpyridinium Chloride, and IPTG stress.

Author Contributions: Conceptualization, S.Z., H.S. and J.C.; Methodology, S.Z., H.S. and Z.Z.; Software, S.Z. and Z.L.; Validation, S.Z. and G.L.; Formal Analysis, S.Z.; Investigation, H.S. and J.C.; Resources, H.S. and Q.S.; Data Curation, S.Z.; Writing—Original Draft Preparation, S.Z., G.L. and Z.Z.; Writing—Review and Editing, S.Z., H.S. and Q.S.; Visualization, S.Z.; Supervision, Q.S.; Project Administration, H.S. and Q.S.; Funding Acquisition, H.S. and Q.S. All authors have read and agreed to the published version of the manuscript.

Funding: This work was supported by the Chengdu Food Safety Risk Research Project (2020SPFX02), the National Key Research and Development Program of China (2019YFE0103800-5) and the International Research and Development Program of Sichuan (2021YFH0060).

Data Availability Statement: The sequencing data generated from this study have been uploaded to the NCBI GenBank database, as detailed in the Materials and Methods section.

Conflicts of Interest: The authors declare no conflict of interest.

References

1. Hora, P.I.; Pati, S.G.; McNamara, P.J.; Arnold, W.A. Increased Use of Quaternary Ammonium Compounds during the SARS-CoV-2 Pandemic and Beyond: Consideration of Environmental Implications. *Environ. Sci. Technol. Lett.* **2020**, *7*, 622–631. [CrossRef]
2. Zheng, G.; Filippelli, G.M.; Salamova, A. Increased Indoor Exposure to Commonly Used Disinfectants during the COVID-19 Pandemic. *Environ. Sci. Technol. Lett.* **2020**, *7*, 760–765. [CrossRef]
3. Butucel, E.; Balta, I.; Ahmadi, M.; Dumitrescu, G.; Morariu, F.; Pet, I.; Stef, L.; Corcionivoschi, N. Biocides as Biomedicines against Foodborne Pathogenic Bacteria. *Biomedicines* **2022**, *10*, 379. [CrossRef] [PubMed]
4. Vereshchagin, A.N.; Frolov, N.A.; Egorova, K.S.; Seitkalieva, M.M.; Ananikov, V.P. Quaternary Ammonium Compounds (QACs) and Ionic Liquids (ILs) as Biocides: From Simple Antiseptics to Tunable Antimicrobials. *Int. J. Mol. Sci.* **2021**, *22*, 6793. [CrossRef]
5. Marple, B.; Roland, P.; Benninger, M. Safety review of benzalkonium chloride used as a preservative in intranasal solutions: An overview of conflicting data and opinions. *Otolaryngol. Head Neck Surg.* **2004**, *130*, 131–141. [CrossRef]
6. Mao, X.; Auer, D.L.; Buchalla, W.; Hiller, K.-A.; Maisch, T.; Hellwig, E.; Al-Ahmad, A.; Cieplik, F. Cetylpyridinium Chloride: Mechanism of Action, Antimicrobial Efficacy in Biofilms, and Potential Risks of Resistance. *Antimicrob. Agents Chemother.* **2020**, *64*, e00576-20. [CrossRef]
7. Merchel Piovesan Pereira, B.; Tagkopoulos, I. Benzalkonium Chlorides: Uses, Regulatory Status, and Microbial Resistance. *Appl. Environ. Microbiol.* **2019**, *85*, e00377-19. [CrossRef]
8. Buffet-Bataillon, S.; Branger, B.; Cormier, M.; Bonnaure-Mallet, M.; Jolivet-Gougeon, A. Effect of higher minimum inhibitory concentrations of quaternary ammonium compounds in clinical *E. coli* isolates on antibiotic susceptibilities and clinical outcomes. *J. Hosp. Infect.* **2011**, *79*, 141–146. [CrossRef]
9. Kim, M.; Weigand, M.R.; Oh, S.; Hatt, J.K.; Krishnan, R.; Tezel, U.; Pavlostathis, S.G.; Konstantinidis, K.T.; Dozois, C.M. Widely Used Benzalkonium Chloride Disinfectants Can Promote Antibiotic Resistance. *Appl. Environ. Microbiol.* **2018**, *84*, e01201-18. [CrossRef]
10. Russell, A.D. Biocide use and antibiotic resistance: The relevance of laboratory findings to clinical and environmental situations. *Lancet Infect. Dis.* **2003**, *3*, 794–803. [CrossRef]
11. Zhang, A.; He, X.; Meng, Y.; Guo, L.; Long, M.; Yu, H.; Li, B.; Fan, L.; Liu, S.; Wang, H.; et al. Antibiotic and Disinfectant Resistance of Escherichia coli Isolated from Retail Meats in Sichuan, China. *Microb. Drug Resist.* **2016**, *22*, 80–87. [CrossRef] [PubMed]
12. Biswas, S.; Brunel, J.M.; Dubus, J.C.; Reynaud-Gaubert, M.; Rolain, J.M. Colistin: An update on the antibiotic of the 21st century. *Expert Rev. Anti. Infect. Ther.* **2012**, *10*, 917–934. [CrossRef] [PubMed]
13. Sheu, C.C.; Chang, Y.T.; Lin, S.Y.; Chen, Y.H.; Hsueh, P.R. Infections Caused by Carbapenem-Resistant Enterobacteriaceae: An Update on Therapeutic Options. *Front. Microbiol.* **2019**, *10*, 80. [CrossRef] [PubMed]
14. Li, J.; Nation, R.L.; Turnidge, J.D.; Milne, R.W.; Coulthard, K.; Rayner, C.R.; Paterson, D.L. Colistin: The re-emerging antibiotic for multidrug-resistant Gram-negative bacterial infections. *Lancet Infect. Dis.* **2006**, *6*, 589–601. [CrossRef]
15. Sun, H.; Wan, Y.; Du, P.; Liu, D.; Li, R.; Zhang, P.; Wu, Y.; Fanning, S.; Wang, Y.; Bai, L. Investigation of tigecycline resistant Escherichia coli from raw meat reveals potential transmission among food-producing animals. *Food Control* **2021**, *121*, 107633. [CrossRef]
16. Tartor, Y.H.; Abd El-Aziz, N.K.; Gharieb, R.M.A.; El Damaty, H.M.; Enany, S.; Soliman, E.A.; Abdellatif, S.S.; Attia, A.S.A.; Bahnass, M.M.; El-Shazly, Y.A.; et al. Whole-Genome Sequencing of Gram-Negative Bacteria Isolated From Bovine Mastitis and Raw Milk: The First Emergence of Colistin mcr-10 and Fosfomycin fosA5 Resistance Genes in Klebsiella pneumoniae in Middle East. *Front. Microbiol.* **2021**, *12*, 770813. [CrossRef]
17. Ling, Z.; Yin, W.; Shen, Z.; Wang, Y.; Shen, J.; Walsh, T.R. Epidemiology of mobile colistin resistance genes mcr-1 to mcr-9. *J. Antimicrob. Chemother.* **2020**, *75*, 3087–3095. [CrossRef]
18. Wang, C.; Feng, Y.; Liu, L.; Wei, L.; Kang, M.; Zong, Z. Identification of novel mobile colistin resistance gene mcr-10. *Emerg. Microbes Infect.* **2020**, *9*, 508–516. [CrossRef]
19. Xu, T.; Zhang, C.; Ji, Y.; Song, J.; Liu, Y.; Guo, Y.; Zhou, K. Identification of mcr-10 carried by self-transmissible plasmids and chromosome in Enterobacter roggenkampii strains isolated from hospital sewage water. *Environ. Pollut.* **2021**, *268*, 115706. [CrossRef]
20. Edgar, R.; Bibi, E. MdfA, an Escherichia coli multidrug resistance protein with an extraordinarily broad spectrum of drug recognition. *J. Bacteriol.* **1997**, *179*, 2274–2280. [CrossRef]
21. Kümmerle, N.; Feucht, H.H.; Kaulfers, P.M. Plasmid-mediated formaldehyde resistance in Escherichia coli: Characterization of resistance gene. *Antimicrob. Agents Chemother.* **1996**, *40*, 2276–2279. [CrossRef] [PubMed]

22. Yang, J.; Liu, L.; Feng, Y.; He, D.; Wang, C.; Zong, Z. Potential Mobilization of mcr-10 by an Integrative Mobile Element via Site-Specific Recombination in Cronobacter sakazakii. *Antimicrob. Agents Chemother.* **2021**, *65*, e01717-20. [CrossRef] [PubMed]
23. Lei, C.W.; Zhang, Y.; Wang, Y.T.; Wang, H.N. Detection of Mobile Colistin Resistance Gene mcr-10.1 in a Conjugative Plasmid from Enterobacter roggenkampii of Chicken Origin in China. *Antimicrob. Agents Chemother.* **2020**, *64*, e01191-20. [CrossRef] [PubMed]
24. Shi, Y.; Hua, X.; Xu, Q.; Yang, Y.; Zhang, L.; He, J.; Mu, X.; Hu, L.; Leptihn, S.; Yu, Y. Mechanism of eravacycline resistance in Acinetobacter baumannii mediated by a deletion mutation in the sensor kinase adeS, leading to elevated expression of the efflux pump AdeABC. *Infect. Genet. Evol.* **2020**, *80*, 104185. [CrossRef] [PubMed]
25. Xu, Q.; Hua, X.; He, J.; Zhang, D.; Chen, Q.; Zhang, L.; Loh, B.; Leptihn, S.; Wen, Y.; Higgins, P.G.; et al. The distribution of mutations and hotspots in transcription regulators of resistance-nodulation-cell division efflux pumps in tigecycline non-susceptible Acinetobacter baumannii in China. *Int. J. Med. Microbiol.* **2020**, *310*, 151464. [CrossRef]
26. Gerson, S.; Nowak, J.; Zander, E.; Ertel, J.; Wen, Y.; Krut, O.; Seifert, H.; Higgins, P.G. Diversity of mutations in regulatory genes of resistance-nodulation-cell division efflux pumps in association with tigecycline resistance in Acinetobacter baumannii. *J. Antimicrob. Chemother.* **2018**, *73*, 1501–1508. [CrossRef]
27. Tong, C.; Hu, H.; Chen, G.; Li, Z.; Li, A.; Zhang, J. Disinfectant resistance in bacteria: Mechanisms, spread, and resolution strategies. *Environ. Res.* **2021**, *195*, 110897. [CrossRef]
28. Zou, L.; Meng, J.; McDermott, P.F.; Wang, F.; Yang, Q.; Cao, G.; Hoffmann, M.; Zhao, S. Presence of disinfectant resistance genes in Escherichia coli isolated from retail meats in the USA. *J. Antimicrob. Chemother.* **2014**, *69*, 2644–2649. [CrossRef]
29. Liu, Y.Y.; Wang, Y.; Walsh, T.R.; Yi, L.X.; Zhang, R.; Spencer, J.; Doi, Y.; Tian, G.; Dong, B.; Huang, X.; et al. Emergence of plasmid-mediated colistin resistance mechanism MCR-1 in animals and human beings in China: A microbiological and molecular biological study. *Lancet Infect. Dis.* **2016**, *16*, 161–168. [CrossRef]
30. Wilksch, J.J.; Yang, J.; Clements, A.; Gabbe, J.L.; Short, K.R.; Cao, H.; Cavaliere, R.; James, C.E.; Whitchurch, C.B.; Schembri, M.A.; et al. MrkH, a novel c-di-GMP-dependent transcriptional activator, controls Klebsiella pneumoniae biofilm formation by regulating type 3 fimbriae expression. *PLoS Pathog.* **2011**, *7*, e1002204. [CrossRef]
31. Huang, Y.-J.; Liao, H.-W.; Wu, C.-C.; Peng, H.-L. MrkF is a component of type 3 fimbriae in Klebsiella pneumoniae. *Res. Microbiol.* **2009**, *160*, 71–79. [CrossRef] [PubMed]
32. Xu, Y.; Zhang, J.; Wang, M.; Liu, M.; Liu, G.; Qu, H.; Liu, J.; Deng, Z.; Sun, J.; Ou, H.Y.; et al. Mobilization of the nonconjugative virulence plasmid from hypervirulent Klebsiella pneumoniae. *Genome Med.* **2021**, *13*, 119. [CrossRef] [PubMed]
33. Furuya, N.; Nisioka, T.; Komano, T. Nucleotide sequence and functions of the oriT operon in IncI1 plasmid R64. *J. Bacteriol.* **1991**, *173*, 2231–2237. [CrossRef] [PubMed]
34. Xiaomin, S.; Yiming, L.; Yuying, Y.; Zhangqi, S.; Yongning, W.; Shaolin, W. Global impact of mcr-1-positive Enterobacteriaceae bacteria on "one health". *Crit. Rev. Microbiol.* **2020**, *46*, 565–577. [CrossRef]
35. Yang, X.; Ye, L.; Chan, E.W.-C.; Zhang, R.; Chen, S. Characterization of an IncFIB/IncHI1B Plasmid Encoding Efflux Pump TMexCD1-TOprJ1 in a Clinical Tigecycline-and Carbapenem-Resistant Klebsiella pneumoniae Strain. *Antimicrob. Agents Chemother.* **2021**, *65*, e02340-20. [CrossRef]
36. Lin, D.L.; Traglia, G.M.; Baker, R.; Sherratt, D.J.; Ramirez, M.S.; Tolmasky, M.E. Functional Analysis of the Acinetobacter baumannii XerC and XerD Site-Specific Recombinases: Potential Role in Dissemination of Resistance Genes. *Antibiotics* **2020**, *9*, 405. [CrossRef]
37. Santos Costa, S.; Viveiros, M.; Rosato, A.E.; Melo-Cristino, J.; Couto, I. Impact of efflux in the development of multidrug resistance phenotypes in Staphylococcus aureus. *BMC Microbiol.* **2015**, *15*, 232. [CrossRef]
38. LaBreck, P.T.; Bochi-Layec, A.C.; Stanbro, J.; Dabbah-Krancher, G.; Simons, M.P.; Merrell, D.S. Systematic Analysis of Efflux Pump-Mediated Antiseptic Resistance in Staphylococcus aureus Suggests a Need for Greater Antiseptic Stewardship. *Msphere* **2020**, *5*, e00959-19. [CrossRef]
39. Knapp, L.; Rushton, L.; Stapleton, H.; Sass, A.; Stewart, S.; Amezquita, A.; McClure, P.; Mahenthiralingam, E.; Maillard, J.Y. The effect of cationic microbicide exposure against Burkholderia cepacia complex (Bcc); the use of Burkholderia lata strain 383 as a model bacterium. *J. Appl. Microbiol.* **2013**, *115*, 1117–1126. [CrossRef]
40. Kampf, G. Biocidal Agents Used for Disinfection Can Enhance Antibiotic Resistance in Gram-Negative Species. *Antibiotics* **2018**, *7*, 110. [CrossRef]
41. Short, F.L.; Lee, V.; Mamun, R.; Malmberg, R.; Li, L.; Espinosa, M.I.; Venkatesan, K.; Paulsen, I.T. Benzalkonium chloride antagonises aminoglycoside antibiotics and promotes evolution of resistance. *EBioMedicine* **2021**, *73*, 103653. [CrossRef] [PubMed]
42. Luo, Q.; Wang, Y.; Xiao, Y. Prevalence and transmission of mobilized colistin resistance (mcr) gene in bacteria common to animals and humans. *Biosaf. Health* **2020**, *2*, 71–78. [CrossRef]
43. Anyanwu, M.U.; Jaja, I.F.; Nwobi, O.C. Occurrence and Characteristics of Mobile Colistin Resistance (mcr) Gene-Containing Isolates from the Environment: A Review. *Int. J. Environ. Res. Public Health* **2020**, *17*, 1028. [CrossRef] [PubMed]
44. Shridhar, P.B.; Worley, J.N.; Gao, X.; Yang, X.; Noll, L.W.; Shi, X.; Bai, J.; Meng, J.; Nagaraja, T.G. Analysis of virulence potential of Escherichia coli O145 isolated from cattle feces and hide samples based on whole genome sequencing. *PLoS ONE* **2019**, *14*, e0225057. [CrossRef]
45. Fernández Márquez, M.L.; Burgos, M.J.; Pulido, R.P.; Gálvez, A.; López, R.L. Biocide Tolerance and Antibiotic Resistance in Salmonella Isolates from Hen Eggshells. *Foodborne Pathog. Dis.* **2017**, *14*, 89–95. [CrossRef]

46. Bankevich, A.; Nurk, S.; Antipov, D.; Gurevich, A.A.; Dvorkin, M.; Kulikov, A.S.; Lesin, V.M.; Nikolenko, S.I.; Pham, S.; Prjibelski, A.D.; et al. SPAdes: A new genome assembly algorithm and its applications to single-cell sequencing. *J. Comput. Biol.* **2012**, *19*, 455–477. [CrossRef]
47. Wick, R.R.; Judd, L.M.; Gorrie, C.L.; Holt, K.E. Unicycler: Resolving bacterial genome assemblies from short and long sequencing reads. *PLoS Comput. Biol.* **2017**, *13*, e1005595. [CrossRef]
48. Seemann, T. Prokka: Rapid prokaryotic genome annotation. *Bioinformatics* **2014**, *30*, 2068–2069. [CrossRef]
49. Thomsen, M.C.; Ahrenfeldt, J.; Cisneros, J.L.; Jurtz, V.; Larsen, M.V.; Hasman, H.; Aarestrup, F.M.; Lund, O. A Bacterial Analysis Platform: An Integrated System for Analysing Bacterial Whole Genome Sequencing Data for Clinical Diagnostics and Surveillance. *PLoS ONE* **2016**, *11*, e0157718. [CrossRef]
50. Hsiao, W.; Wan, I.; Jones, S.J.; Brinkman, F.S. IslandPath: Aiding detection of genomic islands in prokaryotes. *Bioinformatics* **2003**, *19*, 418–420. [CrossRef]
51. Li, X.; Xie, Y.; Liu, M.; Tai, C.; Sun, J.; Deng, Z.; Ou, H.Y. oriTfinder: A web-based tool for the identification of origin of transfers in DNA sequences of bacterial mobile genetic elements. *Nucleic Acids Res.* **2018**, *46*, W229–W234. [CrossRef] [PubMed]
52. Carattoli, A.; Zankari, E.; García-Fernández, A.; Voldby Larsen, M.; Lund, O.; Villa, L.; Møller Aarestrup, F.; Hasman, H. In silico detection and typing of plasmids using PlasmidFinder and plasmid multilocus sequence typing. *Antimicrob. Agents Chemother.* **2014**, *58*, 3895–3903. [CrossRef] [PubMed]
53. Siguier, P.; Perochon, J.; Lestrade, L.; Mahillon, J.; Chandler, M. ISfinder: The reference centre for bacterial insertion sequences. *Nucleic Acids Res.* **2006**, *34*, D32–D36. [CrossRef] [PubMed]
54. Sullivan, M.J.; Petty, N.K.; Beatson, S.A. Easyfig: A genome comparison visualizer. *Bioinformatics* **2011**, *27*, 1009–1010. [CrossRef]
55. Alikhan, N.F.; Petty, N.K.; Ben Zakour, N.L.; Beatson, S.A. BLAST Ring Image Generator (BRIG): Simple prokaryote genome comparisons. *BMC Genom.* **2011**, *12*, 402. [CrossRef]
56. Kozlov, A.M.; Darriba, D.; Flouri, T.; Morel, B.; Stamatakis, A. RAxML-NG: A fast, scalable and user-friendly tool for maximum likelihood phylogenetic inference. *Bioinformatics* **2019**, *35*, 4453–4455. [CrossRef]
57. Letunic, I.; Bork, P. Interactive Tree Of Life (iTOL) v5: An online tool for phylogenetic tree display and annotation. *Nucleic Acids Res.* **2021**, *49*, W293–W296. [CrossRef]

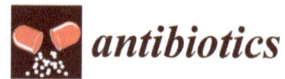

Article

Effects of Typical Antimicrobials on Growth Performance, Morphology and Antimicrobial Residues of Mung Bean Sprouts

Jing Cao [1], Yajie Wang [1], Guanzhao Wang [1], Pingping Ren [1], Yongning Wu [2] and Qinghua He [1,3,*]

1. Department of Food Science and Engineering, College of Chemistry and Environmental Engineering, Shenzhen University, Shenzhen 518060, China; caojing2020@email.szu.edu.cn (J.C.); wangyajie2020@email.szu.edu.cn (Y.W.); wangguanzhao2020@email.szu.edu.cn (G.W.); coolbear001@163.com (P.R.)
2. Food Safety Research Unit (2019RU014), Chinese Academy of Medical Science, NHC Key Laboratory of Food Safety Risk Assessment, China National Center for Food Safety Risk Assessment, Beijing 100021, China; wuyongning@cfsa.net.cn
3. Shenzhen Key Laboratory of Food Macromolecules Science and Processing, Shenzhen University, Shenzhen 518060, China
* Correspondence: qinghua.he@szu.edu.cn

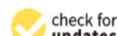

Citation: Cao, J.; Wang, Y.; Wang, G.; Ren, P.; Wu, Y.; He, Q. Effects of Typical Antimicrobials on Growth Performance, Morphology and Antimicrobial Residues of Mung Bean Sprouts. *Antibiotics* **2022**, *11*, 807. https://doi.org/10.3390/antibiotics11060807

Academic Editor: Carlos M. Franco

Received: 7 May 2022
Accepted: 13 June 2022
Published: 15 June 2022

Publisher's Note: MDPI stays neutral with regard to jurisdictional claims in published maps and institutional affiliations.

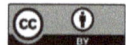

Copyright: © 2022 by the authors. Licensee MDPI, Basel, Switzerland. This article is an open access article distributed under the terms and conditions of the Creative Commons Attribution (CC BY) license (https://creativecommons.org/licenses/by/4.0/).

Abstract: Antimicrobials may be used to inhibit the growth of micro-organisms in the cultivation of mung bean sprouts, but the effects on mung bean sprouts are unclear. In the present study, the growth performance, morphology, antimicrobial effect and antimicrobial residues of mung bean sprouts cultivated in typical antimicrobial solutions were investigated. A screening of antimicrobial residues in thick-bud and rootless mung bean sprouts from local markets showed that the positive ratios of chloramphenicol, enrofloxacin, and furazolidone were 2.78%, 22.22%, and 13.89%, respectively. The cultivating experiment indicated that the production of mung bean sprouts in antimicrobial groups was significantly reduced over 96 h ($p < 0.05$). The bud and root length of mung bean sprouts in enrofloxacin, olaquindox, doxycycline and furazolidone groups were significantly shortened ($p < 0.05$), which cultivated thick-bud and rootless mung bean sprouts similar to the 6-benzyl-adenine group. Furthermore, linear regression analysis showed average optical density of 450 nm in circulating water and average production had no obvious correlation in mung bean sprouts ($p > 0.05$). Antimicrobial residues were found in both mung bean sprouts and circulating water. These novel findings reveal that the antimicrobials could cultivate thick-bud and rootless mung bean sprouts due to their toxicity. This study also proposed a new question regarding the abuse of antimicrobials in fast-growing vegetables, which could be a potential food safety issue.

Keywords: *Vigna radiata*; mung bean sprouts; antimicrobials; production; morphology; residues

1. Introduction

As a common food in China for more than 2000 years, mung bean (*Vigna radiata*), containing protein and dietary fiber, is known for alleviating heatstroke and reducing swelling in summer [1]. During the germination process of mung beans, biochemical reactions not only produce active compounds including polyphenols, saponins and vitamin C [2], but also decrease phytate content, which can form harmful phytate–protein and phytate–mineral–protein complexes that decrease the bio-availability of essential minerals and affect the use of proteins [3]. Mung bean sprouts also have better nutrition and function than mung beans, e.g., the content and bio-availability of zinc and iron [3]. Previous studies have shown that mung bean sprouts are proven to prevent the increase of total cholesterol, low-density lipoprotein and triglyceride, and to transform inorganic Se compounds into organic Se compounds through bio-transformation, which can improve bio-availability [4]. Moreover, the sprouting of mung beans facilitates the generation of total phenolic compounds to improve anti-oxidant capacity [5,6]. Both the antibacterial activity for meat bacteria and the antiviral activity for the respiratory syncytial and herpes simplex viruses were found in extracts from mung beans and its sprouts [7]. Due to the germination process, mung bean sprouts have high bio-availability, anti-oxidant capacity and antiviral activity. Therefore, mung bean sprouts rich in bioactive compounds can be consumed as functional food.

Although there are many nutritional and functional merits for humans, food safety issues often occur in the cultivating process of mung bean sprouts. The existing evidence demonstrates that mung bean sprouts might be contaminated by *Escherichia coli* and *Salmonella*. For example, the occurrence of *Salmonella* in bean sprouts was reported in Germany and the Netherlands in October and November in 2011 [8], and in England and Northern Ireland from January to March in 2011 [9]. Basically, mung bean sprouts are a suitable medium for food-borne pathogens due to their frequent exposure to "water baths" [10]. Food-borne microbial contamination is likely to occur during the production process, which is likely to result in damage to human health. European regulations stipulate that sprout manufacturers are obliged to detect sprout samples for pathogenic bacteria [11]. In addition to the government's regulatory requirements, consumers also pay attention to the safety of edible mung bean sprouts. As a common method to remove microbials in the cooking process, washing treatments are proven to be incompletely effective [12]. The growth of micro-organisms may not only cause food hygiene problems, but also impair the production of mung bean sprouts. Therefore, it is important for food safety practices to control the growth of pathogenic bacteria and to supervise food-borne microbial contamination in mung bean sprouts.

A variety of methods have been applied to regulate the quality of mung bean sprouts due to microbial contamination. For example, physical treatments including hot water and ethanol vapors have been evaluated for the quality and storage life of sprouts [13]. Chemical treatment such as biocontrol with endophytic *Bacillus subtilis* [14] has also gained increasing attention in microbial contamination. Combination treatments have good application prospects regarding microbial quality including ultrasound and aqueous chlorine dioxide [15], and plasma-activated water [16], which have an additional effect on seed germination and the seedling growth of mung bean [17]. Although the methods of controlling microbial contamination in mung bean sprouts are becoming more diverse, antimicrobials that inhibit the growth of micro-organisms are still the common antibacterial method in the mung bean sprout industry due to low cost and simple operation. Therefore, antimicrobials are often used to protect the growth of mung bean sprouts in agriculture [18]. In addition, plant growth regulators (PGRs) have been widely used to accelerate plant growth, which can cause food safety risks [19]. For example, two sample surveys showed that the positive rates of 6-benzyl adenine (6-BA) were 1.1% and 2.4% in Gwangju in South Korea. The concentration was 0.01–0.02 mg/kg [20,21]. Similarly, although 6-BA is banned in China, it was still detected in some mung bean sprout samples, which contained 0.11 mg/kg of 6-BA [19]. Even though antimicrobials and PGRs are potentially harmful to human health, they may be still used to enhance the growth performance of mung bean sprouts. Consequently, the contamination of antimicrobials and PGRs has become a problem that needs to be solved.

According to existing research, antimicrobial contamination in mung bean sprouts poses a potential risk to food safety. However, the existing information mainly focuses on the methods for detecting antimicrobials in mung bean sprouts. Few studies have been conducted to research the specific effect of antimicrobials in the cultivation of mung bean sprouts. This study aimed to investigate the role of antimicrobials in the growth of mung bean sprouts, and to clarify antimicrobial residues in the cultivation of mung bean sprouts. First, commercial mung bean sprout samples were collected from local markets and screened by antimicrobial residues. Second, mung beans were cultivated in typical antimicrobial solutions for 96 h using automatic bean sprout machines. Through the experimental cultivation of mung bean sprouts, the effects of typical antimicrobials on production, growth performance and morphology during the growth of mung bean sprouts are explored and the antimicrobial residues in mung bean sprouts are measured.

2. Methods

2.1. Materials and Reagents

Newly harvested mung bean seeds (*Vigna radiata*) were purchased from a local supermarket in Shenzhen (Guangdong, China). In the market sample survey, a total of 36 samples of short-rooted mung bean sprouts were randomly purchased from local shopping malls, supermarkets, or farmers' markets in Shenzhen (Guangdong, China). Four samples each were taken from nine districts, namely Futian, Nanshan, Luohu, Baoan, Yantian, Guangming, Longhua, Pingshan, and Dapeng in Shenzhen.

Chloramphenicol, enrofloxacin, olaquindox, doxycycline, furazolidone and 6-BA, formic acid, sodium chloride, ethylenediaminetetraacetic acid (EDTA) and EDTA disodium salt were purchased from Aladdin Industrial Co. Ltd. (Shanghai, China). Chromatographic-grade acetonitrile was obtained from Merck & Co. Inc. (Darmstadt, Germany). All antimicrobial standards were purchased from Sigma–Aldrich (St. Louis, MO, USA). MAS-QuEChERS extraction package was bought from Angela Technologies Co. Ltd. (Tianjin, China).

2.2. Germination and Cultivation of Mung Bean Sprouts

Tap water, distilled water, 5 mg/L 6-BA solution, 100 mg/L chloramphenicol solution, 100 mg/L enrofloxacin solution, 50 mg/L olaquindox solution, 50 mg/L doxycycline solution and 500 mg/L furazolidone solution were added into automatic bean sprout machines (Bear Electric Appliance Co. Ltd., Foshan, China). These antimicrobial solutions were prepared with tap water to simulate the actual situation. After the 24 h of germination-accelerating operation, eight portions of 200 g mung bean seeds were placed into individual automatic bean sprout machines. The setting temperature was 30 °C in the dark environment. The sprout period was 96 h, and all experiments were repeated five times. Each bean sprout machine was fixed in the same treatment to avoid cross-contamination.

2.3. Growth Performance Measurement

The sprouts were weighed in dark conditions with closed doors and windows after 24 h, 48 h, 72 h and 96 h, respectively. Total length, bud length and root length were measured after 24 h, 48 h, 72 h and 96 h, respectively. The sprouts were photographed using an iPhone 6 (Apple Inc., Cupertino, CA, USA) with black laboratory benches as the background and a ruler as the standard.

2.4. Microbial Reproduction Measurement in Circulating Water

An optical density of 450 nm (OD450) was used to represent the turbidity of circulating water so that it can infer the microbial concentration in the circulating water [22]. During the growth of the mung bean sprouts, 1 mL of the circulating solution was taken every 24 h and was taken to the spectrophotometer to measure the OD450 value of the circulating water.

2.5. Sample Collection

At the end of experiment, sprouts were collected and were crushed using a grinder (Bear Electric Appliance Co. Ltd., Foshan, China). The grinder was cleaned completely to avoid cross-contamination. Crushed sprout samples and 10 mL of circulating water were collected with sealed bags and EP tubes, respectively. All samples were stored at −80 °C for inspection.

2.6. Sample Extraction and Purification

Sprout samples (5 ± 0.01 g) were weighed into 50 mL centrifuge tubes with a stopper. A total of 9 mL acetonitrile and 1 mL EDTA solution were added into tubes. First, samples were vortexed for 30 s using a vortex mixer (IKA Works GmbH & Co, Germany). Second, the products were put into the ultrasonic cleaner for 15 s and were centrifuged at 8000 rpm for 5 min. Third, 5 mL of supernatant was taken and added into the MAS-QuEChERS extraction package with shaking for 1 min. After centrifugation at 8000 rpm for 5 min, 4 mL of supernatant was taken and was blown to nearly dry with nitrogen using N-EVAP-24 temovap sample concentrator (Organomaition Associates Inc., Berlin, NH, USA). Finally, the above products were diluted to 1 mL with 30% acetonitrile solution and were filtered with a 0.22 μm polyether sulfone filter membrane. In addition, 10 μL circulating water samples were diluted to 10 mL with 30% acetonitrile solution and 1 mL was taken to be filtered with a 0.22 μm polyether sulfone filter membrane. The antimicrobial residues in sprout and circulating water samples were detected using high-performance liquid chromatography-tandem mass spectrometry (HPLC-MS).

2.7. Screening of Antimicrobial Residues in Commercial Mung Bean Sprouts

In the market sample survey, antimicrobial residues were screened by a HPLC-Triple Quad^{TM} 4500 mass spectrometer (AB Sciex, Framingham, MA, USA) with an electrospray ionization (ESI) probe. An analytical column (Phenomenex C_{18}, 50 × 3.0 mm, 2.6 μm particle size) was employed. Mobile phases were water containing 0.1% formic acid (phase A) and acetonitrile containing 0.1% formic acid (phase B). The flow rate of the mobile phase was 0.4 mL/min, 0.3 mL/min and 0.5 mL/min, which represented the flow rates of positive ion gradient A, positive ion gradient B and negative ion gradient A, respectively. The column temperature was 25 °C and the injection volume was 5 μL. Detailed conditions are listed in Tables S1–S3. Multiple reaction monitoring mode was used to detect antimicrobials in the positive and negative electrospray ionization mode. Nitrogen was employed as a nebulizer and drying gas at 50 psi and 600 °C. The ion spray voltage was set to 5500 V and −4500 V in the positive and negative modes, respectively. Detailed conditions are listed in Table S4. Concentrations of the antimicrobial residues in commercial mung bean sprouts were calculated.

2.8. Detection of Antimicrobial Residues in Sprouts and Circulating Water

The corresponding antimicrobial residues in sprout and circulating water samples collected from chloramphenicol, enrofloxacin, olaquindox, doxycycline and furazolidone groups were determined using an HPLC-Triple Quad^{TM} 4500 mass spectrometer (AB Sciex, Framingham, MA, USA), respectively. The HPLC and MS conditions were as referred to in the method described in the previous section. The concentrations of the antimicrobials and relevant metabolite were calculated.

2.9. Statistical Analysis

Data were expressed as mean ± standard deviation (SD). Statistical significance was determined by Student's *t*-test using the SPSS 23 software (IBM SPSS Statistics, Chicago, IL, USA). The correlation analysis between OD450 values and production was analyzed by Pearson linear regression. A difference where $p < 0.05$ was considered to be statistically significant.

3. Results and Discussion

3.1. Antimicrobial Screening of Commercial Mung Bean Sprouts

To investigate the status of antimicrobial residues in mung bean sprouts sold in local shopping malls, supermarkets, or farmers' markets, randomly purchased commercial mung bean sprouts were prospected for antimicrobial residues. Twenty-eight antimicrobials, including chloramphenicol, nitrofuran and quinolones from the sampled bean sprouts, were screened by HPLC-MS [22]. As shown in Table 1, the positive ratios of chloramphenicol, enrofloxacin, and furazolidone were 2.78%, 22.22%, and 13.89% in all samples, respectively.

Table 1. Concentration (μg/kg) of antimicrobial and metabolite residues in mung bean sprouts from market survey (n = 36, mean ± standard deviation).

Residues	Positive Samples	Positive Ratio	Concentration
Chloramphenicol	1	2.78%	9.31
Enrofloxacin	8	22.22%	193.23 ± 98.42
AOZ	5	13.89%	2.88 ± 1.93

The occurrence of antimicrobials in commercial mung bean sprouts might be associated with the addition of antimicrobials by manufacturers. It is similar to the antibacterial effect of fungicides in mung bean sprouts. Previous studies have reported that adding fungicides during cultivation can cause harmful residues in the edible parts of plants, which can adversely affect food and the environment [20]. *Salmonella, E. coli* and other anaerobic bacteria were the common contaminations affecting the growth of mung bean sprouts. The use of chloramphenicol, enrofloxacin and furazolidone in the cultivation of mung bean sprouts is due to their strong antibacterial properties, which can effectively inhibit the reproduction of bacteria [23,24]. It can greatly increase the economic value of mung bean sprouts. Moreover, antimicrobial pollution of the water used to cultivate mung bean sprouts might be another cause of antimicrobial residue. To save costs, manufacturers use surface water or reclaimed water instead of tap water or purified water in the cultivation process. Surface water for planting might be contaminated by antimicrobials when flowing through soil during agricultural production. After the sewage treatment system, there are still antimicrobial residues in reclaimed water [25]. This can cause plants to be exposed to antimicrobials at a concentration of up to 1 mg/L [26]. Furthermore, the increased bacterial resistance to antimicrobials might lead to an increase in the amount of antimicrobials added during the cultivation process, which can have a harmful impact on food safety [27]. Therefore, antimicrobial abuse and pollution might be the main reasons for antimicrobial residues in commercial mung bean sprouts, which poses a great potential risk to human health. However, the actual effect of antimicrobials on mung bean sprouts is unclear. It is crucial that the cultivated experiments on mung bean sprouts be conducted to clarify the role and residue of antimicrobials in the growth of mung bean sprouts.

3.2. Microbial Content in Circulating Water

The inhibitory effects of antimicrobials on micro-organisms were investigated using OD450 values of circulating water. According to Figure 1, the largest OD450 value was found in the tap water group, which was related to the largest turbidity. Turbidity and OD value proved that growth and reproduction of micro-organisms existed in circulating water [28]. OD450 values of circulating water after 96 h in chloramphenicol, enrofloxacin, olaquindox, doxycycline and furazolidone groups were significantly lower than those of tap water, distilled water and 6-BA groups after 96 h ($p < 0.05$). It is suggested that antimicrobials have significant inhibitory effects on the growth of micro-organisms. In agriculture, antimicrobials are used to inhibit the growth of micro-organisms due to the antibacterial effect [18]. In terms of PGRs, the OD450 value of the 6-BA group was not significantly different to that in the tap water group ($p > 0.05$), which indicates that 6-BA had no obvious inhibitory effect on micro-organisms. As mentioned above, microbial growth existed in the cultivation of mung bean sprouts. The growth of micro-organisms is significantly inhibited by the addition of antimicrobials.

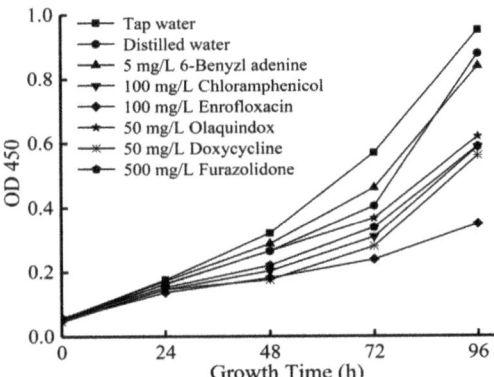

Figure 1. OD450 value of circulating water across 96 h.

3.3. Effects of Typical Antimicrobials on Production of Mung Bean Sprouts

The production of mung bean sprouts grown in typical antimicrobial solutions across 96 h is shown in Table 2. The production of mung bean sprouts in all groups increased with growth time across 96 h. Production in the tap water group was the highest at 1012.1 g and production in the furazolidone group was the lowest, at 563.4 g after 96 h. There was no significant difference in the productions of tap water, distilled water and chloramphenicol groups after 96 h ($p > 0.05$). Productions in the 6-BA, enrofloxacin, olaquindox, doxycycline and furazolidone groups were significantly lower than those in the tap water group after 96 h ($p < 0.05$).

Table 2. Growth performance of mung bean sprouts within 96 h (n = 5, mean ± standard deviation).

Groups	Growth Time			
	24 h	48 h	72 h	96 h
Production (g)				
Tap water	382.9 ± 9.2 a	585.2 ± 10.3 a	858.1 ± 60.1 a	1012.1 ± 95.6 a
Distilled water	379.8 ± 16.0 a	567.6 ± 21.7 ab	763.4 ± 115.4 abc	873.9 ± 162.2 abcd
6-Benzyl adenine	371.7 ± 18.9 a	494.9 ± 42.0 cde	629.8 ± 65.3 def	786.5 ± 98.0 cde
Chloramphenicol	381.9 ± 9.4 a	569.4 ± 10.7 ab	811.4 ± 89.5 ab	971.2 ± 142.0 abc
Enrofloxacin	375.0 ± 8.6 a	528.4 ± 19.6 bcd	697.1 ± 77.0 bcd	806.3 ± 143.6 bcd
Olaquindox	348.7 ± 37.0 b	484.1 ± 92.4 def	643.9 ± 199.1 cde	761.9 ± 266.8 de
Doxycycline	360.5 ± 11.6 ab	451.4 ± 20.9 ef	538.9 ± 53.2 ef	595.3 ± 87.4 ef
Furazolidone	359.3 ± 6.9 ab	436.7 ± 24.6 f	512.0 ± 69.1 f	563.4 ± 108.3 f
Total length (cm)				
Tap water	2.83 ± 1.10	9.12 ± 2.23 a	17.94 ± 3.85 a	23.73 ± 1.89 a
Distilled water	2.97 ± 0.28	8.49 ± 1.74 a	17.30 ± 1.39 a	22.21 ± 2.12 a
6-Benzyl adenine	2.41 ± 0.43	3.49 ± 0.68 d	4.66 ± 1.16 c	6.47 ± 1.27 c
Chloramphenicol	2.91 ± 0.54	7.34 ± 1.39 ab	16.88 ± 2.21 a	22.41 ± 1.94 a
Enrofloxacin	2.57 ± 0.35	5.95 ± 0.52 bc	10.40 ± 3.63 b	13.59 ± 5.26 b
Olaquindox	2.34 ± 0.24	4.87 ± 1.13 cd	8.70 ± 5.06 bc	12.72 ± 6.83 b
Doxycycline	2.39 ± 0.18	4.11 ± 1.05 cd	6.29 ± 1.41 bc	8.61 ± 1.94 bc
Furazolidone	2.27 ± 0.52	3.18 ± 0.79 d	4.45 ± 1.81 c	5.77 ± 2.88 c
Bud length (cm)				
Tap water	0.97 ± 0.15 de	3.77 ± 0.21 ab	11.33 ± 0.32 a	17.17 ± 0.95 b
Distilled water	1.67 ± 0.12 a	3.53 ± 0.64 b	10.67 ± 0.45 a	15.10 ± 0.40 a
6-Benzyl adenine	1.10 ± 0.10 cd	2.10 ± 0.10 de	3.80 ± 0.44 d	4.47 ± 0.55 e
Chloramphenicol	1.53 ± 0.15 ab	4.33 ± 0.29 a	10.97 ± 0.32 a	15.63 ± 1.40 ab
Enrofloxacin	1.17 ± 0.15 cd	3.50 ± 0.36 bc	7.33 ± 0.21 b	12.50 ± 0.53 c

Table 2. Cont.

Groups	Growth Time			
	24 h	48 h	72 h	96 h
Olaquindox	1.30 ± 0.10 [bc]	2.47 ± 0.25 [d]	5.00 ± 0.44 [c]	8.60 ± 0.82 [d]
Doxycycline	1.03 ± 0.21 [cd]	2.80 ± 0.44 [cd]	5.57 ± 0.76 [c]	8.53 ± 0.21 [d]
Furazolidone	0.70 ± 0.10 [e]	1.63 ± 0.32 [e]	3.53 ± 0.30 [d]	4.47 ± 0.93 [e]
Root length (cm)				
Tap water	1.20 ± 0.10 [ab]	6.67 ± 0.65 [a]	11.03 ± 0.68 [a]	9.83 ± 0.55 [a]
Distilled water	1.40 ± 0.36 [ab]	5.97 ± 0.50 [a]	8.80 ± 0.70 [b]	9.50 ± 2.86 [a]
6-Benzyl adenine	0.97 ± 0.06 [bc]	2.07 ± 0.25 [de]	2.67 ± 0.21 [d]	2.83 ± 0.25 [bc]
Chloramphenicol	1.43 ± 0.15 [a]	4.70 ± 0.78 [b]	8.13 ± 0.85 [b]	9.33 ± 0.67 [a]
Enrofloxacin	1.10 ± 0.10 [abc]	3.20 ± 0.66 [c]	3.97 ± 0.67 [c]	4.17 ± 0.95 [b]
Olaquindox	1.17 ± 0.38 [ab]	2.50 ± 0.20 [cd]	2.83 ± 0.35 [d]	2.87 ± 0.29 [bc]
Doxycycline	0.97 ± 0.25 [bc]	1.60 ± 0.36 [de]	2.17 ± 0.40 [d]	2.20 ± 0.36 [bc]
Furazolidone	0.67 ± 0.12 [c]	1.17 ± 0.21 [e]	0.73 ± 0.06 [e]	1.10 ± 0.20 [c]

Values with different letters within a column are significantly different ($p < 0.05$).

Production in the tap water group was higher than that in the distilled water group, which was associated with the presence of Na^+, Cl^-, K^- and Mg^{2+} in tap water. A previous study proved that Na^+ and $K-$ facilitated plant growth in agricultural production by participating in the cellular mechanisms [29]. In the antimicrobial groups, the production in the chloramphenicol group was the largest, which might be ascribed to the fact that Cl^- could regulate osmotic pressure in plants and cause the guard cells to swell [30]. Production in the furazolidone group was the smallest, which might relate to the toxicity of furazolidone. It was proved that furazolidone affected the absorption of water and soluble nutrients in mung bean sprouts [31].

Interestingly, treatments of antimicrobials showed no improvement on the production of mung bean sprouts compared with tap water. The previous study showed that furazolidone and nifuroxazide containing derivatives of 5-nitrofurfural prevented a fresh matter of oats and radishes from weight gain [32], which was similar to the present experiment. It was suggested that this side effect of antimicrobials might inhibit the proliferation and growth of cells, which reduces the production of mung bean sprouts. Moreover, linear regression results of correlation analysis showed that there is no distinct correlation between average OD450 values and average production across 96 h ($p > 0.05$) (Figure S1). It demonstrates that the concentration of micro-organisms in the circulating water has no obvious relationship with production of mung bean sprouts. These new findings indicate that the use of antimicrobials has no improvement on the production of mung bean sprouts. This might be attributed to the effect of antimicrobials on the types of micro-organisms in circulating water, resulting in reduced production. Previous studies have proved that the bio-diversity of key flora in the soil determines crop production [33]. The influence of specific micro-organisms in circulating water on the production of mung bean sprouts might be cause for further research.

3.4. Effects of Antimicrobials on Morphology of Mung Bean Sprouts

The morphology of mung bean sprouts is shown in Figure 2. Long and fine roots are seen on mung bean sprouts in the distilled water and tap water groups from 48 h to 96 h. Extremely short roots or rootless specimens can be seen on mung bean sprouts in the 6-BA group from 48 h to 96 h. Mung bean sprouts in the chloramphenicol and enrofloxacin groups had long roots similar to those of the tap water and distilled water groups. Interestingly, extremely short roots or rootless specimens were also observed on mung bean sprouts in the olaquindox, doxycycline and furazolidone groups, which were similar to rootless mung bean sprouts of the 6-BA group. In addition, thicker and shorter buds were seen on mung bean sprouts in the furazolidone group from 48 h to 96 h, which was similar to those in the 6-BA group from a morphological aspect.

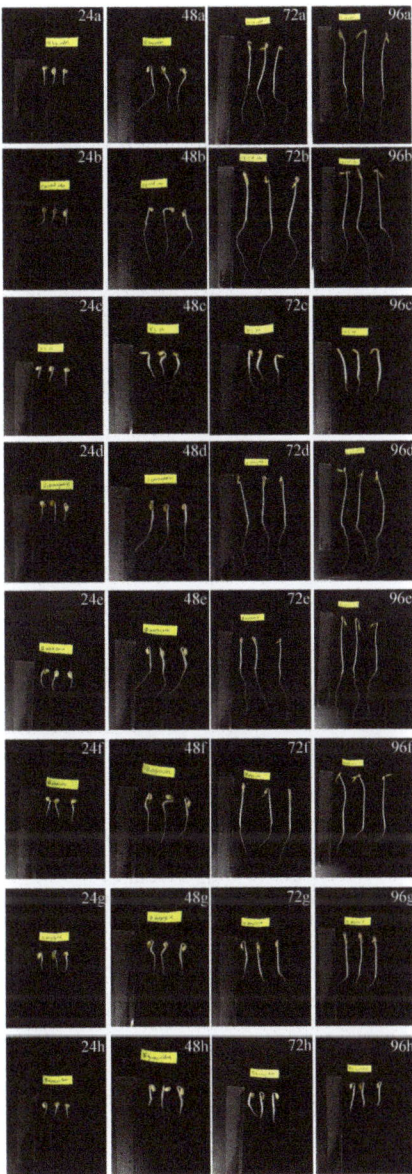

Figure 2. Morphological changes in mung bean sprouts in tap water (**a**), distilled water (**b**), 5 mg/L 6-benzyl adenine (**c**), 100 mg/L chloramphenicol (**d**), 100 mg/L enrofloxacin (**e**), 50 mg/L olaquindox (**f**), 50 mg/L doxycycline (**g**) and 500 mg/L furazolidone (**h**) groups across 96 h. (Group 24, 48, 72 and 96 were the morphologies of mung bean sprouts at 24, 48, 72 and 96 h, respectively. Group (**a**–**h**) represent different antibacterial groups, respectively).

The total lengths, bud lengths and root lengths of the mung bean sprouts are shown in Table 2 and Figure 3. The total length, bud length and root length of mung bean sprouts in the tap water group were the longest of all groups. The total length, bud length and root length of the distilled water and chloramphenicol groups were not significantly different from those of the tap water group ($p > 0.05$). However, the bud lengths of the 6-BA, enrofloxacin, olaquindox, doxycycline and furazolidone groups were significantly shortened ($p < 0.05$). Compared with the tap water group, the root lengths of mung bean sprouts in the enrofloxacin, olaquindox, doxycycline and furazolidone groups were significantly decreased after 96 h ($p < 0.05$). The root lengths of mung bean sprouts in the enrofloxacin, olaquindox, doxycycline and furazolidone groups were not significantly different to the 6-BA group ($p > 0.05$).

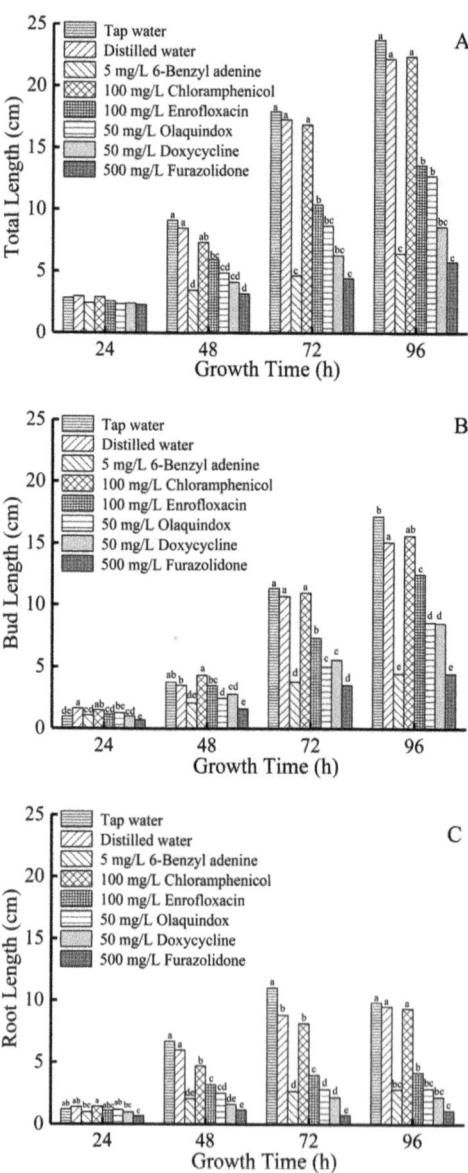

Figure 3. Total length (**A**), bud length (**B**) and root length (**C**) of mung bean sprouts within 96 h. Values with different letters within a column are significantly different ($p < 0.05$).

It is suggested that the use of antimicrobials affects root length and the morphology of mung bean sprouts. Commercially, a longer root affects appearance and reduces the retail price of mung bean sprouts. Since buds are the edible part of mung bean sprouts, short-rooted or rootless mung bean sprouts are more attractive to consumers. The economic benefit of rootless mung bean sprouts might motivate illegal businesses to abuse 6-BA in China. As a PGR, 6-BA is commonly used to cultivate rootless mung bean sprouts in some countries. However, 6-BA has been banned by the State Administration for Market Regulation of China since 2015 due to its irritation of the esophagus and gastric mucosa [34]. In the present study, 6-BA and furazolidone induced a similar appearance of mung bean sprouts as rootless and thick-bud, which would attract consumers and be sold at a higher price. It is suggested that the reason for the abuse of antimicrobials might be to produce rootless and thick mung bean sprouts to increase illegal profit. Therefore, these new findings demonstrate that antimicrobials might be used by illegal manufacturers to replace 6-BA to cultivate rootless mung bean sprouts.

The significant difference between the chloramphenicol group and the other antimicrobial groups might be due to the presence of Cl^-. Cl^- is an indispensable micro-nutrient for plant growth, which can facilitate elongation growth [35]. Therefore, it might reduce the shortening effect of antimicrobials on the lengths of mung bean sprouts. The lengths of mung bean sprouts in the furazolidone group were the smallest, which might be associated with the toxicity of furazolidone in mung bean sprouts [31]. The bud and root lengths of mung bean sprouts in the enrofloxacin, olaquindox, doxycycline and furazolidone groups were obviously shortened, similar to those in the 6-BA group. This suggests that these antimicrobials exhibit harmful effects on plant growth, which inhibit germ and radicle growth, and shorten the length of bud and root. In addition, the degree of root length shortening in mung bean sprouts in antimicrobial groups was greater than that of bud length shortening. This might be related to the stronger sensitivity of roots to the toxicity of antimicrobials compared to buds during plant growth [36]. These results indicate that antimicrobials can shorten the root and bud length of mung bean sprouts. Significant shortening of root length can bring greater benefits to manufacturers. However, it might also lead to the abuse of antimicrobials and potential food safety risks.

3.5. Antimicrobial Residues in Mung Bean Sprouts

Antimicrobial residue in mung bean sprouts and circulating water of antimicrobial groups after 96 h were determined and shown in Table 3. Antimicrobial residues existed in both mung bean sprouts and circulating water in the chloramphenicol, enrofloxacin, olaquindox, doxycycline and furazolidone groups. In addition, a metabolite of furazolidone called 3-amino-2-oxazolidinone (AOZ) was detected in mung bean sprouts and circulating water in the furazolidone group.

Table 3. Concentration (μg/kg) of antimicrobial and metabolite residues in mung bean sprouts and circulating water from cultivating experiment ($n = 5$, mean ± standard deviation).

Groups	Antimicrobial Residues	Mung Bean Sprouts	Circulating Water
Chloramphenicol	Chloramphenicol	45.6 ± 4.8	82.9 ± 6.9
Enrofloxacin	Enrofloxacin	93.1 ± 2.8	84.2 ± 2.9
Olaquindox	Olaquindox	17.6 ± 4.9	41.6 ± 2.9
Doxycycline	Doxycycline	37.7 ± 2.0	44.1 ± 3.0
Furazolidone	Furazolidone	388.6 ± 18.1	458.9 ± 29.9
	AOZ	24.1 ± 3.6	19.3 ± 3.7

Residues of antimicrobial prototypes and metabolite in mung bean sprouts indicate that antimicrobials can be absorbed and metabolized by mung bean sprouts. However, residues of antimicrobial prototypes in circulating water show that antimicrobials cannot be completely absorbed by mung bean sprouts, and a considerable amount of antimicrobials remains in circulating water, causing pollution. The overuse of antimicrobials has caused the occurrence of antimicrobial residue and pollution in plants and soil. Previous studies have shown that furazolidone and nitrofurantoin are efficiently metabolized and produce highly persistent metabolites in plants [37]. Ciprofloxacin and oxytetracycline used in planting vegetables also remain in the soil and the residence time is related to half-life [38]. In addition, AOZ residue in circulating water demonstrates that antimicrobials can be excreted into circulating water after being metabolized by micro-organisms or mung bean sprouts. The metabolic pathway of furazolidone was mainly a reduction of the nitro group in organisms, which might contribute to the generation of reactive metabolites and cause adverse effects [39]. AOZ had a higher stability and longer residence time [40]. Thus, residues of antimicrobials and their metabolites in mung bean sprouts and circulating water might not only cause food safety issues but also induce longer-lasting pollution in surface water and soil.

4. Conclusions

Results of this study indicated that antimicrobials not only affect the production and morphology of mung bean sprouts, but also bring on antimicrobial residue. A novel and unexpected observation is that antimicrobials cultivated thick-bud and rootless mung bean sprouts and decreased production, which is a similar effect to 6-BA. Despite the growth inhibition of micro-organisms, antimicrobials cannot increase the production of mung bean sprouts. Additionally, the cultivation study reveals that antimicrobial residues exist in mung bean sprouts and circulating water. Chloramphenicol, enrofloxacin, and furazolidone residue was also found in commercial mung bean sprouts. These findings indicate that the abuse of antimicrobials might increase potential food safety risks in fast-growing vegetables, and the monitoring of antimicrobial residues might be necessary to guarantee food safety.

Supplementary Materials: The following supporting information can be downloaded at: https://www.mdpi.com/article/10.3390/antibiotics11060807/s1, Table S1. Positive ion A gradient elution conditions; Table S2. Positive ion B gradient elution conditions; Table S3. Negative ion gradient elution conditions; Table S4. Mass spectrometry conditions in MRM mode; Figure S1. Correlation between production of mung bean sprouts and OD450 in circulating water in 96 h.

Author Contributions: J.C.: investigation, formal analysis, writing—original draft. Y.W. (Yajie Wang) and G.W.: investigation. P.R.: writing—review and editing. Y.W. (Yongning Wu): experimental design, conceptualization methodology. Q.H.: experimental design, conceptualization methodology, writing—review and editing. All authors have read and agreed to the published version of the manuscript.

Funding: This research was funded by the Basic Research Program of Shenzhen Municipal Government (JCYJ20200109114242138), the National Natural Science Foundation of China (22193064, 22078198), the Government's Plan of Science and Technology (ZDSYS20210623100800001), the Natural Science Foundation of Guangdong Province (2021A1515010687) and the Special Commissioner for Rural Science and Technology of Guangdong Province (KTP20210345).

Data Availability Statement: All data generated or analyzed during the study appear in the submitted article.

Acknowledgments: The authors thank the Instrumental Analysis Center of Shenzhen University for their assistance in the works.

Conflicts of Interest: The authors declare no conflict of interest.

Abbreviations

6-BA—6-benzyl-adenine; PGRs—plant growth regulators; EDTA—ethylene diamine tetra acetic acid; HPLC-MS—high-performance liquid chromatography–mass spectrometry; OD450—optical density on 450 nm; AOZ—3-amino-2-oxazolidinone.

References

1. Xu, H.; Zhou, Q.; Liu, B.; Cheng, K.W.; Chen, F.; Wang, M. Neuroprotective potential of mung bean (*Vigna radiata* L.) polyphenols in Alzheimer's disease: A review. *J. Agric. Food Chem.* **2021**, *69*, 11554–11571. [CrossRef] [PubMed]
2. Kanatt, S.R.; Arjun, K.; Sharma, A. Antioxidant and antimicrobial activity of legume hulls. *Food Res. Int.* **2011**, *44*, 3182–3187. [CrossRef]
3. Luo, Y.; Xie, W. Effect of soaking and sprouting on iron and zinc availability in green and white faba bean (*Vicia faba* L.). *J. Food Sci. Technol.* **2014**, *51*, 3970–3976. [CrossRef] [PubMed]
4. Tie, M.; Gao, Y.; Xue, Y.; Zhang, A.; Yao, Y.; Sun, J.; Xue, S. Determination of selenium species and analysis of methyl-seleno-l-cysteine in Se-enriched mung bean sprouts by HPLC-MS. *Anal. Methods* **2016**, *8*, 3102–3108. [CrossRef]
5. Aguilera, Y.; Rebollo-Hernanz, M.; Herrera, T.; Cayuelas, L.T.; Rodriguez-Rodriguez, P.; de Pablo, A.L.; Arribas, S.M.; Martin-Cabrejas, M.A. Intake of bean sprouts influences melatonin and antioxidant capacity biomarker levels in rats. *Food Funct.* **2016**, *7*, 1438–1445. [CrossRef] [PubMed]
6. Tiwari, U.; Servan, A.; Nigam, D. Comparative study on antioxidant activity, phytochemical analysis and mineral composition of the mung bean (*Vigna radiata*) and its sprouts. *J. Pharmacogn. Phytochem.* **2017**, *6*, 336–340.
7. Hafidh, R.R.; Abdulamir, A.S.; Bakar, F.A.; Sekawi, Z.; Jahansheri, F.; Jalilian, F.A. Novel antiviral activity of mung bean sprouts against respiratory syncytial virus and herpes simplex virus-1: An in vitro study on virally infected Vero and MRC-5 cell lines. *BMC Complement. Med. Ther.* **2015**, *15*, 179. [CrossRef] [PubMed]
8. Bayer, C.; Bernard, H.; Prager, R.; Rabsch, W.; Hiller, P.; Malorny, B.; Pfefferkorn, B.; Frank, C.; Jong, D.A.; Friesema, I.; et al. An outbreak of *Salmonella* Newport associated with mung bean sprouts in Germany and the Netherlands, October to November 2011. *Eurosurveillance* **2014**, *19*, 20665. [CrossRef] [PubMed]
9. Sadler-Reeves, L.; Aird, H.; de Pinna, E.; Elviss, N.; Fox, A.; Kaye, M.; Jorgensen, F.; Lane, C.; Willis, C.; McLauchlin, J. The occurrence of *Salmonella* in raw and ready-to-eat bean sprouts and sprouted seeds on retail sale in England and Northern Ireland. *Lett. Appl. Microbiol.* **2016**, *62*, 126–129. [CrossRef]
10. Iacumin, L.; Comi, G. Microbial quality of raw and ready-to-eat mung bean sprouts produced in Italy. *Food Microbiol.* **2019**, *82*, 371–377. [CrossRef]
11. Kim, S.H.; Rhee, M.S. Environment-friendly mild heat and relative humidity treatment protects sprout seeds (radish, mung bean, mustard, and alfalfa) against various foodborne pathogens. *Food Control* **2018**, *93*, 17–22. [CrossRef]
12. Baker, K.A.; Beecher, L.; Northcutt, J.K. Effect of irrigation water source and post-harvest washing treatment on the microflora of alfalfa and mung bean sprouts. *Food Control* **2019**, *100*, 151–157. [CrossRef]
13. Gui, M.; He, H.; Li, Y.; Chen, X.; Wang, H.; Wang, T.; Li, J. Effect of UV-B treatment during the growth process on the postharvest quality of mung bean sprouts (*Vigna radiata*). *Int. J. Food Sci. Technol.* **2018**, *53*, 2166–2172. [CrossRef]
14. Shen, Z.; Mustapha, A.; Lin, M.; Zheng, G. Biocontrol of the internalization of *Salmonella enterica* and Enterohaemorrhagic *Escherichia coli* in mung bean sprouts with an endophytic *Bacillus subtilis*. *Int. J. Food Microbiol.* **2017**, *250*, 37–44. [CrossRef]
15. Millan-Sango, D.; Sammut, E.; Van Impe, J.F.; Valdramidis, V.P. Decontamination of alfalfa and mung bean sprouts by ultrasound and aqueous chlorine dioxide. *LWT* **2017**, *78*, 90–96. [CrossRef]
16. Xiang, Q.; Liu, X.; Liu, S.; Ma, Y.; Xu, C.; Bai, Y. Effect of plasma-activated water on microbial quality and physicochemical characteristics of mung bean sprouts. *Innov. Food Sci. Emerg. Technol.* **2019**, *52*, 49–56. [CrossRef]
17. Zhou, R.; Li, J.; Zhou, R.; Zhang, X.; Yang, S. Atmospheric-pressure plasma treated water for seed germination and seedling growth of mung bean and its sterilization effect on mung bean sprouts. *Innov. Food Sci. Emerg. Technol.* **2019**, *53*, 36–44. [CrossRef]
18. Shi, Z.; Chen, D.; Chen, T.T.; Wei, G.; Yin, C.Y.; Xu, H.; Yang, G.F. In vivo analysis of two new fungicides in mung bean sprouts by solid phase microextraction-gas chromatography-mass spectrometry. *Food Chem.* **2019**, *275*, 688–695. [CrossRef]
19. Wang, M.; Liang, S.; Bai, L.; Qiao, F.; Yan, H. Green protocol for the preparation of hydrophilic molecularly imprinted resin in water for the efficient selective extraction and determination of plant hormones from bean sprouts. *Anal. Chim. Acta* **2019**, *1064*, 47–55. [CrossRef]
20. Cho, S.K.; Abd El-Aty, A.M.; Park, K.H.; Park, J.H.; Assayed, M.E.; Jeong, Y.M.; Park, Y.S.; Shim, J.H. Simple multiresidue extraction method for the determination of fungicides and plant growth regulator in bean sprouts using low temperature partitioning and tandem mass spectrometry. *Food Chem.* **2013**, *136*, 1414–1420. [CrossRef]
21. Kim, K.G.; Park, D.W.; Kang, G.R.; Kim, T.S.; Yang, Y.; Moon, S.J.; Choi, E.A.; Ha, D.R.; Kim, E.S.; Cho, B.S. Simultaneous determination of plant growth regulator and pesticides in bean sprouts by liquid chromatography-tandem mass spectrometry. *Food Chem.* **2016**, *208*, 239–244. [CrossRef]
22. Chen, J.; He, L.X.; Cheng, Y.X.; Ye, P.; Wu, D.L.; Fang, Z.Q.; Li, J.; Ying, G.G. Trace analysis of 28 antibiotics in plant tissues (root, stem, leaf and seed) by optimized QuEChERS pretreatment with UHPLC-MS/MS detection. *J. Chromatogr. B* **2020**, *1161*, 122450. [CrossRef]
23. Li, X.; Tang, Z.; Wen, L.; Jiang, C.; Feng, Q. Matrine: A review of its pharmacology, pharmacokinetics, toxicity, clinical application and preparation researches. *J. Ethnopharmacol.* **2021**, *269*, 113682. [CrossRef]
24. Phanwilai, S.; Piyavorasakul, S.; Noophan, P.L.; Daniels, K.D.; Snyder, S.A. Inhibition of anaerobic ammonium oxidation (anammox) bacteria by addition of high and low concentrations of chloramphenicol and comparison of attached- and suspended-growth. *Chemosphere* **2020**, *238*, 124570. [CrossRef] [PubMed]

25. Tong, C.; Zhuo, X.; Guo, Y. Occurrence and risk assessment of four typical fluoroquinolone antibiotics in raw and treated sewage and in receiving waters in Hangzhou, China. *J. Agric. Food Chem.* **2011**, *59*, 7303–7309. [CrossRef] [PubMed]
26. Rocha, D.C.; da Silva Rocha, C.; Tavares, D.S.; de Morais Calado, S.L.; Gomes, M.P. Veterinary antibiotics and plant physiology: An overview. *Sci. Total Environ.* **2021**, *767*, 144902. [CrossRef] [PubMed]
27. Zhang, H.; Li, X.; Yang, Q.; Sun, L.; Yang, X.; Zhou, M.; Deng, R.; Bi, L. Plant growth, antibiotic uptake, and prevalence of antibiotic resistance in an endophytic system of pakchoi under antibiotic exposure. *Int. J. Environ. Res. Public Health* **2017**, *14*, 1336. [CrossRef] [PubMed]
28. Ambalavanan, N.; Kavitha, M.; Jayakumar, S.; Raj, A.; Nataraj, S. Comparative evaluation of bactericidal effect of silver nanoparticle in combination with Nd-YAG laser against enterococcus faecalis: An *in vitro* study. *J. Contemp. Dent. Pract.* **2020**, *21*, 1141–1145. [PubMed]
29. Khan, I.; Raza, M.A.; Awan, S.A.; Shah, G.A.; Rizwan, M.; Ali, B.; Tariq, R.; Hassan, M.J.; Alyemeni, M.N.; Brestic, M.; et al. Amelioration of salt induced toxicity in pearl millet by seed priming with silver nanoparticles (AgNPs): The oxidative damage, antioxidant enzymes and ions uptake are major determinants of salt tolerant capacity. *Plant Physiol. Biochem.* **2020**, *156*, 221–232. [CrossRef]
30. Li, C.L.; Wang, M.; Ma, X.Y.; Zhang, W. NRGA1, a putative mitochondrial pyruvate carrier, mediates ABA regulation of guard cell Ion channels and drought stress responses in arabidopsis. *Mol. Plant* **2014**, *7*, 1508–1521. [CrossRef]
31. Lewkowski, J.; Rogacz, D.; Rychter, P. Hazardous ecotoxicological impact of two commonly used nitrofuran-derived antibacterial drugs: Furazolidone and nitrofurantoin. *Chemosphere* **2019**, *222*, 381–390. [CrossRef]
32. Lewkowski, J.; Morawska, M.; Karpowicz, R.; Rychter, P.; Rogacz, D.; Lewicka, K. Novel (5-nitrofurfuryl)-substituted esters of phosphonoglycine- their synthesis and phyto- and ecotoxicological properties. *Chemosphere* **2017**, *188*, 618–632. [CrossRef]
33. Fan, K.; Delgado-Baquerizo, M.; Guo, X.; Wang, D.; Zhu, Y.G.; Chu, H. Biodiversity of key-stone phylotypes determines crop production in a 4-decade fertilization experiment. *ISME J.* **2021**, *15*, 550–561. [CrossRef]
34. Wang, D.; Liang, F.; Ma, P.; Yang, Q.; Gao, D.; Song, D.; Wang, X. Determination of 6-benzylaminopurine and Hg^{2+} in bean sprouts and drinking mineral water by surface-enhanced raman spectroscopy. *Food Anal. Methods* **2015**, *9*, 934–941. [CrossRef]
35. Geilfus, C.M. Review on the significance of chlorine for crop yield and quality. *Plant Sci.* **2018**, *270*, 114–122. [CrossRef]
36. Min, P.; Chu, L.M. Phytotoxicity of veterinary antibiotics to seed germination and root elongation of crops. *Ecotoxicol. Environ. Saf.* **2016**, *126*, 228–237. [CrossRef]
37. Wang, D.; Chan, K.K.J.; Chan, W. Plant uptake and metabolism of nitrofuran antibiotics in spring onion grown in nitrofuran-contaminated soil. *J. Agric. Food Chem.* **2017**, *65*, 4255–4261. [CrossRef]
38. Sun, Y.; Guo, Y.; Shi, M.; Qiu, T.; Gao, M.; Tian, S.; Wang, X. Effect of antibiotic type and vegetable species on antibiotic accumulation in soil-vegetable system, soil microbiota, and resistance genes. *Chemosphere* **2021**, *263*, 128099. [CrossRef]
39. EFSA. Scientific opinion on nitrofurans and their metabolites in food. *EFSA J.* **2015**, *13*, 4140. [CrossRef]
40. Gong, J.; Li, J.; Yuan, H.; Chu, B.; Lin, W.; Cao, Q.; Zhao, Q.; Fang, R.; Li, L.; Xiao, G. Determination of four nitrofuran metabolites in gelatin Chinese medicine using dispersive solid phase extraction and pass-through solid phase extraction coupled to ultra high performance liquid chromatography-tandem mass spectrometry. *J. Chromatogr. B* **2020**, *1146*, 122018. [CrossRef]

MDPI
St. Alban-Anlage 66
4052 Basel
Switzerland
www.mdpi.com

Antibiotics Editorial Office
E-mail: antibiotics@mdpi.com
www.mdpi.com/journal/antibiotics

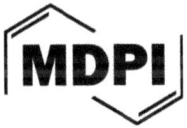

Disclaimer/Publisher's Note: The statements, opinions and data contained in all publications are solely those of the individual author(s) and contributor(s) and not of MDPI and/or the editor(s). MDPI and/or the editor(s) disclaim responsibility for any injury to people or property resulting from any ideas, methods, instructions or products referred to in the content.